Implant Dentistry: Clinical Cases

Implant Dentistry: Clinical Cases

Editor: Isobel Cole

AMERICAN
MEDICAL PUBLISHERS
www.americanmedicalpublishers.com

AMERICAN
MEDICAL PUBLISHERS
www.americanmedicalpublishers.com

Cataloging-in-Publication Data

Implant dentistry: clinical cases / edited by Isobel Cole.
p. cm.
Includes bibliographical references and index.
ISBN 979-8-88740-644-2
1. Dental implants. 2. Dentistry. I. Cole, Isobel.
RK667.I45 M63 2023
617.693--dc23

American Medical Publishers,
41 Flatbush Avenue,
1st Floor, New York,
NY 11217, USA

ISBN 979-8-88740-644-2 (Hardback)

Contents

Preface

Dental implants refer to artificial tooth roots which are made of a biocompatible material such as titanium. These are surgically placed into the jawbone and are used to support a dental prosthesis. Implant dentistry is a specialized field of dentistry that aims to replace missing teeth or stabilize dentures using dental implants. They offer a wide variety of benefits for restoring appearance and improving the quality of life of patients. It also helps in promoting the health of the surrounding bone and gums, and preventing the shrinkage of the jawbone which may be caused by bone loss. Most of the topics introduced in this book cover new techniques and the applications of implant dentistry. From theories to research to practical applications, case studies related to all contemporary topics of relevance to this field have been included herein. This book is a vital tool for all researching and studying this field.

The researches compiled throughout the book are authentic and of high quality, combining several disciplines and from very diverse regions from around the world. Drawing on the contributions of many researchers from diverse countries, the book's objective is to provide the readers with the latest achievements in the area of research. This book will surely be a source of knowledge to all interested and researching the field.

In the end, I would like to express my deep sense of gratitude to all the authors for meeting the set deadlines in completing and submitting their research chapters. I would also like to thank the publisher for the support offered to us throughout the course of the book. Finally, I extend my sincere thanks to my family for being a constant source of inspiration and encouragement.

Editor

1

Partial Extraction Therapy with Early Implant Placement in the Esthetic Zone: A Clinical Case Report

Saleh N. Almohammed,[1] **Reem S. Abdel-Hafez**,[2] **and Duaa D. Ailabouni**[1]

[1]*Department of Prosthodontics, Jordan University of Science and Technology, Irbid, Jordan*
[2]*Department of Preventive Dentistry, Jordan University of Science and Technology, Irbid, Jordan*

Correspondence should be addressed to Saleh N. Almohammed; snalmohammed@just.edu.jo

Academic Editor: Darko Macan

Immediate replacement of teeth designated for extraction is an appealing treatment rationale for both the patient and the operator. However, it has been associated with a greater risk of facial recession and compromised soft-tissue esthetics. Partial extraction therapy (PET) or synonymously socket shield technique (SST) or root membrane technique (RMT) has been proposed to conserve the facial alveolar contour and soft-tissue esthetics. In this article, a special case is described where a root membrane was used to prevent the modeling of the facial aspect of the extraction socket. Partial extraction was performed allowing the socket with the facial root membrane in situ to partially heal for 8 weeks before implant placement. Successful integration and restoration were achieved with very minimal hard- and soft-tissue changes, accentuating satisfactory esthetic results as dictated by objective esthetic assessment. PET with early implant placement may be considered a viable treatment option for selected cases.

1. Introduction

Immediate implant placement has the advantage of reducing the overall treatment time and providing patients with expeditious replacement of extracted teeth. However, placing a dental implant in the alveolar socket does not prevent ridge dimensional changes associated with the extraction of teeth [1, 2]. The disruption of the periodontal ligament upon extraction is associated with modeling/remodeling of the alveolar bone which is considered a tooth-dependent structure [3, 4]. The facial alveolar bone is more pronouncedly affected in this resorptive process being predominantly composed of bundle bone [3, 5]. This explains the greater horizontal loss on the facial aspect compared to the lingual. These alveolar changes are also associated with soft-tissue changes that might compromise the treatment outcome and soft-tissue esthetics [3, 6].

Several studies demonstrated that immediate implant placement is associated with a greater percentage of facial recession [7, 8]; nevertheless, a minimum of intact 1 mm thickness facial plate and a thick gingival phenotype were associated with a lower risk [9]. However, these features are missing in most of the cases [10, 11], which makes it difficult to guarantee predictable esthetic outcomes.

Retaining roots was described by several authors [12, 13] in an attempt to reduce the undesirable remodeling of the alveolar bone. In 2010, Professor Hürzeler described PET (SST) for immediate implant placement based on retaining a facial root fragment at the coronal third of the alveolar socket. This was proposed to result in more favorable soft- and hard-tissue esthetics and greater patients' satisfaction [14, 15]. Beagle dog histology [14] and human histology [16] were provided as proof of bone formation between the implant surface and the root fragment. A few studies were published to demonstrate the success of this technique [17–20].

2. Materials and Methods

This article demonstrates the clinical and radiographic outcomes of an esthetic implant case treated utilizing the concept of PET in a modified manner, in an attempt to

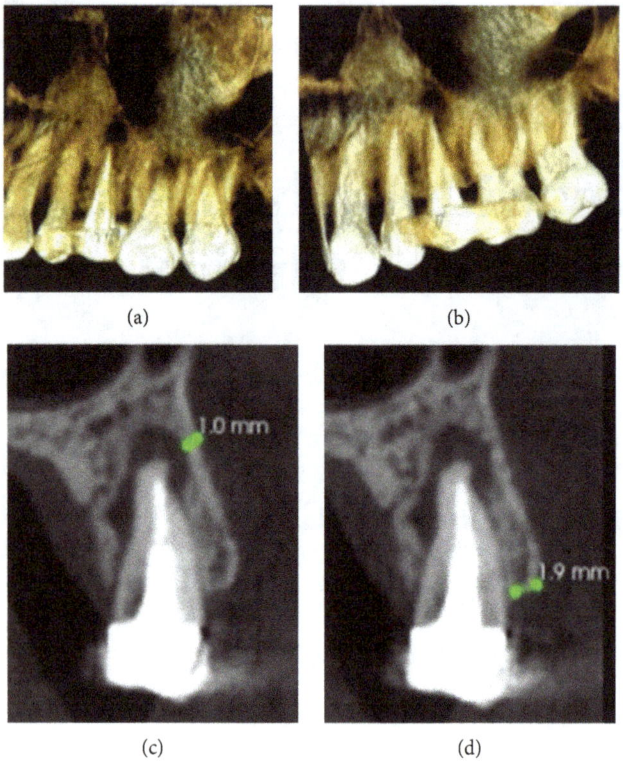

FIGURE 1: Palatal (a) and facial (b) views of M-D radiographic sections and facial plate thicknesses (c and d).

maintain the facial ridge contours around the installed dental implant. A descriptive report will be presented; a case with early, rather than immediate, implant placement with an overall follow-up period of 19 months. Pink and White Esthetic Scores (PES and WES) [21] were recorded to objectively assess the restoration and the related facial tissues. The patient was treated in the authors' private clinics.

3. The Case

A 43-year-old medically fit female patient presented with mild chronic pain and a mobile crown of the upper left second premolar. Upon clinical and radiographic assessment, the tooth had root canal treatment and a cast-post/core with a metal-ceramic crown which had been in service for about 8 months. CBCT assessment revealed a frank periapical lesion extending close to the floor of the maxillary sinus with a facial bony plate thickness of 1.9 mm at the crest and 1.0 mm at the level of the root apex. The crown was mobile and a small manual force was enough to dislodge the post-crown leaving a root with no ferrule effect, hence designated as hopeless (Figures 1(a), 1(b), 1(c), and 1(d)). Bone sounding revealed an intact buccal plate with a normal supracrestal attachment level at the facial and interproximal areas.

Upon esthetic risk assessment [22], it was evident that the patient had a high lip line with a thin phenotype (Figure 2(a)), aggravated by the patient's high esthetic demands. Different treatment options were discussed with the patient and the decision was to proceed with an implant-supported restoration. The case failed to fulfill the criteria for immediate implantation as there was no sufficient apical bone to place the implant with predictable primary stability; thus, a decision to perform partial extraction of the root and wait for 4–8 weeks before implant placement [23] was adopted in an attempt to combine the benefits of both PET and early implant placement. All details were discussed with the patient and consent was obtained.

—Partial extraction and early implant placement.

After administration of the local anesthetic agent, a straight fissured carbide bur (Meisinger HM33IL/Implant burs, Surgical Carbide X-Cut Taper RA-L-010, Morris Dental, Ireland) in a surgical straight handpiece (NSK, Japan) was used to section the root in a mesiodistal direction and then section the apical portion of facial root wall, leaving a coronal fragment of the facial root wall of about 1.5–2 mm in thickness and 6–8 mm in length. This facial fragment was shortened using a flame-shaped diamond red-band bur (Jota diamond burs, Switzerland) into a "c" shape which was just coronal (about 0.5 mm) to the facial alveolar bone crest to help avoid jeopardizing the bony crest during preparation. The facial margin of the fragment was beveled to help avoid external shield exposure, and the palatal margin of the fragment was thinned and concavely shaped to avoid internal shield exposure and to provide prosthetic space. The palatal root wall and the apical part of the facial wall were extracted using periotomes and Coupland's elevators followed by debridement of the socket and disinfection using chlorhexidine gluconate 0.2%. The socket was left to heal without implant placement, socket grafting, or interim prosthesis.

After 8 weeks (Figure 2(b)), another CBCT was taken to check the root fragment and the socket healing (Figure 2(c)). It was evident that the socket had significant but incomplete bone healing with the facial root membrane stable in situ; thus, early implant placement was decided. Using the flapless soft-tissue punch technique, sequential preparation of the osteotomy was carefully performed to allow a prosthetically driven 3D implant placement (4.1 × 12mm SLActive®, Roxolid® BLT implant, Straumann®, Switzerland). To increase the amount of "press fit" and improve the implant primary stability, the last osteotomy drill (Ø 3.5 mm) to be used before implant placement was inserted for a depth of 7 mm rather than 12 mm and the countersinking step was skipped. The insertion torque achieved was 35 Ncm and the ISQ was 68 labiolingually and 72 mesiodistally. After that, a Ø 4.7 mm bottle-shaped gingival former was attached and no interim prosthesis was provided based on the patient's preference (Figures 2(d) and 2(e)). Postoperative instructions were given, and indicated medications were prescribed. This was followed by a re-evaluation visit 2 weeks after the implant placement and the patient was asked to attend after 3 months for further assessment and proceeding with the restorative phase.

—Restorative phase.

After verification of clinically successful osseointegration using periapical X-ray and ISQ test (a reading of about 84); an open-tray, implant-level definitive impression was made, implant analog attached, and impression poured to fabricate a definitive working cast. A titanium abutment (Variobase® abutment, Ø 4.5 mm, GH = 3 mm, AH = 5.5 mm, Straumann®,

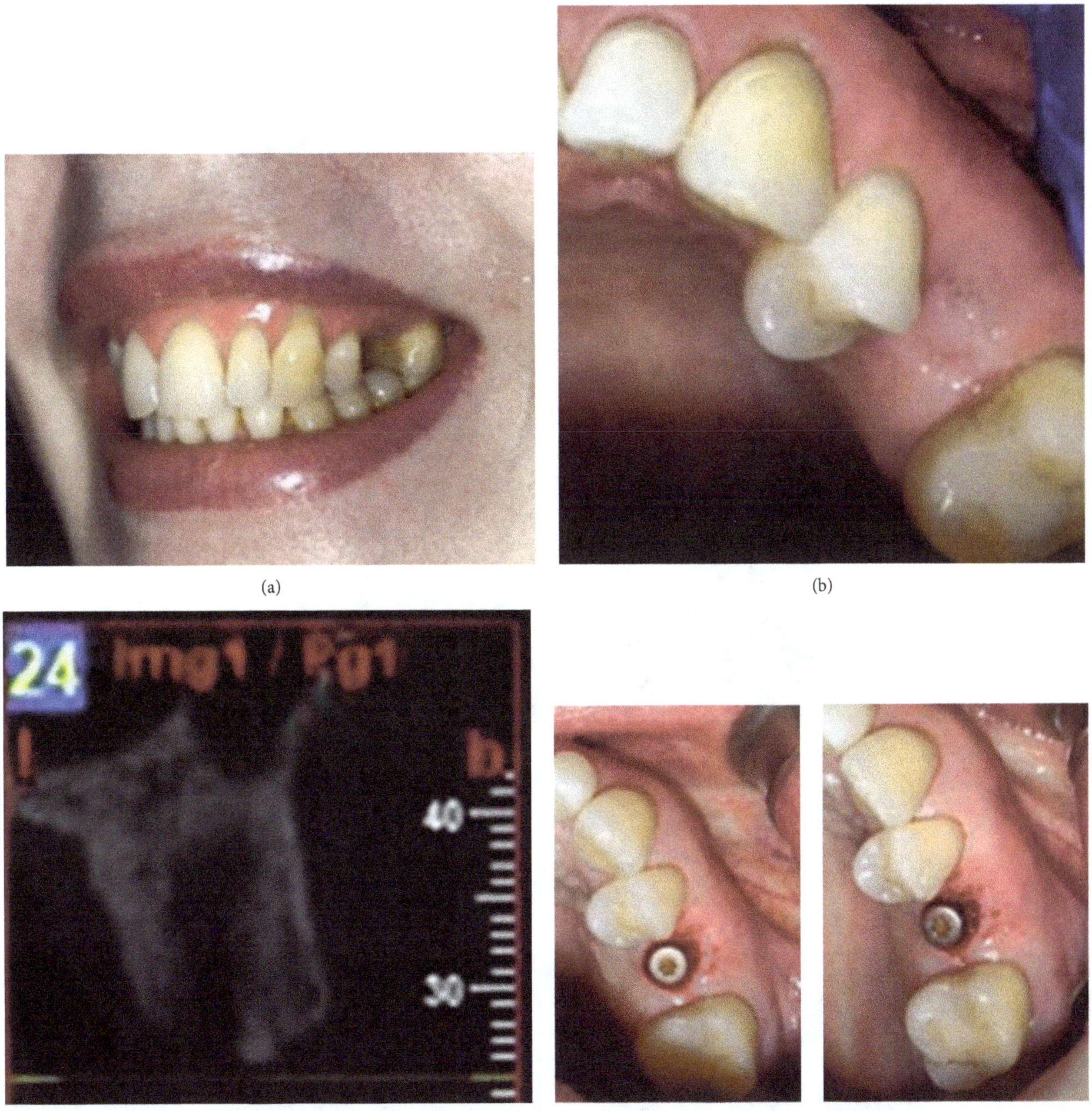

Figure 2: Lateral view upon smiling (a), occlusal view of extraction site of tooth 25 after 8 weeks (b), B–P radiographic section with root fragment in situ (c), and occlusal and buccal views of the healing abutment and remaining root shield immediately following implant placement (d and e).

Switzerland) was selected and screwed into the analog, then CAD-CAM lab technology (Ceramill map400, Ceramill motion2; Amanngirrbach, Koblach, Austria) was utilized to fabricate an occlusally vented zirconia core that precisely fits the Variobase® abutment. The dental technician built up the veneering ceramic onto the core fabricating a veneered-zirconia crown. After the laboratory work was finalized and checked on the dental cast, the definitive veneered-zirconia crown was cemented onto the abutment using dual-cured resin cement (TotalCem, ITENA, France) (Figures 3(a) and 3(b)), and then the abutment-crown assembly was transferred to the patient's mouth, tried-in and screwed into the implant using an insertion torque of 35 Ncm. Occlusal adjustment was performed, and the screw access hole was filled with composite resin, finished, and polished.

The first follow-up was performed after 2 weeks, then after 1, 3, 6, and 16 months; an overall follow-up period of 19 months since implant placement. After 16 months of loading, the PES and WES were collectively about18 of 20, indicative of an acceptable esthetic outcome with very minimal volumetric ridge changes, confirming the patient's satisfaction (Figures 3(c) and 3(d)). Also, PA and CBCT

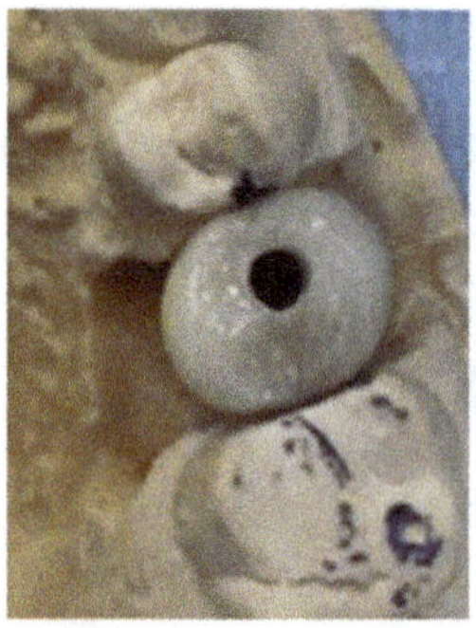

(a)

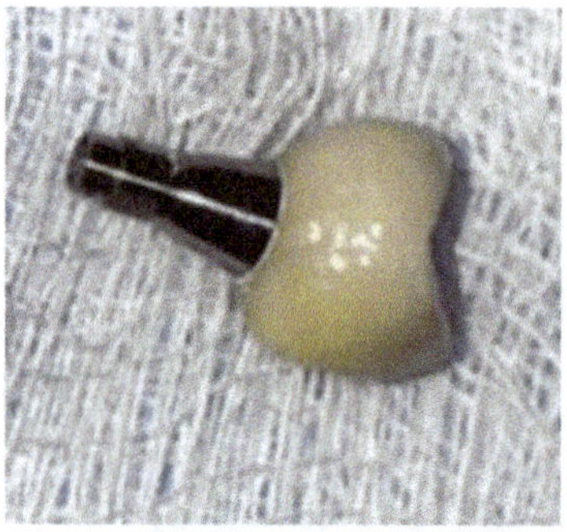

(b)

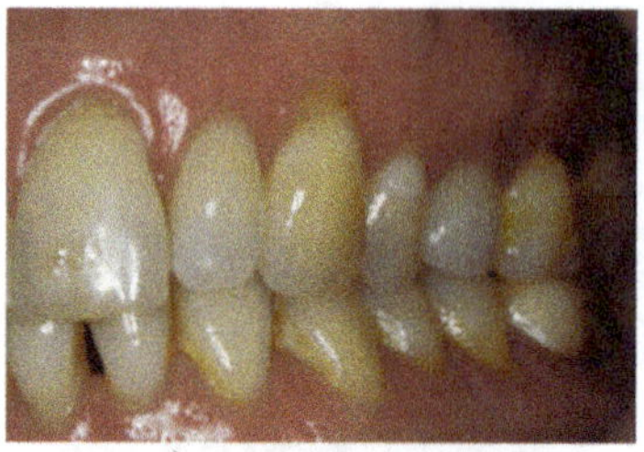

(c)

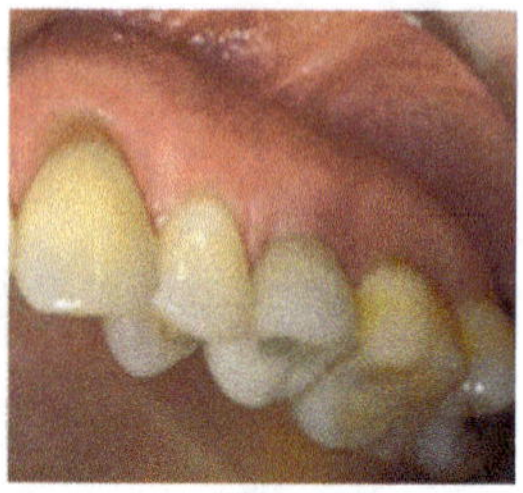

(d)

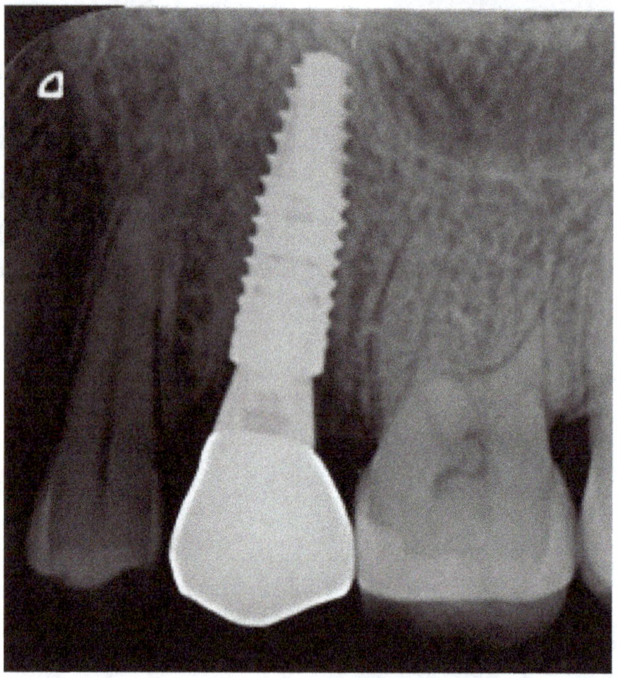

(e)

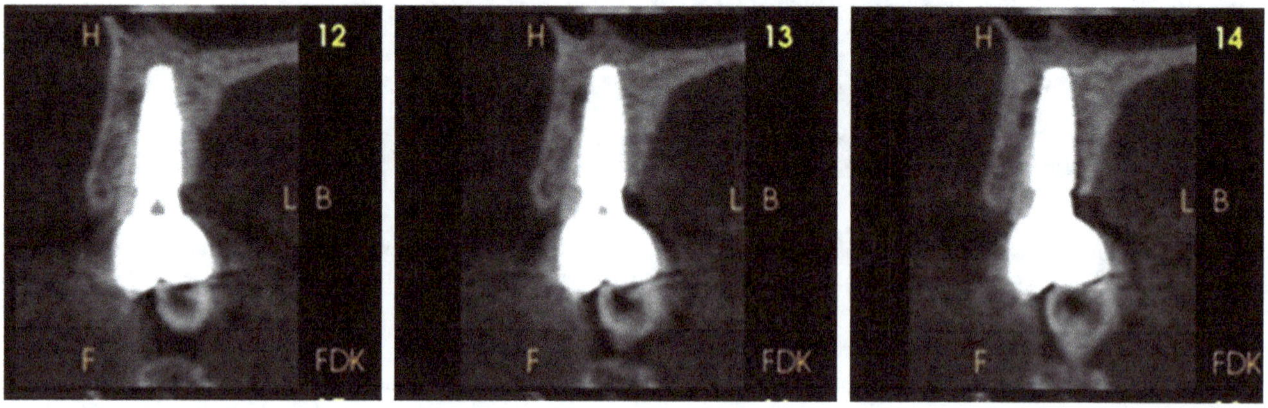

(f)

FIGURE 3: Continued.

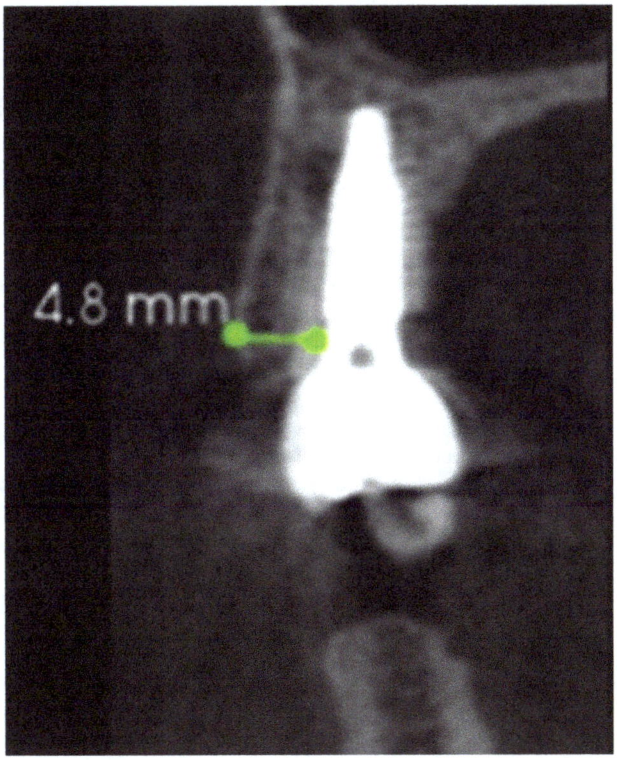

(g)

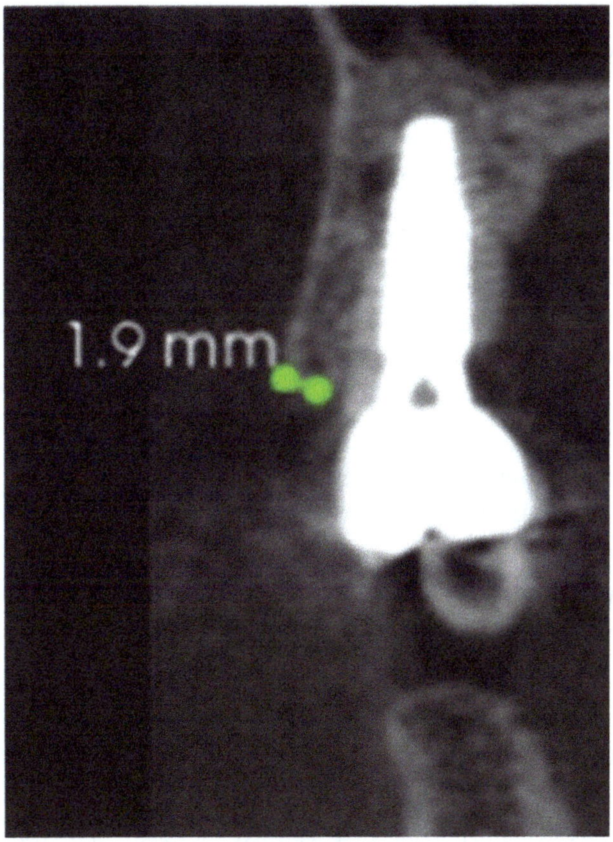

(h)

FIGURE 3: Zirconia crown cemented onto titanium abutment (a) and (b), lateral and occlusal views of crown screwed into the implant (c) and (d), postoperative PA (e), F–L radiographic sections (f), F–L section verifying width of hard facial tissues (g), and F–L section verifying width of facial plate crest (h).

radiographs were taken; the crestal facial bony plate thickness was very similar to that before partial extraction (~1.9 mm) with a total distance of 4.8 mm from the bony crest to the implant platform. A significant bone fill between the root fragment and the implant was verified (Figures 3(e), 3(f), 3(g), and 3(h)).

4. Discussion

Providing patients with immediate replacement of extracted teeth with optimum soft-tissue esthetics is a desirable treatment outcome. Several techniques have been proposed to counteract the volumetric changes associated with the extraction of a tooth, such as site preservation and hard- and/or soft-tissue grafting [24, 25].

Leaving a facial portion of the root has been demonstrated to prevent or reduce the unfavorable modeling of the facial plate of bone following extraction of a tooth in what is known as PET or synonymously SST or RMT [14].

The case reported in this article provided different insights into the application of PET; the implant was placed 8 weeks following partial extraction rather than immediately.

To the extent of the authors' knowledge, in almost all reported cases of implantation using PET, implant placement was performed at the time of partial tooth extraction [19, 26]. In the case reported in this article, the decision was to prepare the root fragment and leave the socket to partially heal for 8 weeks before implant placement and without any grafting material. This protocol was selected once the assessment revealed that immediate implant placement with good primary stability was not feasible.

Successful early implant placement following soft- and hard-tissue healing was recently reported by Oliveira and his co-workers [27]. In their report, a connective tissue graft and the shield were used to preserve the socket, and the implant was placed 100 days following the extraction. In contrast, the root shield without a soft- or hard-tissue graft was used to preserve the socket in the case reported in this article. The root fragment remained stable and succeeded at maintaining the facial alveolar ridge contour during the 19-month follow-up period.

Bäumer and his co-workers in a retrospective clinical study, prepared the osteotomy through the root of the tooth to be replaced followed by the removal of the remaining root fragments except for the one on the labial aspect [19]. In contrast, in this case, the root was separated, the facial segment was prepared, and the lingual segment was extracted before the later preparation of the osteotomy. This was in an attempt to reduce the risk of dislodgment of the facial fragment and to ensure that all other parts of the root were removed.

Adequate space between the coronal edge of the shield and the subgingival contour of the crown was recommended by Gluckman et al. [26] to reduce the risk of exposure and inflammation of the root fragment. In this study, the root fragment was trimmed just coronal to the alveolar bone crest to allow for adequate soft-tissue thickness and help prevent exposure from occurring.

Different studies reported different loading protocols. Most studies provided immediate provisional restorations [19, 20, 26, 28] and a few had a delayed approach [29, 30]. In this case, the decision was to install the healing abutment and postpone restoration until osseointegration is clinically verified. This approach was adopted to allow peri-implant soft-tissue healing and supracrestal attachment formation, postulating that this might reduce the possibilities for fragment exposure.

In this case, the space between the root fragment and the implant was not filled with any biomaterial. Bäumer et al. [19], on the other hand, used an enamel matrix protein which was hypothesized to induce cementum formation and prevent resorption of the root fragment. Others reported the use of bone grafts [29]. So far, there is no evidence to support any added benefit for the use of any biomaterial.

This report and a few other reports and case series demonstrated the preliminary success of this technique in preserving the facial contour following extraction. The benefits of preserving extraction sites with less morbidity and cost cannot be emphasized enough. However, further extensive research regarding the complication rate, technique sensitivity, and longer-term follow-up is of great value to validate such a delicate and case-specific technique. Until fulfilled, PET remains a controversy.

Additional Points

Patient's Consent. The patient signed an informed consent stating that "I declare that all the information regarding the treatment options, treatment plan, sequence of treatment, and possible complications were thoroughly discussed and approved by me before the commencement of treatment".

References

[1] M. G. Araújo, F. Sukekava, J. L. Wennström, and J. Lindhe, "Ridge alterations following implant placement in fresh extraction sockets: an experimental study in the dog," *Journal of Clinical Periodontology*, vol. 32, no. 6, pp. 645–652, 2005.

[2] D. Botticelli, T. Berglundh, and J. Lindhe, "Hard-tissue alterations following immediate implant placement in extraction sites," *Journal of Clinical Periodontology*, vol. 31, no. 10, pp. 820–828, 2004.

[3] M. G. Araújo and J. Lindhe, "Dimensional ridge alterations following tooth extraction. An experimental study in the dog," *Journal of Clinical Periodontology*, vol. 32, no. 2, pp. 212–218, 2005.

[4] M. G. Araújo, C. O. Silva, M. Misawa, and F. Sukekava, "Alveolar socket healing: what can we learn?," *Periodontology*, vol. 2015, no. 68, pp. 122–134, 2015.

[5] L. Schropp, A. Wenzel, L. Kostopoulos, and T. Karring, "Bone healing and soft tissue contour changes following single-tooth extraction: a clinical and radiographic 12-month prospective study," *The International Journal of Periodontics & Restorative Dentistry*, vol. 23, no. 4, pp. 313–323, 2003.

[6] D. Cardaropoli, L. Tamagnone, A. Roffredo, and L. Gaveglio, "Evaluation of dental implants placed in preserved and non-preserved Postextraction ridges: a 12-month Postloading study," *The International Journal of Periodontics & Restorative Dentistry*, vol. 35, no. 5, pp. 677–685, 2015, PMID: 26357697.

[7] S. T. Chen and D. Buser, "Clinical and esthetic outcomes of implants placed in postextraction sites," *The International Journal of Oral & Maxillofacial Implants*, vol. 24 Suppl, pp. 186–217, 2009.

[8] S. T. Chen and D. Buser, "Esthetic outcomes following immediate and early implant placement in the anterior maxilla— a systematic review," *The International Journal of Oral & Maxillofacial Implants*, vol. 29, Supplement, pp. 186–215, 2014.

[9] D. Buser, V. Chappuis, U. C. Belser, and S. Chen, "Implant placement post extraction in esthetic single tooth sites: when immediate, when early, when late?," *Periodontology 2000*, vol. 73, no. 1, pp. 84–102, 2017.

[10] A. L. Januário, W. R. Duarte, M. Barriviera, J. C. Mesti, M. G. Araújo, and J. Lindhe, "Dimension of the facial bone wall in the anterior maxilla: a cone-beam computed tomography study," *Clinical Oral Implants Research*, vol. 22, no. 10, pp. 1168–1171, 2011.

[11] M. Olsson and J. Lindhe, "Periodontal characteristics in individuals with varying form of the upper central incisors," *Journal of Clinical Periodontology*, vol. 18, no. 1, pp. 78–82, 1991.

[12] D. M. Casey and F. R. Lauciello, "A review of the submerged-root concept," *Journal of Prosthetic Dentistry*, vol. 43, no. 2, pp. 128–132, 1980.

[13] M. Salama, T. Ishikawa, H. Salama, A. Funato, and D. Garber, "Advantages of the root submergence technique for pontic site development in esthetic implant therapy," *The International Journal of Periodontics & Restorative Dentistry*, vol. 27, pp. 521–527, 2007.

[14] M. B. Hurzeler, O. Zuhr, P. Schupbach, S. F. Rebele, N. Emmanouilidis, and S. Fickl, "The socket-shield technique: a proof-of-principle report," *Journal of Clinical Periodontology*, vol. 37, no. 9, pp. 855–862, 2010.

[15] H. Gluckman, M. Salama, and J. Du Toit, "Partial extraction therapies (PET) part 1: maintaining alveolar ridge contour at pontic and immediate implant sites," *The International Journal of Periodontics & Restorative Dentistry*, vol. 36, no. 5, pp. 681–687, 2016.

[16] C. Schwimer, G. Pette, H. Gluckman, M. Salama, and J. du Toit, "Human histologic evidence of new bone formation and osseointegration between root dentin (unplanned socket-shield) and dental implant: case report," *The International Journal of Oral & Maxillofacial Implants*, vol. 33, no. 1, pp. e19–e23, 2018.

[17] H. Gluckman, M. Salama, and J. Du Toit, "A retrospective evaluation of 128 socket-shield cases in the esthetic zone and posterior sites: partial extraction therapy with up to 4 years follow-up," *Clinical Implant Dentistry and Related Research*, vol. 20, no. 2, pp. 122–129, 2018.

[18] D. Bäumer, O. Zuhr, S. Rebele, D. Schneider, P. Schupbach, and M. Hürzeler, "The socket-shield technique: first histological, clinical, and volumetrical observations after separation of the buccal tooth segment - a pilot study," *Clinical Implant Dentistry and Related Research*, vol. 17, no. 1, pp. 71–82, 2015.

[19] D. Bäumer, O. Zuhr, S. Rebele, and M. Hurzeler, "Socket shield technique for immediate implant placement - clinical, radiographic and volumetric data after 5 years," *Clinical Oral Implants Research*, vol. 28, no. 11, pp. 1450–1458, 2017.

[20] E. Bramanti, A. Norcia, M. Cicciù et al., "Postextraction dental implant in the aesthetic zone, socket shield technique versus conventional protocol," *The Journal of Craniofacial Surgery*, vol. 29, no. 4, pp. 1037–1041, 2018.

[21] U. C. Belser, L. Grütter, F. Vailati, M. M. Bornstein, H. P. Weber, and D. Buser, "Outcome evaluation of early placed maxillary anterior single-tooth implants using objective esthetic criteria: a cross-sectional, retrospective study in 45 patients with a 2- to 4-year follow-up using pink and white esthetic scores," *Journal of Periodontology*, vol. 80, no. 1, pp. 140–151, 2009.

[22] D. Buser, W. Maritn, and U. C. Belser, "Optimizing esthetics for implant restorations in the anterior maxilla: anatomic and surgical considerations," *International Journal of Oral & Maxillofacial Implants*, vol. 19, SUPPL, pp. 43-61, 2004.

[23] D. Morton, G. Gallucci, W.-S. Lin et al., "Group 2 ITI consensus report: prosthodontics and implant dentistry," *Clinical Oral Implants Research*, vol. 29, Suppl. 16, pp. 215–223, 2018.

[24] A. Barone, M. Ricci, P. Tonelli, S. Santini, and U. Covani, "Tissue changes of extraction sockets in humans: a comparison of spontaneous healing vs. ridge preservation with secondary soft tissue healing," *Clinical Oral Implants Research*, vol. 24, no. 11, pp. 1231–1237, 2012.

[25] G. I. Benic and C. H. F. Hämmerle, "Horizontal bone augmentation by means of guided bone regeneration," *Periodontology 2000*, vol. 2014, no. 66, pp. 13–40, 2014.

[26] H. Gluckman, M. Salama, and J. Du Toit, "Partial extraction therapies (PET) part 2: procedures and technical aspects," *The International Journal of Periodontics & Restorative Dentistry*, vol. 37, no. 3, pp. 377–385, 2017.

[27] G. B. D. Oliveira, M. D. A. Basilio, N. S. Araujo, and P. R. Cury, "The socket-shield technique and early implant placement for tooth rehabilitation: a case report," *Journal of Clinical Images and Medical Case Reports*, vol. 1, no. 3, p. 1118, 2021.

[28] M. E. Mitsias, K. D. Siormpas, G. A. Kotsakis, S. D. Ganz, C. Mangano, and G. Iezzi, "The root membrane technique: human histologic evidence after five years of function," *BioMed Research International*, vol. 2017, 2017.

[29] M. Petsch, B. Spies, and R. J. Kohal, "Socket shield technique for implant placement in the esthetic zone: a case report," *The International Journal of Periodontics & Restorative Dentistry*, vol. 37, no. 6, pp. 853–860, 2017.

[30] R. Saeidi Pour, O. Zuhr, M. Hürzeler et al., "Clinical benefits of the immediate implant socket shield technique," *Journal of Esthetic and Restorative Dentistry*, vol. 29, no. 2, pp. 93–101, 2017.

2

Correction of Vertical Smile Discrepancy through Ceramic Laminate Veneers and Surgical Crown Lengthening

Paula Bernardon,[1] Carlos Estevão Lagustera,[1] Luiz Roberto Coutinho Manhães Junior,[2] Bruno de Castro Figuêiredo,[2] Danielle Shima Luize,[1] Rolando Plumer Pezzini,[1] George Borja de Freitas,[3] and José Luiz Cintra Junqueira[4]

[1]*West State University of Parana, No. 1618 Universitária St., Cascavel, PR 85819-110, Brazil*
[2]*São Leopoldo Mandic College-SP, No. 13 Dr. José Rocha Junqueira St., Campinas, SP 13045-755, Brazil*
[3]*Integrated College of Patos- (FIP-) PB, Horácio Nóbrega St., S/N, Belo Horizonte, Patos, PB 58704-000, Brazil*
[4]*Faculdade São Leopoldo Mandic-SP, No. 13 Dr. José Rocha Junqueira St., Campinas, SP 13045-755, Brazil*

Correspondence should be addressed to Paula Bernardon; paula.bernardon@yahoo.com.br

Academic Editor: Mine Dündar

In cases where malocclusion is associated with intrinsic discoloration and/or discrepancies in tooth size and shape, such as peg-shaped laterals, orthodontics alone may not improve the aesthetics. In these situations, veneers may be considered as an adjunct to orthodontic treatment to improve the overall aesthetics. The aim of this study is to report a clinical case where an uneven occlusal plane was corrected, and the positioning of gingival zeniths, color, shape, and size of the dental elements involved were improved by means of gingivectomy and rehabilitation with 10 ceramic laminate veneers. It was possible to conclude that multidisciplinary treatment, when properly planned and indicated, respecting the limits and established techniques of periodontics, prosthesis, and dentistry, makes small occlusal leveling predictable and possible through these tools.

1. Introduction

Ceramic laminates are a highly conservative treatment when compared to total crowns due to the minimum structure removal required for this procedure, around 0.3 to 0.9 mm. Ideally, the preparation should be restricted to the enamel, although dentin exposure is often unavoidable, especially in the cervical area, as discussed by Gresnigt et al. [1].

The ceramic laminates are restorations that are bonded using adhesive cements that range from the application of phosphoric acid to silanization and the application of the adhesive and the cement itself, which guarantee high predictability, as well as aesthetics, allowing improvements in color, shape, positioning, reestablishment of the vertical dimension of occlusion, and dental exposure (D'Arcangelo et al. [2]). According to Aboushelib et al. [3], "Once properly cemented, ceramic veneers become an integral part of the tooth structure and share part of applied loading stresses during masticatory cycle."

Patients who present significant dental misalignment should have as their first choice of treatment the orthodontic movement as the most conservative option. However, those who have defects in color or shape of the dental elements will already be subject to a more invasive restorative treatment for aesthetic correction. In cases such as this, minor dental corrections can be performed during dental preparation and the gingival zenith may become harmonic through crown lengthening, according to Marchionatti et al. [4].

In order to correct or change the positioning of the gingival zeniths, some periodontal procedures may be necessary, such as surgical clinical crown lengthening or root coverage. These maneuvers will allow a proper new dental height (Patel and Durey [5]; Ganji et al. [6]).

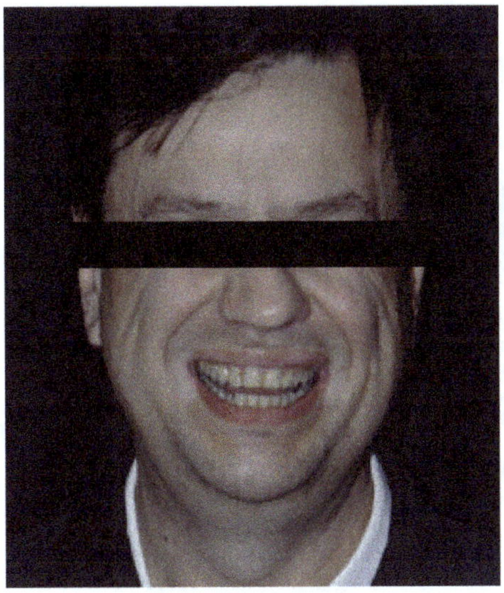

Figure 1: Face photograph.

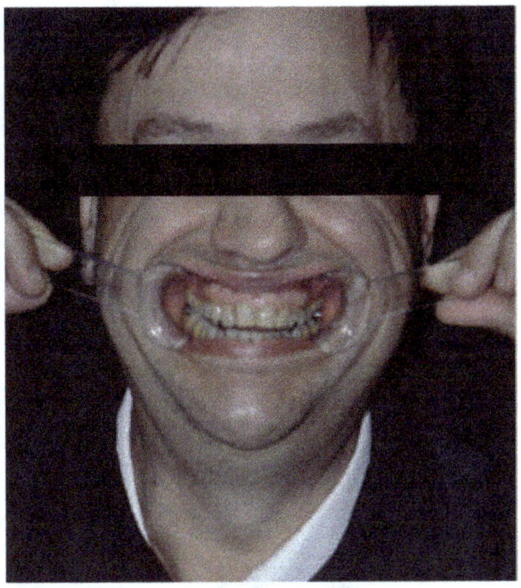

Figure 2: Smile with lip retractors.

The aim of this study is to report a clinical case where an uneven occlusal plane was corrected, the positioning of gingival zeniths, color, shape, and size of the dental elements involved were improved by means of gingivectomy and rehabilitation with 10 ceramic laminate veneers.

2. Case Report

This case involves a 56-year-old male patient with an angle class I occlusion, but with an uneven occlusal plane and dental elements with alterations in color, size, shape, incisal wear, and gingival zenith. Initially, dental impressions from both dental arches (performed with the addition of silicone rubber; Virtual, Ivoclar Vivadent), occlusion record, and digital smile design protocol photos (DSD) were used for the case planning (Figures 1–3). By means of radiographs, it was possible to evaluate the necessity of strategic bone removals to redefine the supracrestal space (Figure 4).

80% of the width to height ratio was applied to define the new design of the dental elements, starting at the central incisor. The possibility of performing this new aesthetic planning was confirmed by radiographic and clinical examinations and subsequent mock-ups (Figures 5(a)–5(c) and 6).

The mock-up with Protemp™ 4 bisacrylic resin was performed in the patient for aesthetic, phonetic, and functional proof of virtual planning by means of CAD/CAM milling diagnostic waxing. A surgical guide was manufactured to increase the clinical crown (gingivectomy and osteotomy) according to the parameters suggested by the virtual design (DSD) (Figure 7). According to Lee's classification system for aesthetic crown lengthening procedures (Lee [7]), all dental elements were classified as type I (sufficient soft tissue allows gingival exposure of the alveolar crest or violation of the biologic width), except for element 23 which was classified as type II (sufficient soft tissue allows gingival excision without the exposure of the alveolar crest but with violation of the biologic width).

In order to perform surgical crown lengthening (Figures 8–11), the surgical guide was used to perform the

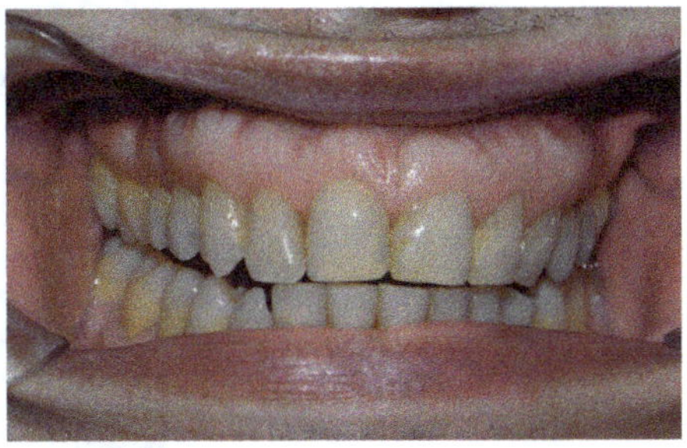

Figure 3: Approximate view of the smile.

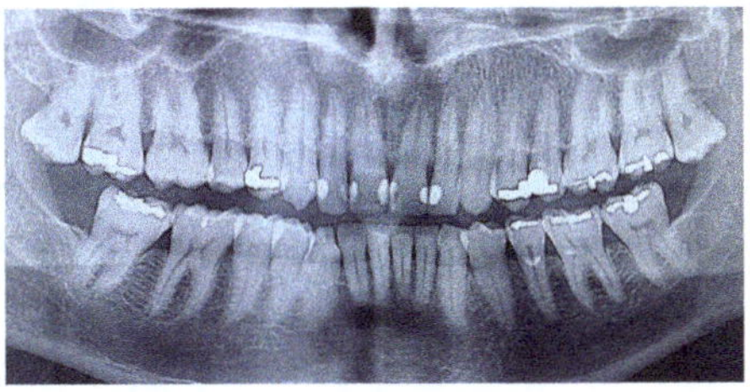

Figure 4: Radiograph aspect.

incisions and the definition of the new gingival zeniths. Osteotomies were performed intrasulcularly with the aid of Ochsenbein's chisels, acquiring a biological space of 3 mm. The patient was followed up postoperatively; because the gingival margin was stable and to avoid the inflammation process, no type of temporary material was used during the healing period. 60 days after the surgical procedure, new dental impressions were obtained, diagnostic waxing was performed under the new periodontal parameters, and a new mock-up with Protemp™ 4 Temporization Material (3M ESPE) bisacrylic resin was realized (Figure 12).

Dental preparations under gingival spacing with retractor cord number 000 Ultrapack (Ultradent) were obtained by means of the selective wear of the tooth structure with a diamond drill in an electric motor under constant irrigation,

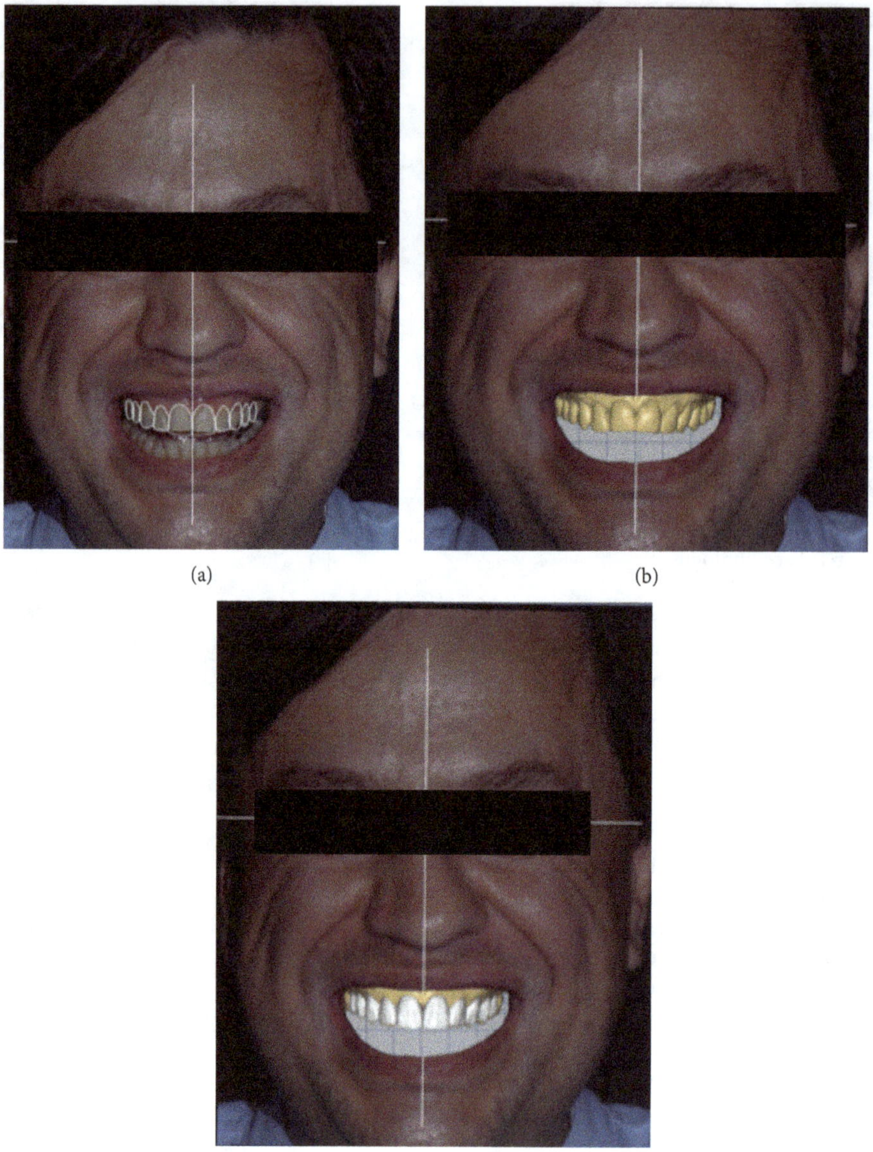

(a) (b) (c)

FIGURE 5: DSD planning.

guided by a condensation silicone rubber index made from the diagnostic waxing, both palatal and incisal and vestibular (in its three-thirds). Measurements of adequate ceramic space (between 0.3 and 0.5 mm) were checked from time to time with the aid of a periodontal probe from the dental enamel to the guide (Figures 13 and 14). Every angle should be rounded, and the preparation should be adequately finished and polished. Care should be taken to keep the tooth reduction inside the thickness of the enamel (Figure 15).

After polishing and finishing the preparation, a number 2 Ultrapack retractor cord (Ultradent) was inserted into all 10 dental elements soaked in hemostatic solution and held for 5 minutes for a horizontal spacing of the gingival tissues (Figure 16).

After the cord removal, the preparations were washed, dried, and scanned using the 3Shape (TRIOS) scanner. The antagonist teeth and the occlusion of the patient were also obtained by means of the scanning. As the preparation was restricted to the dental enamel, dentin was not previously sealed and the provisional restoration was made with the Protemp™ 4 Temporization Material (3M ESPE) bisacrylic resin. The silicone index, obtained from the wax-up, was used to mold a self-curing composite material in the same morphology obtained with the previsualization mock-up. The direct provisional restoration, after intraoral finishing and polishing, was macromechanically retained on the prepared teeth until the luting session.

The ceramic laminate veneers (IPS e.max, Ivoclar Vivadent) were made to CAD/CAM impressions and painted by the technician. At first, the dry test was performed in the mouth, to check the individual adaptation of each one (Figures 17 and 18). This was followed by the wet test with the try-in pastes of the Variolink Esthetic LC System Kit e.max (Ivoclar Vivadent) and cemented under absolute

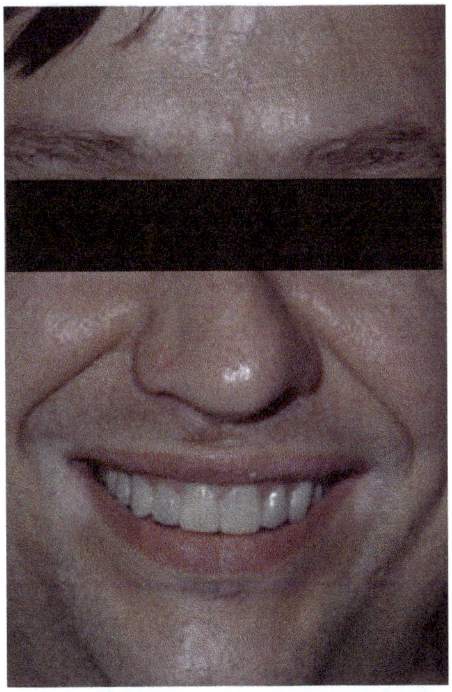

FIGURE 6: Mock-up.

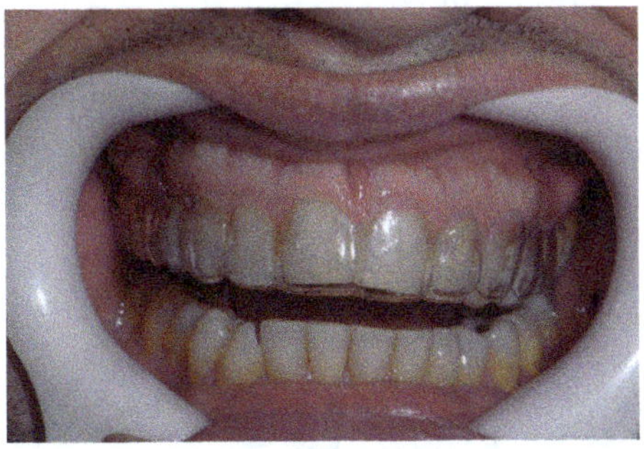

FIGURE 7: Surgical index.

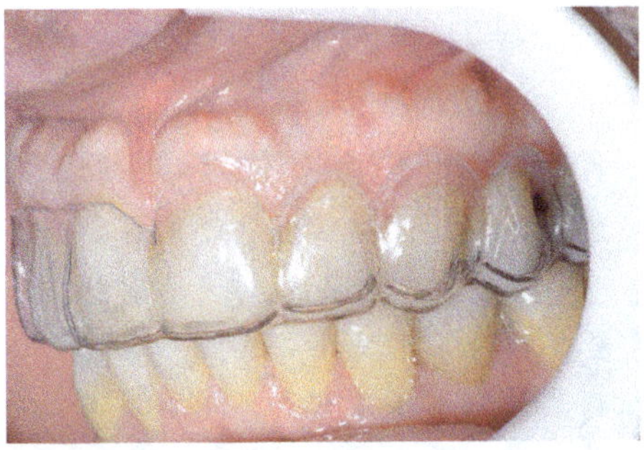

FIGURE 8: Surgical index: lateral view.

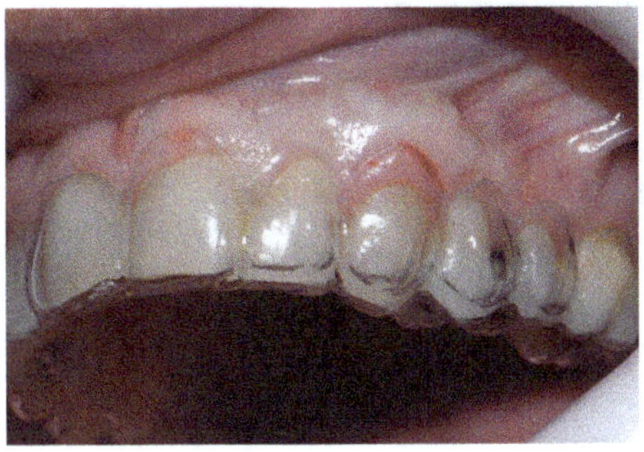

FIGURE 9: Incisions with the guide.

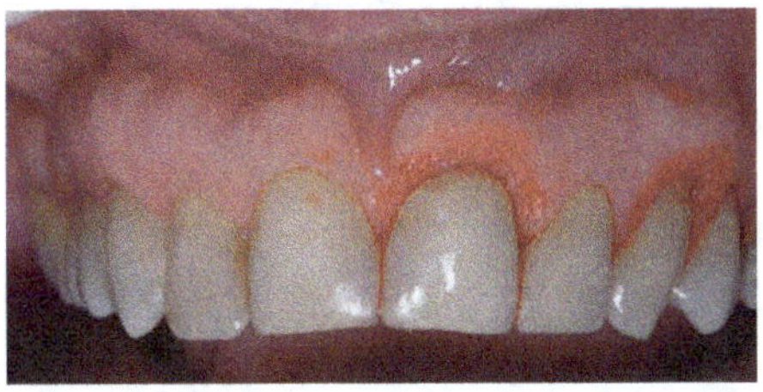

FIGURE 10: Incisions.

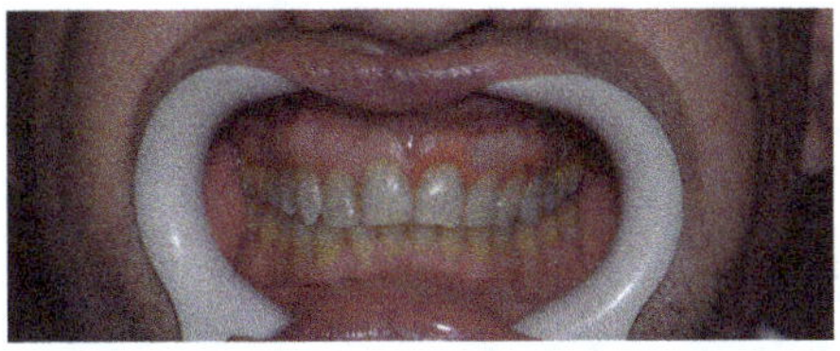

FIGURE 11: Final aspect.

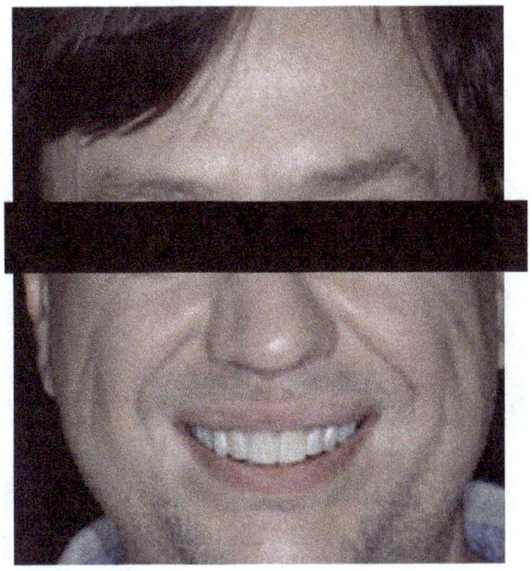

FIGURE 12: Mock up with the new gingival position.

isolation of the operative field and previous prophylaxis of dental elements, starting with the treatment of the lithium disilicate (IPS e.max, Ivoclar Vivadent) pieces with 10% hydrofluoric acid (Dentsply) (Figures 19 and 20) for 20 seconds, washing and drying, followed by the application of phosphoric acid Total Etch 37% (Ivoclar Vivadent) for 30 seconds (Figure 21), Monobond N (Ivoclar Vivadent) silanization (Figure 22) of two layers with heat activation for 1 minute, and application of Tetric N-Bond Universal adhesive (Ivoclar Vivadent) and Variolink Esthetic LC cement (Ivoclar Vivadent) in light color.

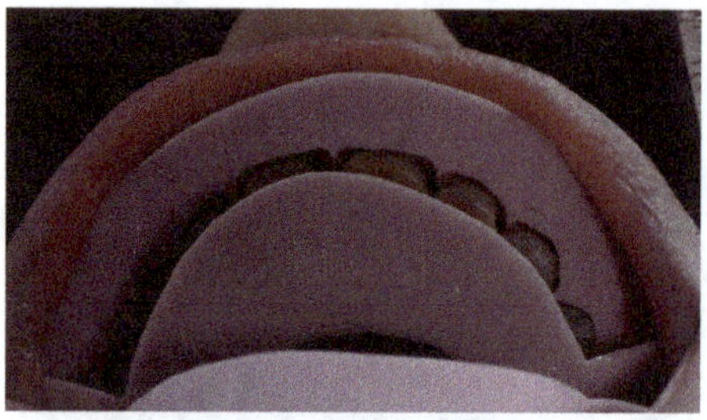

Figure 13: Vestibular guide.

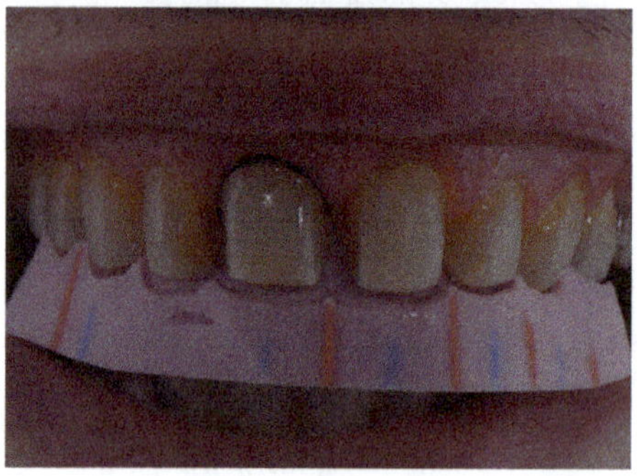

Figure 14: Incisal guide.

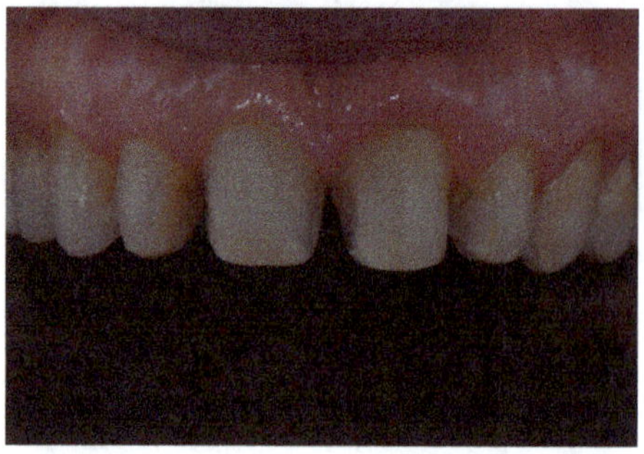

Figure 15: Final aspect of dental preparation.

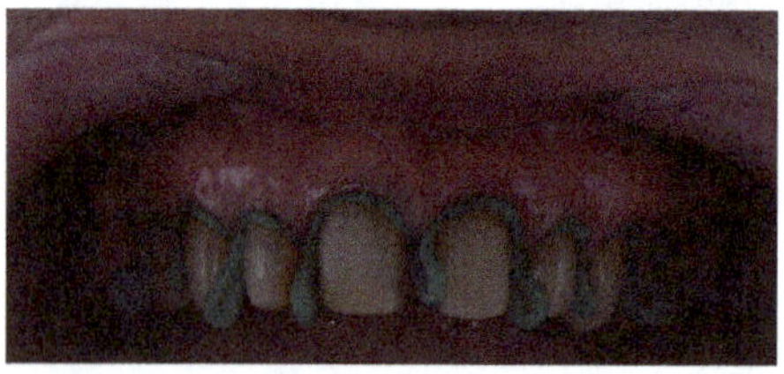

Figure 16: Retractor cord number 2.

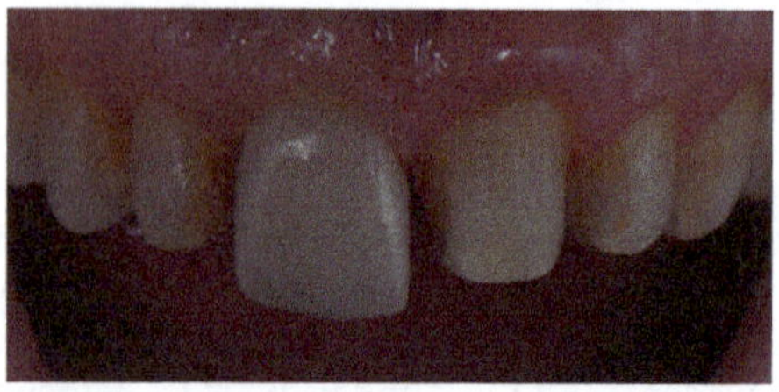

Figure 17: Dry proof in a vestibular view.

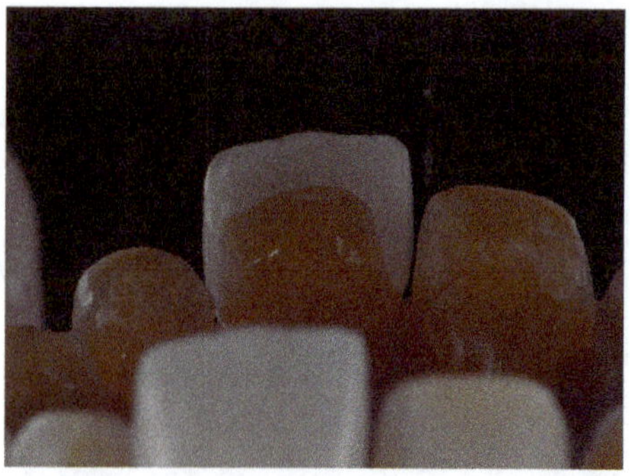

Figure 18: Dry proof in a palatine view.

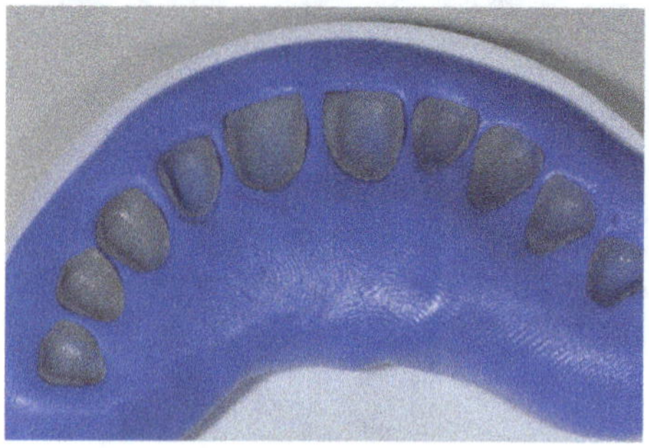

Figure 19: Ceramic laminate veneers.

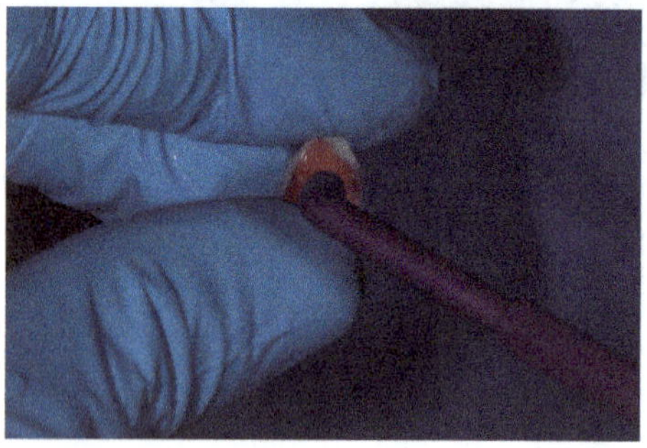

Figure 20: Hydrofluoric acid application for 20 seconds.

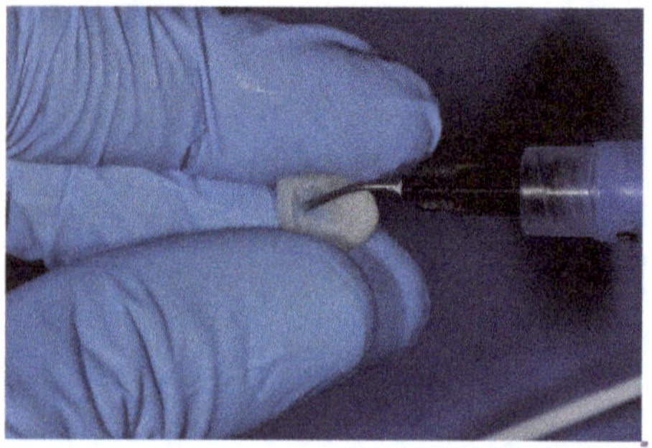

Figure 21: Phosphoric acid application for 30 seconds.

Dental elements were conditioned with 37% Total Etch phosphoric acid (Ivoclar Vivadent) for 30 seconds in enamel (Figure 23) and Tetric N-Bond Universal adhesive (Ivoclar

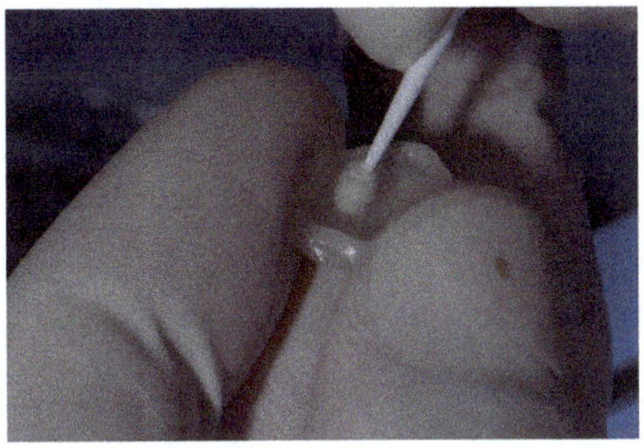

Figure 22: Silanization.

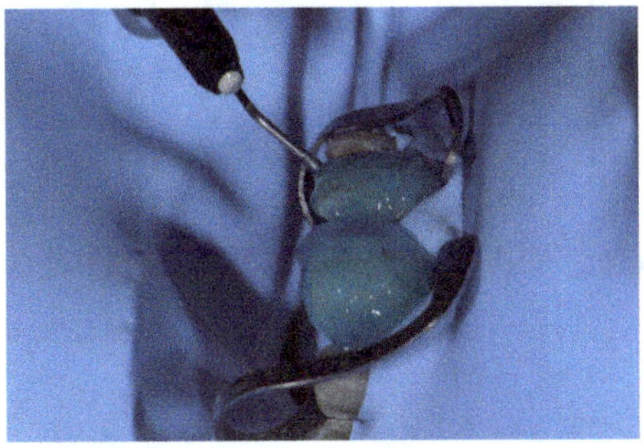

Figure 23: Phosphoric acid application for 30 seconds in enamel.

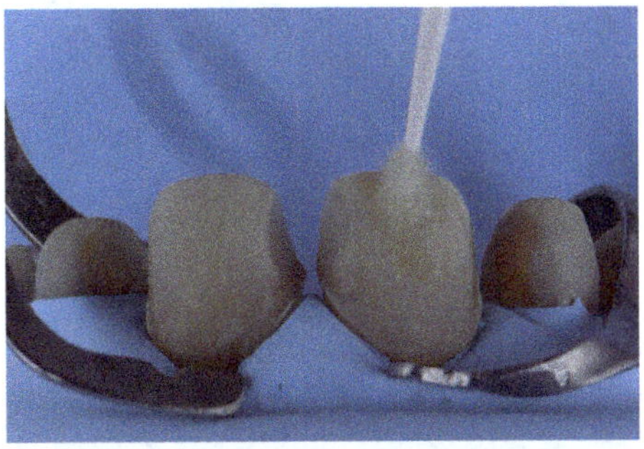

Figure 24: Bond application.

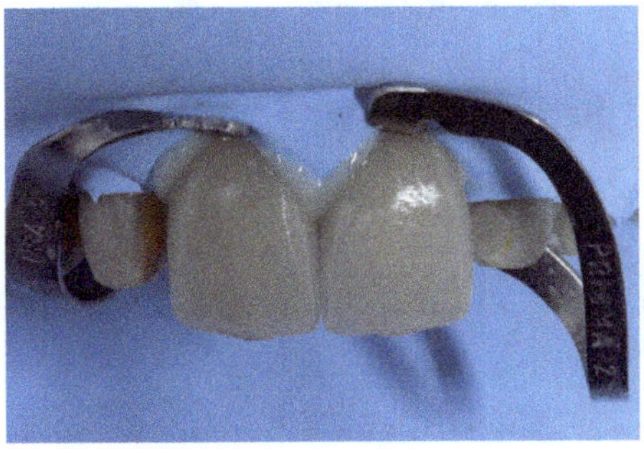

Figure 25: Ceramic laminate veneers with cement.

Vivadent) (Figure 24) was applied followed by air jets for solvent evaporation, laying the laminates in pairs beginning with the central incisors and then ending one side at a time (Figure 25), removal of excesses with the aid of dental floss

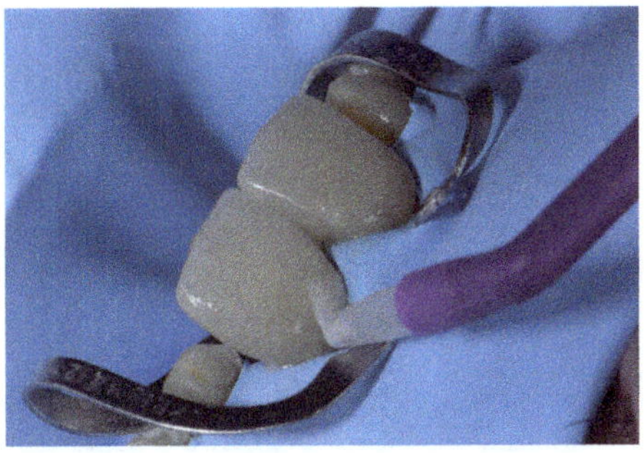

Figure 26: Cement excess removal.

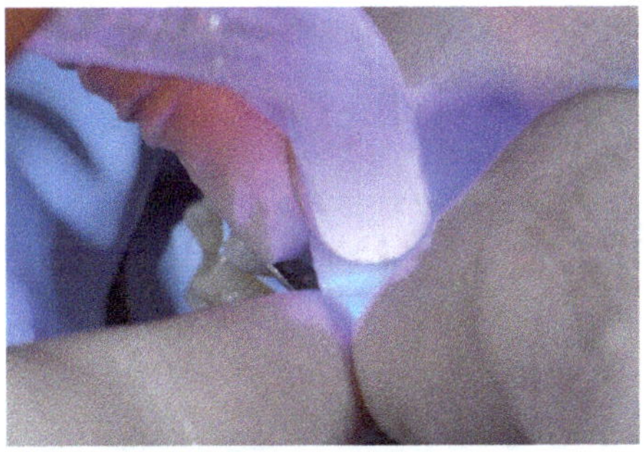

Figure 27: Photopolymerization.

and brushes (Figure 26), photopolymerization for 40 seconds of each face (Figure 27) and followed by the application of Liquid Strip (Ivoclar Vivadent) glycerin on the edges of the restoration and new photopolymerization to inhibit the effect of oxygen in the last layer of cement.

A delicate margin of finishing and polishing was performed (Figure 28). A slight excess was removed with a box carver or a No. 12 scalpel blade; then, if necessary, low-grit diamond burs and flexible blades (40 and 15 μm) were used on a reciprocating handpiece. Finally, composite polishers, cups, and synthetic brushes with diamond paste were used. Once the rubber dam was removed, occlusal relation was checked in maximum intercuspation, then in laterality and during protrusive movements (Figures 29 and 30).

A two-year follow-up was performed, and the pieces did not present fractures, discoloration, or decreased cementation. The margin preparation was sealed and the occlusion was stable. Other dental elements did not present structural wear and tear (Figures 31–34).

3. Discussion

Associated with a high level of dental aesthetics, the occlusal parameters must be stable and must ensure that the temporomandibular joint remains healthy, the teeth are firm, and the support structures are in a suitable condition. Otherwise, the prognosis of restorative treatment becomes unpredictable (Brea et al. [8]). In this case, all the mandibular excursion movements were performed; protrusive, lateral-lateral, and all contacts were checked; and possible premature contacts were removed, in order to guarantee occlusal stability.

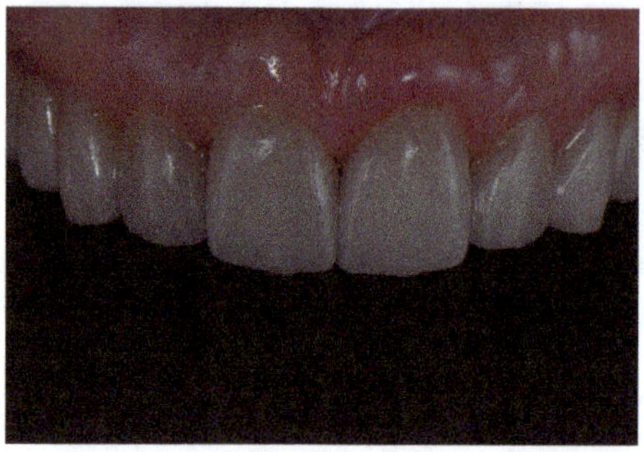

Figure 28: After finishing and polishing.

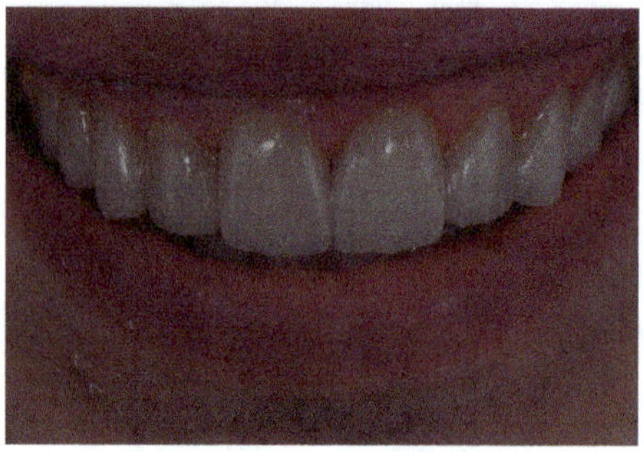

Figure 29: Final aspect of the smile.

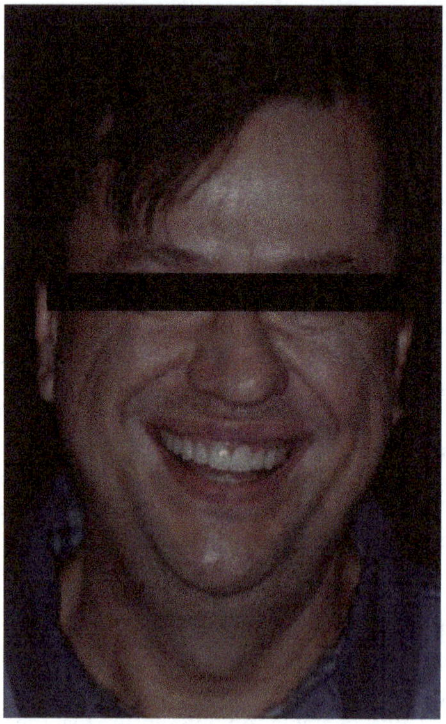

Figure 30: Final aspect of the face.

According to Lee in 2004 [7], conventional protocols require a waiting period of 4 to 6 weeks for sufficient healing of the attachment apparatus prior to initiating restorative endeavors. In this case, a longer period of healing was expected due to patient availability.

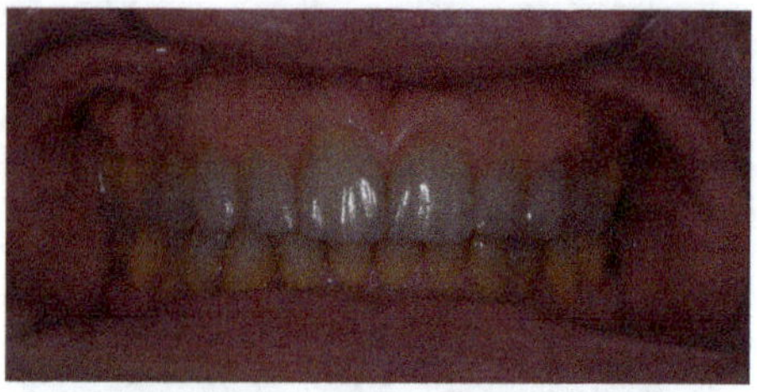

Figure 31: Two-year follow-up period.

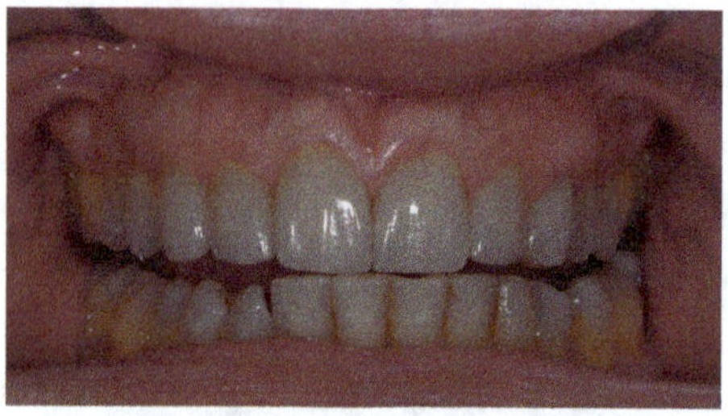

Figure 32: Two-year follow-up period: protrusion movement.

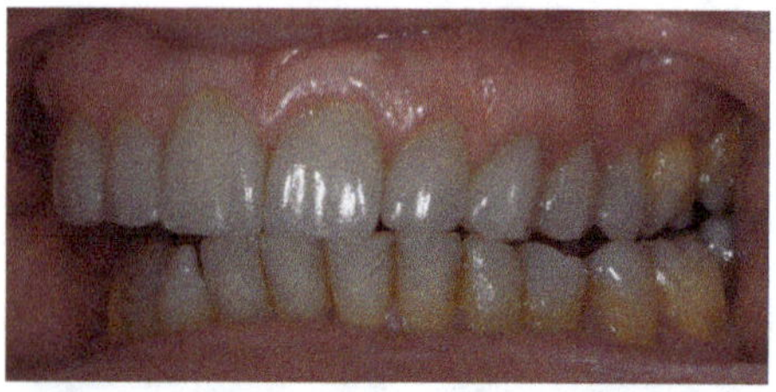

Figure 33: Two-year follow-up period: excursion movement.

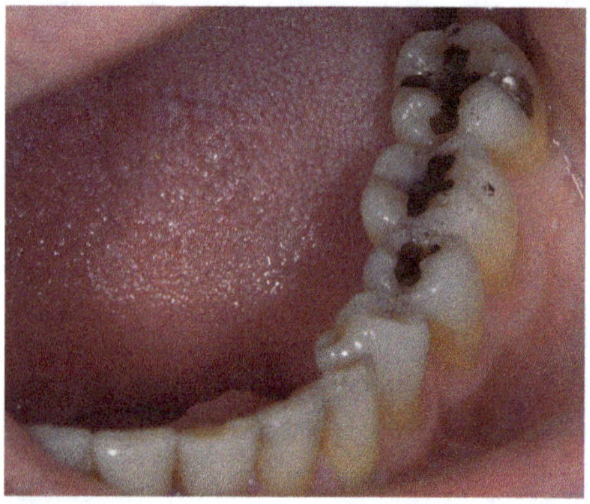

Figure 34: Two-year follow-up period: occlusal points in maximum intercuspidation.

"Minimal tooth reduction, esthetics, and maintenance of healthy tissues are the major advantages of conservative preparation of ceramic laminate veneers. Since ceramic is a translucent material, tooth-colored resin cement under these restorations is mainly reflected from beneath the restoration for optimal esthetics" (Çömlekoğlu et al. [9]). For these reasons, in this study a cement was selected that presented the try-in in its system to allow adequate selection of the final color of the set formed by the dental element, cement, and ceramic laminate.

In a randomized split-mouth clinical trial carried out by Gresnigt et al. [10], a comparison of the indirect resin composite and ceramic laminate veneers was performed. The results presented cover observations up to 120 months of clinical function and showed that ceramic veneers performed significantly better than the indirect composite ones.

Increased fractures and chippings were noticed up to 8 times in studies with composite laminate veneers. Debondings of composite laminate veneers occurred in the same patient whilst all laminate veneers functioned until the end of the study. Indirect resin composite material showed surface degradation and diminished gloss retention. On the other hand, all ceramic restorations remained smooth and their gloss was retained until the final follow-up. In this way, surface quality changes were more frequently observed in the composite veneer material that may require more maintenance over time (Gresnigt et al. [10]). However, despite the results obtained in this study for composites, they should not be discarded as a restorative option, since they have low cost, ease of access, and easy resolution of any intercurrences that may arise.

In agreement with this case, the inadequate periodontal contour of the restorations causes food impaction, making it difficult to control the plaque. For this reason, the alignment of the dental elements, either by means of orthodontic movement or by the association of periodontal restorative and surgical techniques that allow a balance between the white and pink aesthetics, guarantee health in all aspects in cases of mild to moderate discrepancies. In cases of crowding or severe malposition, in which the disharmony of the papillae is present, the treatment indicated is the orthodontic treatment prior to any restorative treatment (Brea et al. [8]).

4. Conclusion

It was possible to conclude that multidisciplinary treatment, when properly planned and indicated, respecting the limits and established techniques of periodontics, prosthesis, and dentistry, makes small occlusal leveling predictable and possible through these tools.

Consent

Informed consent was obtained from the patient.

References

[1] M. M. M. Gresnigt, M. S. Cune, J. G. de Roos, and M. Özcan, "Effect of immediate and delayed dentin sealing on the fracture strength, failure type and Weilbull characteristics of lithiumdisilicate laminate veneers," *Dental Materials*, vol. 32, no. 4, pp. e73–e81, 2016.

[2] C. D'Arcangelo, F. De Angelis, M. Vadini, and M. D'Amario, "Clinical evaluation on porcelain laminate veneers bonded with light-cured composite: results up to 7 years," *Clinical Oral Investigations*, vol. 16, no. 4, pp. 1071–1079, 2012.

[3] M. N. Aboushelib, W. A. M. Elmahy, and M. H. Ghazy, "Internal adaptation, marginal accuracy and microleakage of a pressable versus a machinable ceramic laminate veneers," *Journal of Dentistry*, vol. 40, no. 8, pp. 670–677, 2012.

[4] A. M. E. Marchionatti, V. F. Wandscher, M. M. May, M. A. Bottino, and L. G. May, "Color stability of ceramic laminate veneers cemented with light-polymerizing and dual-polymerizing luting agent: a split-mouth randomized clinical trial," *The Journal of Prosthetic Dentistry*, vol. 118, no. 5, pp. 604–610, 2017.

[5] M. Patel, K. Durey, and P. A. Brunton, "Porcelain laminate veneers. What, when and how?," *Dental Nursing*, vol. 6, no. 10, pp. 556–564, 2010.

[6] K. K. Ganji, V. A. Patil, and J. John, "A comparative evaluation for biologic width following surgical crown lengthening using gingivectomy and ostectomy procedure," *International Journal of Dentistry*, vol. 2012, Article ID 479241, 9 pages, 2012.

[7] E. Lee, "Aesthetic crown lengthening: classification, biologic rationale, and treatment planning considerations," *Practical Procedures & Aesthetic Dentistry*, vol. 16, pp. 769–778, 2004.

[8] L. Brea, A. Oquendo, and S. David, "Dental crowding: the restorative approach," *Dental Clinics of North America*, vol. 55, no. 2, pp. 301–310, 2011.

[9] M. E. Çömlekoğlu, G. Paken, F. Tan et al., "Evaluation of different thickness, die color, and resin cement shade for veneers of multilayered CAD/CAM blocks," *Journal of Prosthodontics*, vol. 25, no. 7, pp. 563–569, 2016.

[10] M. M. M. Gresnigt, M. S. Cune, K. Jansen, S. A. M. van der Made, and M. Ozcan, "Randomized clinical trial on indirect resin composite and ceramic laminate veneers: up to 10-year findings," *Journal of Dentistry*, vol. 86, pp. 102–109, 2019.

3

Bilateral Bone Ridge Splitting in Maxilla with Immediate Implant Placement in a Patient with Osteoporosis: A Clinical Report with 2-Year Follow-up

Rafał Flieger

Private Dental Healthcare, ul. Nacławska 11, 64-000 Kościan, Poland

Correspondence should be addressed to Rafał Flieger; rafal.flieger@wp.pl

Academic Editor: Eugenio Maiorano

Every year, a higher percentage of bisphosphonates is prescribed for osteoporosis treatment which can lead to bone osteonecrosis after several surgical procedures in the oral cavity. This report describes an approach to restore two missing teeth, employing bilateral bone ridge splitting in the maxilla with immediate placement of implants in a patient using bisphosphonates in the management of osteoporosis. Two titanium implants with a width of 3.45 mm and a length of 10 mm were placed in the maxillary ridge with a diameter of 4.4 mm and 3.0 mm in positions 15 and 24 according to the classification of the World Dental Federation. The implants were placed immediately by bone splitting, using a piezosurgery device and guided bone regeneration with an alloplastic material and a collagen membrane. Five months later, the implants were uncovered and the final porcelain crowns were cemented. 24 months later, the control through clinical and radiographical examinations showed no bone loss in the collar part of the implants and the proper status of the peri-implant soft tissue without any signs of inflammation. Piezosurgery is a useful and safe method of ridge splitting in a very thin ridge (4.5 and 3.0 mm).

1. Introduction

The rapid development of implant dentistry has resulted in improvements in the characteristics and design of titanium implants achieving a high level of bone-to-implant contact; therefore, the osseointegration process no longer poses a challenge [1]. The recent literature confirmed that 99.1% of implants in the mandible and 84.9% of implants in the maxilla have become osseointegrated and have allowed for the prosthetic reconstruction of missing teeth in a 5-year follow-up [2]. The complication rate of this treatment varies from 0% to 29% after 5- and 10-year follow-ups, respectively [3, 4]. The essential factor conditioning the implant insertion success is the availability of sufficient amounts of soft and hard tissues [5–7]. In cases of a lack of proper bone thickness of the alveolar ridge, an additional surgical procedure is required. Augmentation of thin alveolar ridges can be accomplished by several techniques, such as by bone block grafting and by ridge splitting [8].

The method of ridge splitting was introduced for the first time by Tatum in 1969 [9]. The study of Sethi and Kaus showed implant survival rates of 97-98.8% after five years [10]. Bone splitting using different devices, such as the piezo saw and osteotome, allows for implant insertion even with a ridge thinner than 3.5 mm with only a minimal risk of a bone plate fracture or perforation. The lateral ridge split augmentation technique, with immediate implant placement, reduces the time of the treatment and the time of the final prosthetic reconstruction. Furthermore, compression of the bone increases its density [11]. Lateral crest splitting can be performed using various surgical tools, e.g., chisels, rotary burs, and saws, or using the piezosurgery unit [8]. The piezosurgery machine produces ultrasounds with a frequency in the range of 22–35 kHz and affords surgical precision and safeness of cutting with minimal bleeding [8]. The relative disadvantage of this technique is the increase in bone temperature during osteotomy; hence, adequate cooling and the high-level skills of the operator are demanded [12, 13].

The success of the implant treatment is affected by the quality and quantity of the soft and hard tissues and the characteristics of the titanium implants [1, 5–8, 14]. However, patient-related factors are also crucial, especially their health status. Every year, a higher percentage of antiresorptive and antiangiogenetic medicines are prescribed for osteoporosis treatment. Specific remedies hinder osteoclastic action, thereby reducing bone turnover, which raises the patients' quality of life [15]. The administration of antiresorptive and antiangiogenetic medicines, especially in oncology, diminishes the incidence of bone fracture for patients with osteoporosis [16]. However, a serious side effect that can develop as a result of this therapy is medication-related osteonecrosis of the jaws (MRONJ) and in particular bisphosphonate-related osteonecrosis of the jaw (BRONJ), the first form of this side effect, described by Marx in 2003 [17].

In 2014, the American Association of Oral and Maxillofacial Surgeons define MRONJ as jawbone osteonecrosis related to antiresorptive and antiangiogenetic drugs, describing its main features as follows: bone exposure in the maxillofacial region that persisted for more than 8 weeks, patient treated with antiresorptive or antiangiogenic medications, no history of radiation, and no traumatic origin of bone exposure [15].

This article describes an approach to restore two missing teeth employing bilateral bone ridge splitting in the maxilla with immediate implant placements in a patient using bisphosphonates in the management of osteoporosis.

2. Case Presentation

2.1. Presurgical Phase. A 56-year old white woman was referred to our clinic for prosthetic crown reconstruction of two missing molars in the maxilla. The patient lost her teeth (15, 24 FDI) 15 months ago because of a deep carious lesion. The patient was not using any dental prostheses post the extractions. Medical history revealed that she suffered from hypertension and osteoporosis, which were all under medical control. For her osteoporosis, the patient used oral bisphosphonate of alendronate (Fosamax) at a dose of 70 mg/week for 24 months. During the time of osteoporosis treatment with alendronate, there were no accidents of bone osteonecrosis following the teeth's extraction.

After a consultation with the medical doctor of the patient and reviewing the literature concerning surgical therapy in patients with osteoporosis, we decided to perform the placement of the implants without stopping the bisphosphonate therapy. However, before the operation the patient was given antibiotic treatment with amoxicillin+clavulanic acid (Amoxiclav, Sandoz, Poland) at a dose of 1000 mg/day for 1 week, and laser photobiomodulation using a diode laser with a wavelength of 635 nm (dose of 4 J per point, 2 points at each site) was performed one day before the procedure.

Intraoral examination using CBCT (Kodak 9000 3D, Carestream/Trophy, Marne-la-Vallée, France) revealed that the volume of the ridge at the right side of the maxilla was 4.5 mm in width and 16.5 mm in height. At the opposite left side of the maxilla, the ridge amounted to 3.0 mm in diameter and 13.5 mm in height (Figure 1). A written informed consent form was signed by the patient before the treatment.

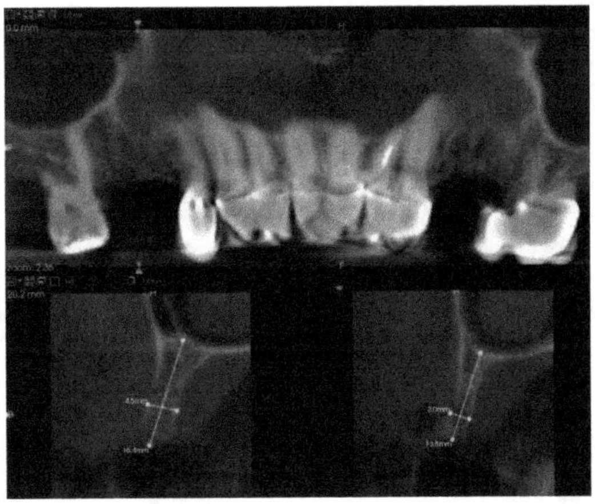

Figure 1: A CBCT scan of the patient with a very thin maxillary alveolar ridge.

2.2. Surgical Phase and Prosthetic Rehabilitation. The surgical procedure was conducted under local infiltrative anesthesia with articaine hydrochloride 4% plus epinephrine (Ubistesin®, 3M, USA). The access to the buccal and lingual part of the maxillary crests on both sides was prepared with a cold blade and a soft tissue elevator. Three cuts were conducted during the proceedings of the ridge splitting: one horizontal cut on the alveolar ridge and two vertical cuts on the buccal bone plate using the piezosurgery unit (Piezotome Solo, Acteon, New Jersey, USA) with a BS1 tip. In the first phase of the implant bed preparation, the Lindemann guide drill with a diameter of 2.2 mm was utilized; then, the ridge was split employing a bone spreader (Meisinger, Colorado, USA). In the last stage, the final drill with a diameter of 2.9 mm was used to prepare the implant bed, and two ICX-plus implants (ICX, Germany, USA) with a width of 3.45 mm and a length of 10 mm were placed. On both surgical sides, the guided bone regeneration was done using an alloplastic material (SinossGraft, Novadento, Italy) and a collagen membrane (SinossMem, Novadento, Italy) with a long disintegration time (5-6 months). The wound was protected using a nonabsorbable monofilament and an uncoated suture made of polyamide (Dafilon, B. Braun, Germany) with a size of 4.0 (Figure 2).

After the surgery, an antiseptic mouth rinse (chlorhexidine gluconate 0.12%, twice a day for 7 days) was directed and the patient was provided with the usual postsurgical indications (cold compresses in the first two days, antibiotic treatment with amoxicillin+clavulanic acid (Amoxiclav, Sandoz, Poland) at a dose of 1000 mg/day for 1 week, and nonsteroidal anti-inflammatory drugs, i.e., ibuprofen 200 mg, 3 times per day for 3 days).

Five months later, the implants were uncovered with use of a scalpel and healing screws were placed for two weeks. Next, the open tray method with prosthetic transfers was used to take the impression of the upper jaw. After ten days, the final porcelain crowns were made by a dental laboratory and cemented onto the implants (Figure 3).

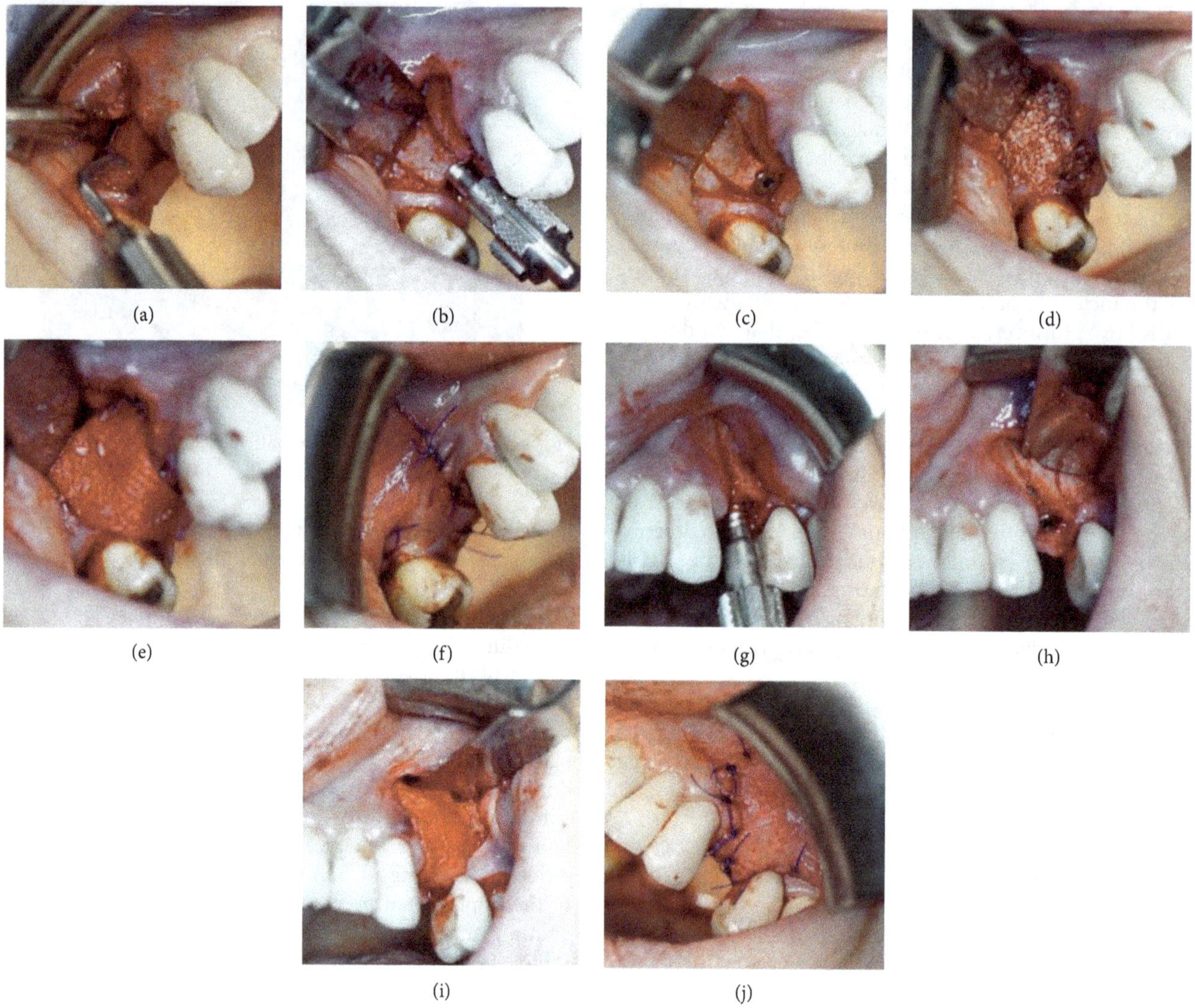

Figure 2: Ridge splitting with immediate placement of implants. (a) Bone osteotomy using piezosurgery. (b) Bone spreading with hand instruments. (c) The implant placement on the right side of the maxilla. (d) Alloplastic material grafting. (e) Collagen membrane placement. (f) Sutures. (g) Bone spreading with hand instruments on the left side of the maxilla. (h) The implant placement on the left side of the maxilla. (i) Placement of alloplastic material and collagen membrane. (j) Sutures.

2.3. Follow-Up Phase. Every six months, the patient was referred for a check-up visit and the last control 24 months after the prosthetic crown placement showed a lack of bone loss in the collar part of both implants and the normal status of the peri-implant soft tissue without any signs of inflammation (Figures 4 and 5).

3. Discussion

Prevention of BRONJ/MRONJ in oral and maxillofacial surgery is critical in patients considered at risk. Proper oral hygiene, mouth rinsing with antibacterial fluids, and antibiotic and laser therapies are crucial factors to decrease the risk of bone necrosis after various surgical procedures in the oral cavities. According to the literature, the risk of BRONJ/MRONJ in patients taking oral bisphosphonates is low [16]. However, the risk of MRONJ for patients exposed to oral bisphosphonates in the management of osteoporosis after endodontic treatment, periodontal surgery, or implant placement is unknown [18]. Thus, the patients who need teeth restoration using dental implants and at the same time are treated with oral and especially intravenous bisphosphonates belong to a group with a higher risk of postsurgical complications.

In a recent systematic review, Khan et al. [16] showed that the incidence of BRONJ/MRONJ in the osteoporotic patient group ranged between 0.001% and 0.01%, similar to the percentage found in the general population (<0.001%). On the other hand, the occurrence of MRONJ/BRONJ is most significant in the oncology patient group that used high doses of bisphosphonates (1% to 15%). In the study conducted by Dodson in 2015 [18], the author concluded that MRONJ is an uncommon disease among patients exposed to antiresorptive or antiangiogenic medications. Furthermore, the risk of MRONJ among patients who are treated for osteoporosis using antiresorptive prescriptions is about 0.1% (range 0.004%–0.2%). The same risk for patients with cancer exposed to antiresorptive or antiangiogenic medicines

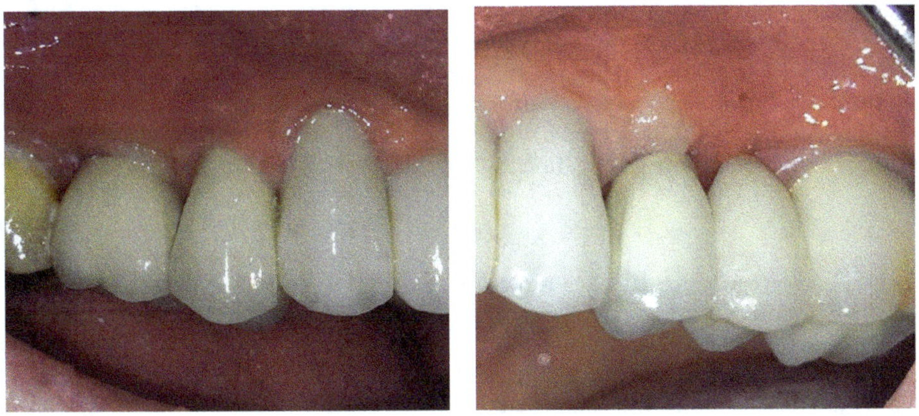

(a) (b)

FIGURE 3: Prosthetic crowns immediately after cementation on the abutments. (a) Right side of the maxilla. (b) Left side of the maxilla.

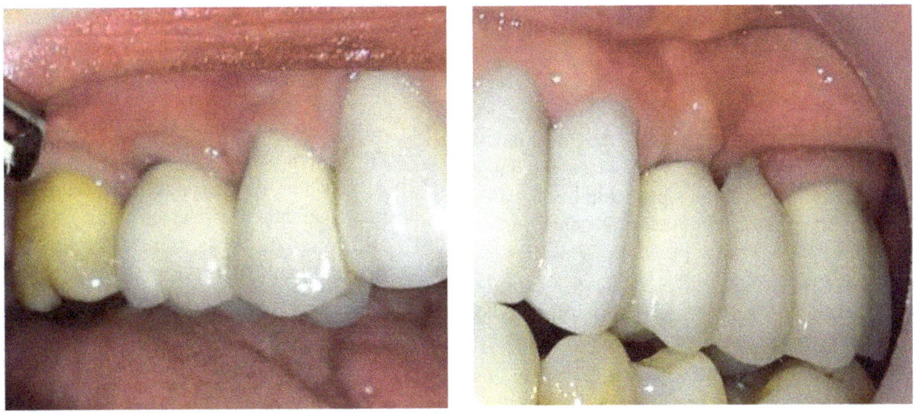

(a) (b)

FIGURE 4: Prosthetic crowns 2 years after the cementation. (a) Right side of the maxilla. (b) Left side of the maxilla.

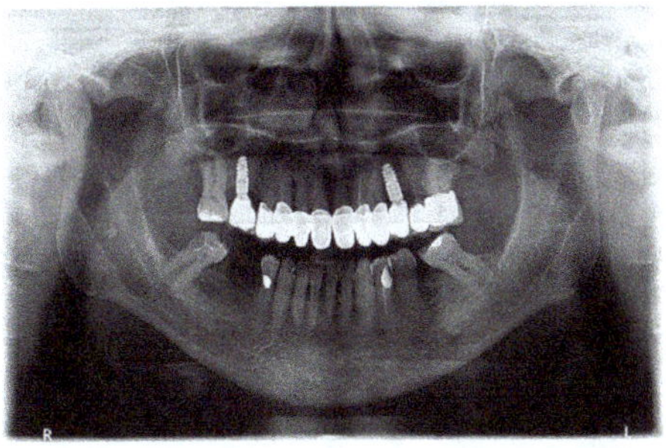

FIGURE 5: OPG 2 years after the treatment.

is approximately 1% (range 0.2%–6.7%). Moreover, the risk of MRONJ for patients exposed to oral bisphosphonates in the management of osteoporosis after tooth extraction has amounted to 0.5% [18].

To know what bisphosphonate patients are taking along with the time duration is essential before any surgical approach in an oral cavity. Grant et al. [19] advised C-terminal telopeptide and collagen type 1 C test (CTx test) for patients receiving treatment for more than three years. The CTx test is a serum blood test allowing the observation of markers of bone turnover, and it may help in the examination and risk estimation to determine if MRONJ is developing.

Multiple methods are utilized for bone tissue augmentation [20]. The crest splitting technique allows placing an implant simultaneously with guided bone regeneration alternatively to horizontal and vertical augmentation procedures. It was proven that this method improves bone volume with a minimal failure rate [8]. The disadvantage of this procedure when using osteotomes for bone expansion is a fracturing of bone trabeculae that results in a decrease in peri-implant bone density and causes delayed secondary stability in contrast to the classical drilling technique. Trisi et al. [21] pointed out some bone necrosis on account of an obstruction of the Havers and Volkmann canals when using osteotomes. Furthermore, the temperature of bone increases by 10°C after using piezosurgery and the laser or surgical saw can lead to bone cell necrosis; thus, a proper cooling system of sufficient quality and experienced surgeons are crucial points if the surgery is to be performed safely [22, 23].

Admittedly, this paper is based on the therapy of an individual patient and does not involve the standardized measurement of a group. Within these limitations, the results imply that the method can be advantageous for patients taking bisphosphonates in the management of osteoporosis and it can be advantageous for an implantologist as well. Future randomized clinical trials considering a longer follow-up period are needed to support the safeness of this treatment.

4. Conclusion

The piezosurgery device has great potential to advance surgical techniques where accuracy in bone preparation is expected. Piezosurgery is useful and has safe tools for ridge splitting surgery on a very thin ridge (4.5 and 3.0 mm). Ridge splitting and guided bone regeneration with immediate implant placement can be safely performed on a patient taking bisphosphonates in the management of osteoporosis.

References

[1] J. Matys, U. Botzenhart, T. Gedrange, and M. Dominiak, "Thermodynamic effects after diode and Er:YAG laser irradiation of grade IV and V titanium implants placed in bone - an ex vivo study. Preliminary report," *Biomedical Engineering/-Biomedizinische Technik*, vol. 61, no. 5, pp. 499–507, 2016.

[2] D. Buser, R. Mericske-Stern, K. Dula, and N. P. Lang, "Clinical experience with one-stage, non-submerged dental implants," *Advances in Dental Research*, vol. 13, no. 1, pp. 153–161, 1999.

[3] D. Tinsley, C. J. Watson, and J. L. Russell, "A comparison of hydroxylapatite coated implant retained fixed and removable mandibular prostheses over 4 to 6 years," *Clinical Oral Implants Research*, vol. 12, no. 2, pp. 159–166, 2001.

[4] A. Binahmed, A. Stoykewych, A. Hussain, B. Love, and V. Pruthi, "Long-term follow-up of hydroxyapatite-coated dental implants–a clinical trial," *International Journal of Oral & Maxillofacial Implants*, vol. 22, no. 6, pp. 963–968, 2007.

[5] J. Matys, K. Swider, and R. Flieger, "Laser instant implant impression method: a case presentation," *Dental and Medical Problems*, vol. 54, no. 1, pp. 101–106, 2017.

[6] M. Dominiak and J. Matys, "Assessment of pain when uncovering implants with Er:YAG laser or scalpel for second stage surgery," *Advances in Clinical and Experimental Medicine*, vol. 25, no. 6, pp. 1179–1184, 2016.

[7] J. Matys, K. Świder, K. Grzech-Leśniak, M. Dominiak, and U. Romeo, "Photobiomodulation by a 635nm diode laser on peri-implant bone: primary and secondary stability and bone density analysis—a randomized clinical trial," *BioMed Research International*, vol. 2019, Article ID 2785302, 8 pages, 2019.

[8] J. Matys, R. Flieger, and M. Dominiak, "Assessment of temperature rise and time of alveolar ridge splitting by means of Er:YAG laser, piezosurgery, and surgical saw: an ex vivo study," *BioMed Research International*, vol. 2016, Article ID 9654975, 8 pages, 2016.

[9] H. Tatum Jr., "Maxillary and sinus implant reconstructions," *Dental Clinics of North America*, vol. 30, no. 2, pp. 207–229, 1986.

[10] A. Sethi and T. Kaus, "Maxillary ridge expansion with simultaneous implant placement: 5-year results of an ongoing clinical study," *International Journal of Oral & Maxillofacial Implants*, vol. 15, no. 4, pp. 491–499, 2000.

[11] A. Stricker, J. Fleiner, S. Stübinger, R. Schmelzeisen, M. Dard, and D. D. Bosshardt, "Bone loss after ridge expansion with or without reflection of the periosteum," *Clinical Oral Implants Research*, vol. 26, no. 5, pp. 529–536, 2015.

[12] Y. L. Tang, J. Yuan, Y. L. Song, W. Ma, X. Chao, and D. H. Li, "Ridge expansion alone or in combination with guided bone regeneration to facilitate implant placement in narrow alveolar ridges: a retrospective study," *Clinical Oral Implants Research*, vol. 26, no. 2, pp. 204–211, 2015.

[13] A. Rahpeyma, S. Khajehahmadi, and V. R. Hosseini, "Lateral ridge split and immediate implant placement in moderately resorbed alveolar ridges: how much is the added width?," *Dental Research Journal*, vol. 10, no. 5, pp. 602–608, 2013.

[14] K. Grzech-Leśniak, J. Matys, K. Jurczyszyn et al., "Histological and thermometric examination of soft tissue de-epithelialization using digitally controlled Er:YAG laser handpiece: an ex vivo study," *Photomedicine and Laser Surgery*, vol. 36, no. 6, pp. 313–319, 2018.

[15] S. L. Ruggiero, T. B. Dodson, J. Fantasia et al., "American Association of Oral and Maxillofacial Surgeons position paper on medication-related osteonecrosis of the jaw—2014 update," *Journal of Oral and Maxillofacial Surgery*, vol. 72, no. 10, pp. 1938–1956, 2014.

[16] A. A. Khan, A. Morrison, D. A. Hanley et al., "Diagnosis and management of osteonecrosis of the jaw: a systematic review and international consensus," *Journal of Bone and Mineral Research*, vol. 30, no. 1, pp. 3–23, 2015.

[17] R. E. Marx, "Pamidronate (Aredia) and zoledronate (Zometa) induced avascular necrosis of the jaws: a growing epidemic," *Journal of Oral and Maxillofacial Surgery*, vol. 61, no. 9, pp. 1115–1117, 2003.

[18] T. B. Dodson, "The frequency of medication-related osteonecrosis of the jaw and its associated risk factors," *Oral and Maxillofacial Surgery Clinics of North America*, vol. 27, no. 4, pp. 509–516, 2015.

[19] B. T. Grant, C. Amenedo, K. Freeman, and R. A. Kraut, "Outcomes of placing dental implants in patients taking oral bisphosphonates: a review of 115 cases," *Journal of Oral and Maxillofacial Surgery*, vol. 66, no. 2, pp. 223–230, 2008.

[20] A. Santarelli, M. Mascitti, G. Orsini et al., "Osteopontin, osteocalcin and OB-cadherin expression in synthetic nanohydroxyapatite vs bovine hydroxyapatite cultured osteoblastic-like cells," *J Biol Regul Homeost Agents.*, vol. 28, no. 3, pp. 523–529, 2014.

[21] P. Trisi, M. Berardini, A. Falco, and M. Podaliri Vulpiani, "Effect of implant thread geometry on secondary stability, bone density, and bone-to-implant contact: a biomechanical and histological analysis," *Implant Dentistry*, vol. 24, no. 4, pp. 384–391, 2015.

[22] J. Matys, J. Hadzik, and M. Dominiak, "Schneiderian membrane perforation rate and increase in bone temperature during maxillary sinus floor elevation by means of Er: YAG laser—an animal study in pigs," *Implant Dentistry*, vol. 26, no. 2, pp. 238–244, 2017.

[23] J. Matys, R. Flieger, G. Tenore, K. Grzech-Leśniak, U. Romeo, and M. Dominiak, "Er:YAG laser, piezosurgery, and surgical drill for bone decortication during orthodontic mini-implant insertion: primary stability analysis—an animal study," *Lasers in Medical Science*, vol. 33, no. 3, pp. 489–495, 2018.

4

Aesthetic Rehabilitation of a Patient with Bruxism using Ceramic Veneers and Overlays Combined with Four-Point Monolithic Zirconia Crowns for Occlusal Stabilization: A 4-Year Follow-Up

André Moreira,[1] Filipe Freitas,[1,2] Duarte Marques,[1,3] and João Caramês[1,4]

[1]*Private practice, Implantology Institute, Lisboa, Portugal*
[2]*Department of Oral Surgery and Oral Medicine, Faculdade de Medicina Dentária da Universidade de Lisboa, Lisbon, Portugal*
[3]*Department of Morfo-Functional Sciences, Faculdade de Medicina Dentária da Universidade de Lisboa, Lisbon, Portugal*
[4]*Department of Oral Surgery and Implant Dentistry, Faculdade de Medicina Dentária da Universidade de Lisboa, Lisbon, Portugal*

Correspondence should be addressed to André Moreira; andregonmoreira@gmail.com

Academic Editor: Tatiana Pereira-Cenci

Management of severe worn dentition in patients with bruxism is challenging as a result of the loss of tooth structure and occlusal vertical dimension, temporomandibular implications, tooth hypersensitivity, and masticatory or aesthetic impairment. This case describes the 4-year follow-up clinical evaluation of a full mouth tooth-supported rehabilitation made on a 66-year-old man with bruxism and tooth wear, with aesthetic complaints and compromised masticatory function. The prosthetic treatment was planned with a digital smile design and a mock-up technique for an aesthetic and minimally invasive approach using lithium disilicate pressed and layered veneers on anterior teeth, posterior CAD/CAM lithium disilicate overlays with facial coverage, and CAD/CAM monolithic zirconia crowns with facial feldspathic ceramic on maxillary and mandibular canines and first molars in order to ensure the occlusal stability at the increased occlusal vertical dimension. After 4 years of function, no complications were registered. The choice of an appropriate material for the rehabilitation of these patients is essential to improve treatment prognosis and should be guided by mechanical and aesthetical properties. The use of four-point occlusal stabilization with CAD/CAM high strength monolithic zirconia crowns combined with ceramic veneers and overlays appears to be a reliable treatment option that enhances aesthetics and minimizes the occurrence of ceramic fractures, ensuring the treatment prognosis and predictability.

1. Introduction

According to the American Academy of Sleep Medicine, bruxism can be defined as the repetitive muscle activity of the jaw characterized by clenching or grinding of teeth and/or bracing or thrusting of the mandible [1]. Although the exact etiology of bruxism is still uncertain and probably multifactorial, the consequences are varied and include temporomandibular disorders, headaches, tooth wear or fracture, implant and restoration failure, tooth hypermobility, periodontal breakdown, occlusal dimpling, exostosis, muscle enlargement, and loss of occlusal vertical dimension. Bruxism is one of the most frequent causes for occlusal tooth wear, with the loss of tooth structure caused by mechanical wear between maxillary and mandibular tooth surfaces [2]. Loss of dental tissue can also result in sensitivity, pulp necrosis, and pain [3].

The prosthodontic rehabilitation of patients with bruxism must take into account the patient's needs and available materials. An appropriate material is essential to improve treatment prognosis and should combine mechanical properties and aesthetics.

The restorative approaches for patients with bruxism and worn dentition may include direct or indirect restorations such as direct resin composites or metal, gold, and ceramic and laboratory composites to make onlays or crowns, alone or in combination [4]. In cases of severely worn dentition, the traditional prosthetic treatment would include tooth preparation for complete crowns and an increase on the occlusal vertical dimension. In these cases, porcelain-fused-to-metal crowns were the traditional prosthetic option. With the introduction of new materials, zirconia has been shown to be a viable alternative to metal [5]. A systematic review about the clinical success of zirconia-based crowns suggests that the success rate of tooth-supported and implant-supported zirconia crowns is adequate, similar, and comparable to that of conventional porcelain-fused-to-metal crowns [6]. Despite the acceptable clinical results of bilayered porcelain-zirconia rehabilitations, the occurrence of ceramic chipping and fractures has been reported as a frequent complication [7].

In order to minimize ceramic fracture and chipping events, the introduction of zirconia computer-aided design and computer-aided manufacturing (CAD/CAM) has provided a new way of producing fixed restorations. A monolithic zirconia treatment option minimizes fracture events and improves structural mechanical properties [8]. Monolithic zirconia with minimal porcelain veneering limited to facial surface presents lower technical complications [9].

On the other hand, to avoid potentially harmful consequences to the teeth, non- or minimally invasive treatment options have emerged. With recent advances in dental adhesion, direct or conservative indirect restorations have become a treatment option. For many decades, ceramics have been used for anterior restorations because of their excellent aesthetic qualities and superior biocompatibility [10]. However, ceramics were brittle, required careful polishing techniques, and were abrasive to the opposite dentition [11]. Some authors suggested that placement of ceramics over the occlusal surfaces can lead to wear of the opposing dentition [12]. The use of traditional ceramic restorations on opposing occlusal surfaces is not a commonly used treatment option.

Based on this, the proposed case report describes a conservative full-mouth treatment modality of worn dentition on a patient with bruxism, using porcelain veneers and overlays combined with monolithic zirconia crowns for occlusal stabilization.

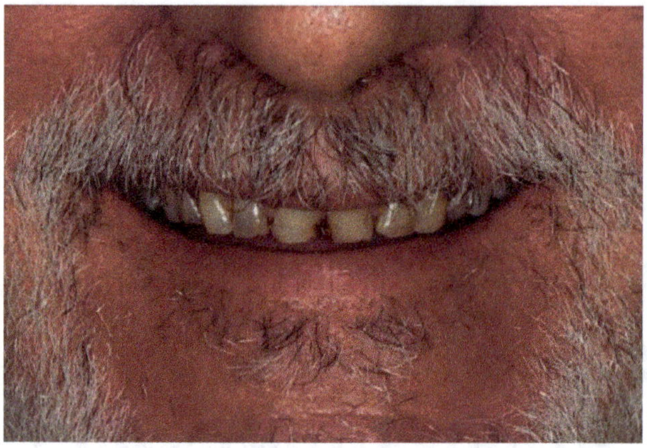

Figure 1: Smile (frontal view).

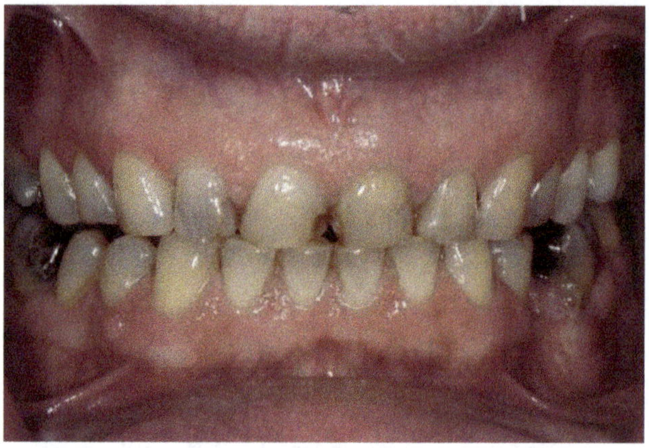

Figure 2: Intraoral frontal view.

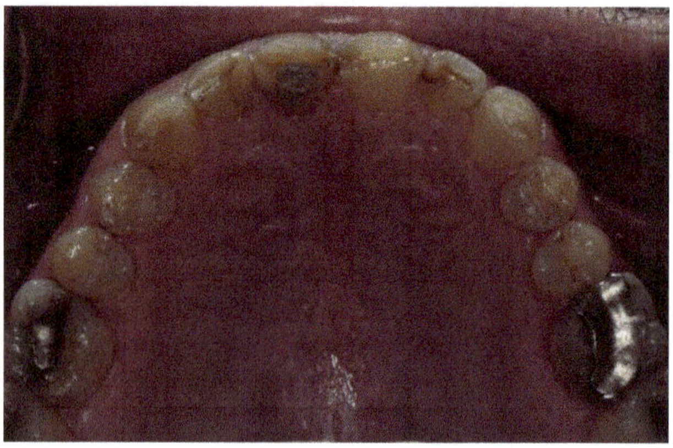

Figure 3: Maxillary occlusal view.

2. Case Report

A 66-year-old man reported to the appointment with complaints related to impaired aesthetics. The intraoral clinical examination revealed the presence of worn maxillary and mandibular dentition, with dentinal craters and sharp edges on the enamel of remaining teeth (Figures 1–4).

Upon extraoral examination, the patient showed bilateral hypertrophy of the masticatory muscles. The radiographic examination revealed the absence of tooth number 20. Teeth number 9 and 19 had previous endodontic treatment and direct composite restorations (Figure 5). Both posterior maxillary and mandibular dentition displayed worn occlusal/incisal surfaces. No anterior or canine guidance for eccentric jaw movements was present. The magnitude of occlusal vertical dimension loss was achieved using the interocclusal rest space with the jaw in rest position that was found to be around 6 mm, greater than the normal value (2 to 4 mm).

The treatment options were explained and a conservative treatment modality was adopted, which included the preparation of maxillary and mandibular canines and first molars for monolithic zirconia crowns in order to obtain four-point occlusal stability on the increased vertical dimension, that would allow to rehabilitate the anterior teeth with porcelain veneers and the remaining posterior teeth with ceramic overlays with facial coverage. In order to improve aesthetics,

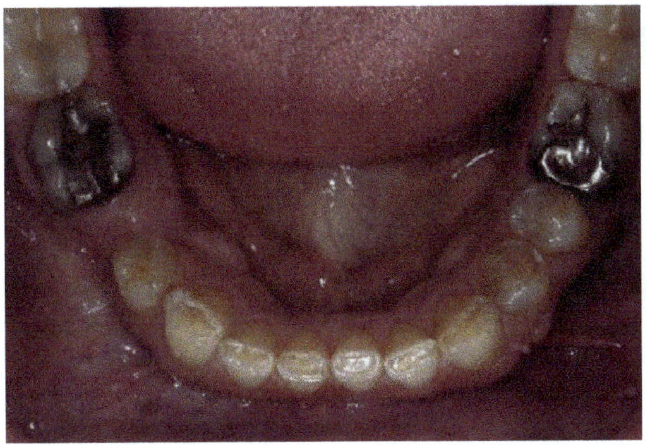

Figure 4: Mandibular occlusal view.

these monolithic zirconia crowns were veneered with porcelain in nonfunctional facial areas. A dental implant was proposed on the region of tooth number 20, but the patient decided to place a fixed bridge.

An informed consent was obtained from the patient. After facial and smile analysis, the photographic sequences were obtained and intraoral impressions were taken with irreversible hydrocolloid (Orthoprint, Zhermack). The digital planning using a digital smile design was complemented with a diagnostic wax-up that was produced on study casts and a direct mock-up with bis-acrylic composite (Protemp Plus, 3M ESPE).

All changes needed were done on the mock-up, and a silicone guide was obtained. Following this, the canines and first molars of both arches were prepared for full crowns. A medium grit diamond bur with rounded edge was used to ensure a minimum axial wall thickness for zirconia of about 1.0 mm to 1.5 mm. At gingival margin, a continuous circumferential chamfer with at least 0.5 mm reduction was made. A minimum of 1.5 to 2 mm incisal/occlusal reduction was ensured, approximately. The vertical and horizontal preparations were performed in order to obtain an angle of approximately 6 to 10 degrees between them. All edges and angles were rounded.

The anterior maxillary and mandibular teeth were minimally prepared for veneers, ensuring a minimum restoration thickness on the cervical and labial area of about 0.5 mm and 0.7 mm on the incisal edge. All other teeth were only softened from the sharp edges of the enamel.

Then, the retraction cords were applied (double retraction cord technique, #000 and #0 Ultrapak, Ultradent) and elastomeric single step impressions were made with putty and low consistency polyvinylsiloxane impression materials (Affinis, Coltene) to obtain the definitive casts. Maxillomandibular records (facebow) with the increased occlusal vertical dimension were obtained, and the master casts were mounted on a semiadjustable articulator. After tooth preparations, provisionals on the anterior teeth and first molars were placed and cemented with noneugenol temporary dental cement (TempBond NE, Kerr).

Digital technologies were then included in the workflow with the laboratory scanning of the master casts and CAD/-CAM manufacturing software, along with computer-controlled machinery (Zirkonzahn).

The casts and the wax-up were scanned into the computer-aided design software in order to produce the monolithic zirconia crowns for the canines and first molar crowns. Facial cutbacks for feldspathic ceramic were made digitally in order to improve aesthetics on these crowns. These crowns were designed in such a way so that the incisal edges of the canines were included and the veneering porcelain was applied only onto nonfunctional labial/buccal areas. The monolithic zirconia frameworks were milled using CAD/CAM software according to the manufacturer's specifications (Prettau Zirkon, Zirkonzahn).

Following framework proof and occlusal adjustments of canines and first molar upper and lower crowns, ceramic was applied on the facial surfaces of the monolithic zirconia frameworks (IPS e.max Ceram, Ivoclar Vivadent) and the feldspathic veneers for the anterior maxillary and mandibular teeth were produced (IPS e.max Press, Ivoclar Vivadent).

The canine and first molar monolithic zirconia crowns were cemented according to the manufacturer's instructions. The crowns were pretreated with aluminum oxide sandblasting (110 μm; 3.5 bar), steam blasted, and dried with compressed air. After the application of the bonder, the excesses were removed by compressed air and the crowns were allowed to dry for 60 seconds. The dual-cured resin cement (RelyX Unicem, 3M ESPE) was applied, and the crowns were finally inserted. After an initial polymerization of 2 seconds of light cure, all the excesses were removed and a glycerin gel was applied before the final polymerization of 120 seconds.

The anterior upper and lower porcelain veneers were cemented with resin cement (RelyX Veneer Cement, 3M ESPE).

Immediately after cementation (Figures 6 and 7), a digital scan of remaining teeth of booth arches and a bite registration was obtained with an intraoral scanner (Trios, 3Shape) (Figure 8). Posterior facial and occlusal lithium disilicate glass-ceramic restorations were that obtained via CAD/CAM (IPS e.max CAD for Cerec and inLab, Ivoclar Vivadent) (Figure 9) and cemented on the same day with composite (Figure 10).

Minor occlusal adjustments were made intraorally and polished with polishing burs. Canine guidance and anterior guidance were also verified for eccentric jaw movements with posterior disclusion. A panoramic radiograph was obtained after cementation (Figures 11–13), and oral hygiene instructions were given to the patient such as an acrylic occlusal mouthguard for nocturnal use. The patient expressed his complete satisfaction with the aesthetics and function value of the final restorations. After 4 years, no complications were found with respect to fracture or cracking of any restoration (Figures 14 and 15).

3. Discussion

The rehabilitation of worn dentition usually includes extensive treatment approaches. Among all the available treatment alternatives, there is a need to identify the modality that

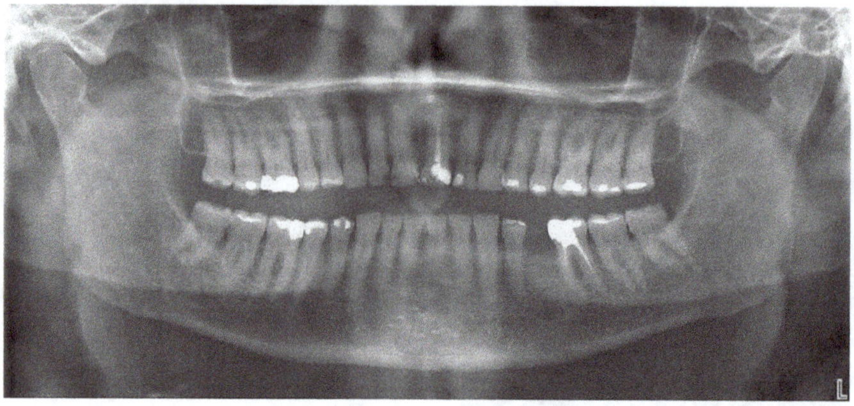

Figure 5: Initial panoramic view.

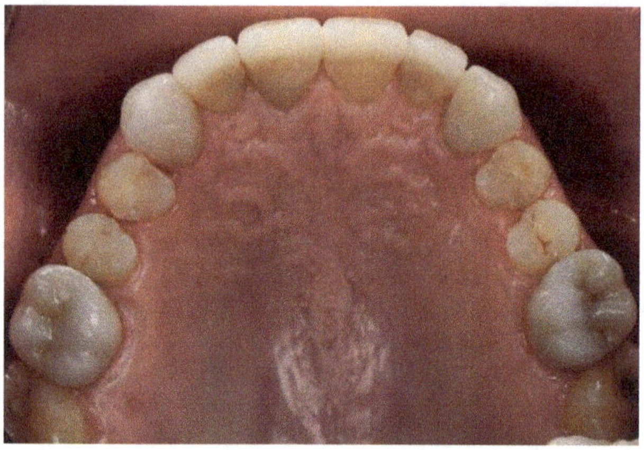

Figure 6: Maxillary occlusal view after initial cementation.

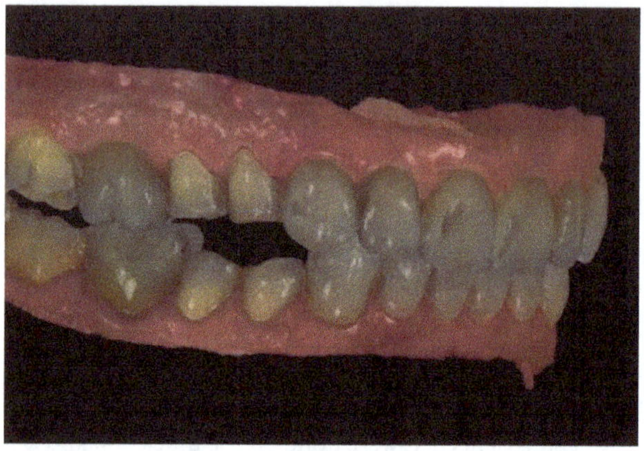

Figure 8: Digital scan.

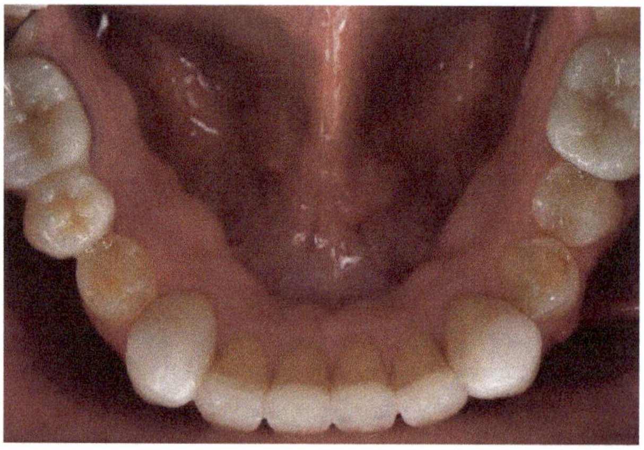

Figure 7: Mandibular occlusal view after initial cementation.

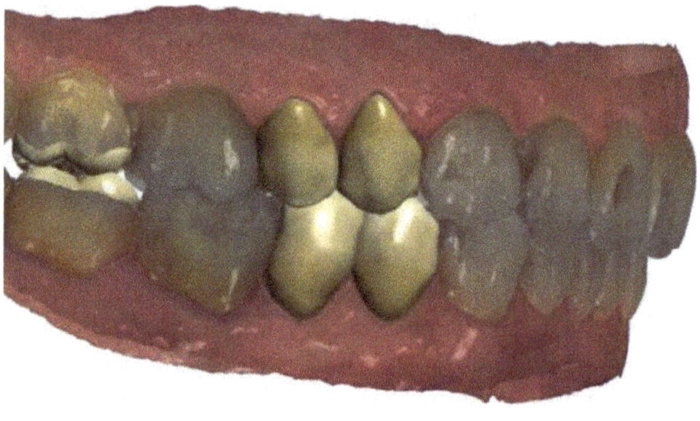

Figure 9: Maxillary and mandibular computer-aided design of lithium disilicate restorations.

combines the best relative cost-effective with the most acceptable longevity and with the greatest benefit to the patient, for the longest period of time [13]. The right choice of the appropriate material, guided by strength and aesthetics, is crucial in determining the life of restorations and the predictability of the treatment.

The case presented showed signs of tooth wear which were attributed to bruxism. Trying to maximize aesthetics without compromising the strength and durability of the restorations and using a conservative clinical protocol, a treatment option using ceramics was proposed.

Unfortunately, for many years, some clinical evidence on ceramic failure for posterior restorations due to fracture has been reported. In addition, the use of ceramic restorations in patients with bruxism would considerably increase the risk of complications and failure [14].

This clinical report illustrates an alternative approach on the rehabilitation of a bruxer patient. Using conventional and digital techniques, maxillary and mandibular canines

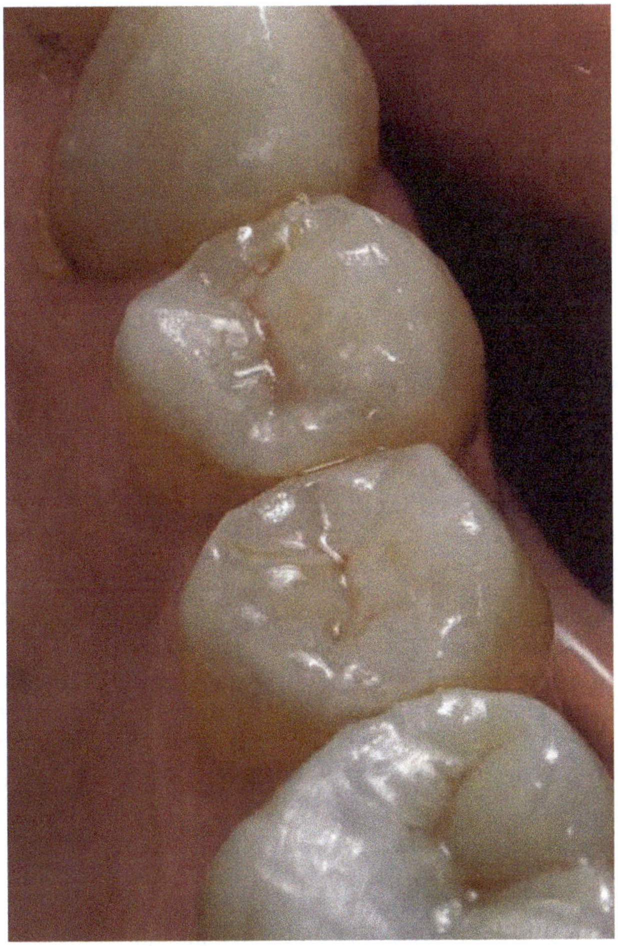

FIGURE 10: Maxillary left occlusal view after cementation of lithium disilicate restorations.

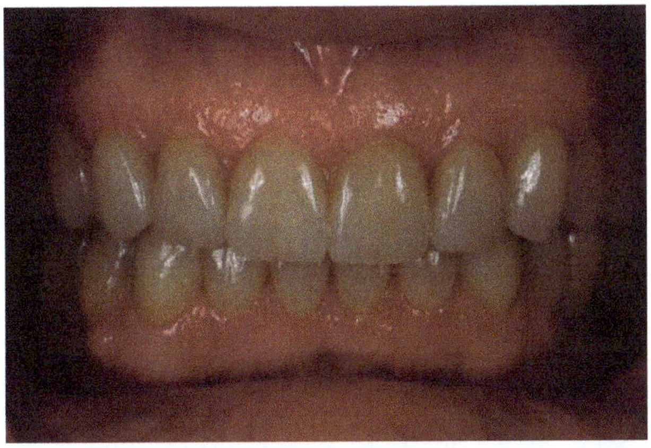

FIGURE 11: Final intraoral frontal view.

and first molars were restored with CAD/CAM monolithic zirconia crowns in order to ensure the occlusal stability at the increased occlusal vertical dimension. This way, the occlusal stability was ensured as well as the canine guidance.

Monolithic zirconia crowns may provide a valid treatment modality in the aesthetic zone in heavy grinders with

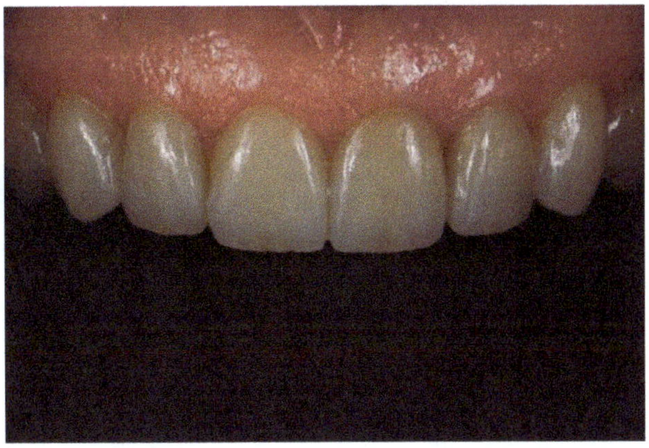

FIGURE 12: Final intraoral maxillary frontal view.

severe tooth wear, with minor clinical complications [15]. However, the monochromic and opaque aesthetic properties of monolithic zirconia can be a limitation. The use of monolithic zirconia crowns with facial porcelain veneers can combine the mechanical strength of monolithic zirconia with the aesthetics of feldspathic ceramics, providing satisfactory clinical results with minimal biologic and mechanical complications [16]. A 1-year follow-up prospective clinical study of tooth-supported monolithic zirconia crowns made with CAD/CAM technology revealed an overall success rate of 98.5% [17].

The occlusal stabilization with high-strength monolithic zirconia crowns allowed the minimally invasive aesthetic rehabilitation of the remaining teeth, with the use of ceramic on increased vertical dimension. Thus, the anterior teeth of both arches were restored with lithium disilicate pressed and layered veneers, on a minimum tooth reduction. Lithium disilicate glass ceramics are commonly selected because of their optical properties and adhesion to the tooth structure. Furthermore, this ceramic presents slower crack propagation, better resistance, and greater biaxial strength and fracture resistance [18].

Finally, all posterior teeth (premolars and remaining molars) were restored with CAD/CAM lithium disilicate overlays with facial coverage, on a digital and noninvasive approach. Monolithic lithium disilicate overlays feature a satisfying 97.7% survival rate, on a mean follow-up of 32 months [19]. The technique allows performing restorations with a minimum thickness, minimal complications, and excellent aesthetical performance.

In order to reduce the deleterious effects of bruxism, the use of different interocclusal appliances such as soft mouthguards or hard occlusal stabilization splints has been proposed. Although there are some controversial results on the efficacy of occlusal splints in the management of bruxism, they have an important role on the prevention and limitation of dental damage caused by this disorder [20]. An acrylic occlusal mouthguard was made for nocturnal use in order to minimize the risk of fractures. The patient was advised on the importance of regular follow-ups on a 6-month recall basis. After a 4-year follow-up, no biological or prosthetic complications were registered.

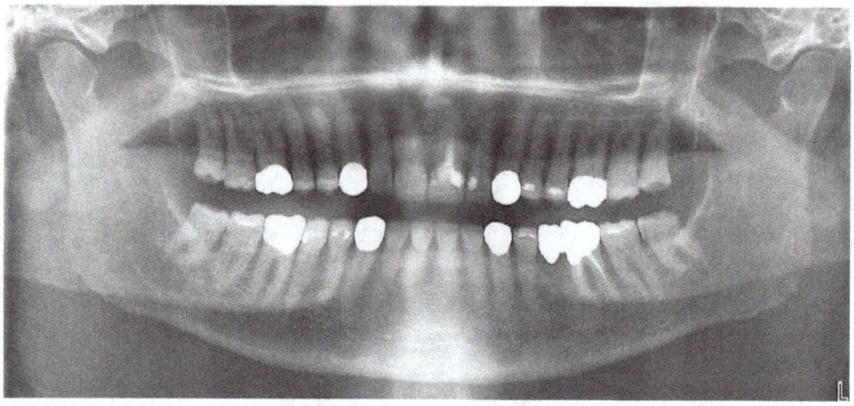

Figure 13: Final panoramic view.

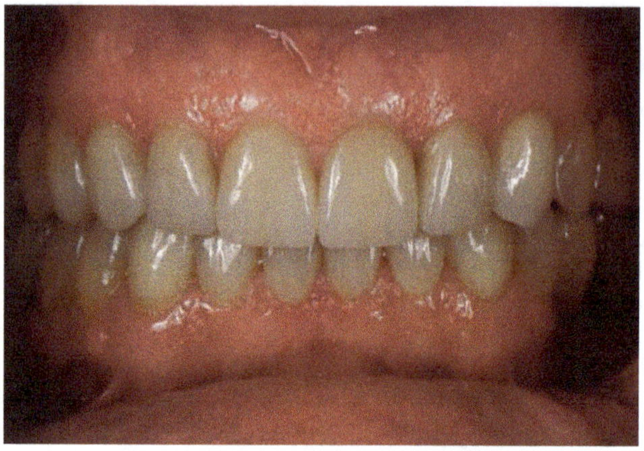

Figure 14: Intraoral frontal view after 48 months.

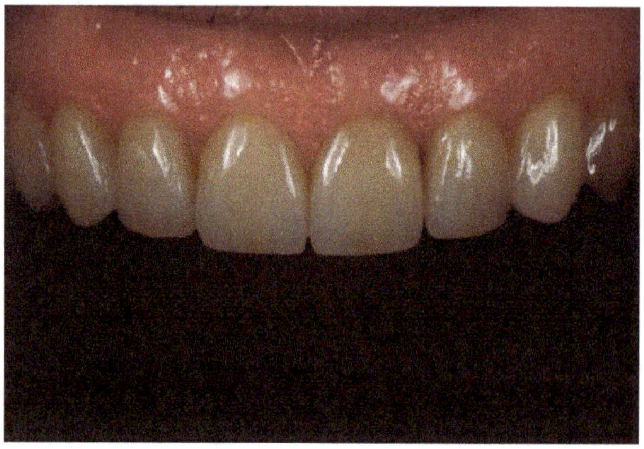

Figure 15: Intraoral maxillary view after 48 months.

4. Conclusion

The management of worn dentition is a major challenge for dental professionals. A correct diagnosis and a multidisciplinary treatment plan are essential to improve the treatment prognosis and patient satisfaction. The treatment decisions taken by the clinician should be based on available materials and patient demand, and the choice of an appropriate material should be guided by strength and aesthetics. Traditional options like metal-ceramic and zirconia-ceramic rehabilitations are found to be more like to chipping and fracture of ceramic.

This treatment approach appears to be a reliable treatment option with high aesthetics and strength and satisfactory clinical results minimizing technical complications. More long-term randomized control studies on the use of ceramics on grinders are necessary in order to evaluate the predictability of this kind of restorations.

Authors' Contributions

This manuscript has been read and approved by all the authors, all the requirements for authorship have been met, and each author believes that the manuscript represents honest work.

References

[1] American Academy of Sleep Medicine, "Sleep related bruxism," in *International Classification of Sleep Disorders*, American Academy of Sleep Medicine, Westchester, Darien, IL, USA, 3rd edition, 2014.

[2] D. W. Bartlett, "The role of erosion in tooth wear: aetiology, prevention and management," *International Dental Journal*, vol. 55, no. S4, pp. 277–284, 2005.

[3] F. Lobbezoo, J. Ahlberg, A. G. Glaros et al., "Bruxism defined and graded: an international consensus," *Journal of Oral Rehabilitation*, vol. 40, no. 1, pp. 2–4, 2013.

[4] D. Hurst, "What is the best way to restore the worn dentition?," *Evidence-Based Dentistry*, vol. 12, no. 2, pp. 55-56, 2011.

[5] P. F. Manicone, P. Rossi Iommetti, and L. Raffaelli, "An overview of zirconia ceramics: basic properties and clinical applications," *Journal of Dentistry*, vol. 35, no. 11, pp. 819–826, 2007.

[6] C. Larsson and A. Wennerberg, "The clinical success of zirconia-based crowns: a systematic review," *The International Journal of Prosthodontics*, vol. 27, no. 1, pp. 33–43, 2014.

[7] I. Sailer, N. A. Makarov, D. S. Thoma, M. Zwahlen, and B. E. Pjetursson, "All-ceramic or metal-ceramic tooth-supported

fixed dental prostheses (FDPs)? A systematic review of the survival and complication rates. Part I: single crowns (SCs)," *Dental Materials*, vol. 31, no. 6, pp. 603–623, 2015.

[8] A. A. Abdulmajeed, K. G. Lim, T. O. Närhi, and L. F. Cooper, "Complete-arch implant-supported monolithic zirconia fixed dental prostheses: a systematic review," *The Journal of Prosthetic Dentistry*, vol. 115, no. 6, pp. 672–677.e1, 2016.

[9] J. Caramês, D. Marques, J. Malta Barbosa, A. Moreira, P. Crispim, and A. Chen, "Full-arch implant-supported rehabilitations: a prospective study comparing porcelain-veneered zirconia frameworks to monolithic zirconia," *Clinical Oral Implants Research*, vol. 30, no. 1, pp. 68–78, 2019.

[10] H. Rashid, Z. Sheikh, S. Misbahuddin, M. Kazmi, S. Qureshi, and M. Uddin, "Advancements in all-ceramics for dental restorations and their effect on the wear of opposing dentition," *European Journal of Dentistry*, vol. 10, no. 4, pp. 583–588, 2016.

[11] M. Etman, M. Woolford, and S. Dunne, "Quantitative measurement of tooth and ceramic wear: in vivo study," *The International Journal of Prosthodontics*, vol. 21, no. 3, pp. 245–252, 2008.

[12] H. Rashid, "Evaluation of the surface roughness of a standard abraded dental porcelain following different polishing techniques," *Journal of Dental Sciences*, vol. 7, no. 2, pp. 184–189, 2012.

[13] M. E. Mesko, R. Sarkis-Onofre, M. S. Cenci, N. J. Opdam, B. Loomans, and T. Pereira-Cenci, "Rehabilitation of severely worn teeth: a systematic review," *Journal of Dentistry*, vol. 48, pp. 9–15, 2016.

[14] M. Granell-Ruíz, R. Granell-Ruiz, A. Fons-Font, J. L. Roman-Rodriguez, and M. F. Sola-Ruiz, "Influence of bruxism on survival of porcelain laminate veneers," *Medicina Oral, Patología Oral y Cirugía Bucal*, vol. 19, no. 5, pp. e426–e432, 2014.

[15] T. L. Hansen, C. Schriwer, M. Øilo, and H. Gjengedal, "Monolithic zirconia crowns in the aesthetic zone in heavy grinders with severe tooth wear – an observational case-series," *Journal of Dentistry*, vol. 72, pp. 14–20, 2018.

[16] P. Venezia, F. Torsello, R. Cavalcanti, and S. D'Amato, "Retrospective analysis of 26 complete-arch implant-supported monolithic zirconia prostheses with feldspathic porcelain veneering limited to the facial surface," *The Journal of Prosthetic Dentistry*, vol. 114, no. 4, pp. 506–512, 2015.

[17] I. Konstantinidis, D. Trikka, S. Gasparatos, and M. Mitsias, "Clinical outcomes of monolithic zirconia crowns with CAD/-CAM Technology. A 1-year follow-up prospective clinical study of 65 patients," *International Journal of Environmental Research and Public Health*, vol. 15, no. 11, p. 2523, 2018.

[18] A. Maluly-Proni, B. Oliveira-Reis, W. Assunção, and P. Dos Santos, "Minimum intervention management of diastema closure using cordless displacement system and laminate veneers: a 2-year follow-up," *European Journal of Dentistry*, vol. 12, no. 3, pp. 446–449, 2018.

[19] M. Luciano, Z. Francesca, S. Michela, M. Tommaso, and A. Massimo, "Lithium disilicate posterior overlays: clinical and biomechanical features," *Clinical Oral Investigations*, pp. 1–8, 2019.

[20] J. Okeson, "The effects of hard and soft occlusal splints on nocturnal bruxism," *The Journal of the American Dental Association*, vol. 114, no. 6, pp. 788–791, 1987.

5

The Placement of Four Short Implants and Full-Arch Early Loading in the Edentulous Patient Suffering from Severe Mandibular Alveolar Ridge Atrophy

Yuri Sedov,[1] Oleg Mordanov,[2] Sergei Grigoriev,[3] Anatoly Avanesov,[1] and Kamil Khabiev[2]

[1]*Department of General and Clinical Dentistry, RUDN University, Medical Institute, Moscow, Russia*
[2]*Private Practice, Moscow, Russia*
[3]*Private Practice, Cheboksary, Russia*

Correspondence should be addressed to Oleg Mordanov; mordanov19@gmail.com

Academic Editor: Mariano A. Polack

One of the treatments of patients with severe bone atrophy is short implants. It is important to position short implants taking into account the prosthetic loading and right position according to vital anatomical structures. In the presented case report, a seventy-one-year-old female patient underwent the rehabilitation with four short dental implants placed in the anterior mandibula with fully guided surgery to avoid mandibular incisive canal. It solves all the problems in the planning stage when you determine the osteotomy protocol in advance and the prognosis of future restoration according to patient requirements. This clinical case demonstrates the efficiency of patient rehabilitation with the use of short implants in difficult clinical situations.

1. Introduction

Dental implants are recommended as a high-quality rehabilitation method for edentulous patients [1, 2]. The survival rates of short dental implants are quite high, on average 91-97% in patients with generalized aggressive periodontitis and 100% in periodontally healthy patients [1]. Not so long ago, there were restrictions on using short implants associated with its stability and prognosis [3]. However, today, there is an evidence-based scientific basis for the effectiveness of the use of short implants in the rehabilitation of patients with severe ridge atrophy [1, 4]. It is often possible not to do additional surgery to augment the tissue volume because of the design of these implants [5, 6]. It is important to note that previously there were age limits, for patients who required implant placement, but at the moment, due to technological improvement of the method, it is not a contraindication to the procedure [7, 8]. Severe bone atrophy makes doctors apply various augmentation methods, but in some clinical situations [9], it is necessary to manage only the available bone [10]. This implies the need for a thorough clinical and radiological examination of the patient in order to be able to place implants and ensure the prosthodontic restoration function [11], especially if the short implants are planned [12].

It has become possible to comply with a specific treatment protocol and improve outcome quality using dental implants even in difficult situations with the development of digital technologies in dentistry. Also, it is possible to reduce the number of possible complications and achieve favorable clinical outcomes through such approach [13].

The aim of this clinical report is to demonstrate the rehabilitation of the patient using four immediate short implants after extraction of all teeth and early prosthetics.

2. Case Report

A seventy-one-year-old female patient came to the dental practice because of poor denture fixation on the mandible. Previously, the denture was corrected and adjusted, but it was ineffective. The maxilla also had a complete removable prosthesis, which was suited to the patient. The patient noted the occurrence of pain in the projection of the

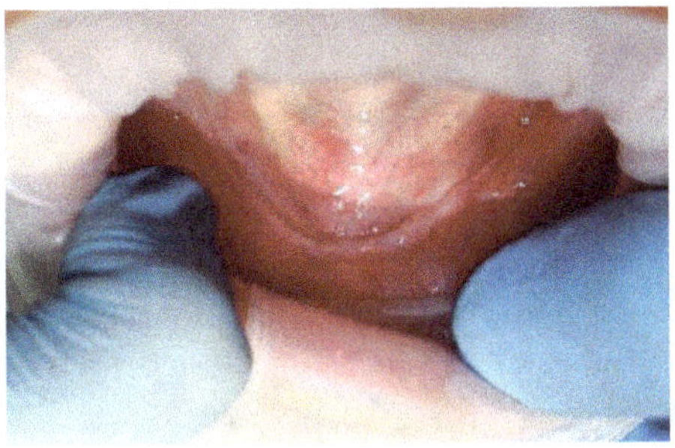

FIGURE 1: Oral cavity examination. Severe atrophy of the alveolar mandible.

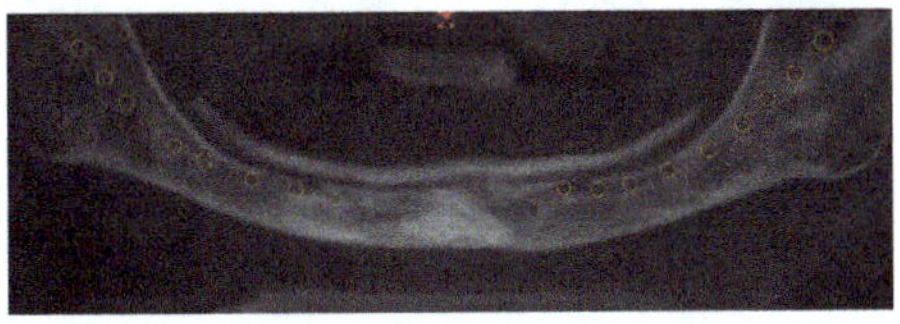

FIGURE 2: Panoramic view of the CBCT scan. The mandibular canal is traced. The opening of a neurovascular bundle under soft tissue is noted.

mental foramens during the closing of the jaws with the prostheses.

The absence of the border between vestibule and oral cavity proper was noted during the clinical examination (Figure 1). There was a marked deficiency of the mandibular alveolar ridge.

The CBCT scan showed a close position of the mandibular canal with the opening of the inferior alveolar nerve from the mental foramens under soft tissues, which was confirmed by the patient's complaints (Figure 2). She was offered treatment options with dental implants and bone augmentation. The patient refused bone augmentation and chose the option with the short implant placement in the anterior mandible. A strict treatment plan was individually prescribed, which included the following points:

(1) Impressions and cast models fabrication

(2) Making a radiopaque mould for CBCT

(3) CBCT examination along with the individual radiopaque mould

(4) Scanning of cast models and the radiopaque mould

(5) Comparison of scan and tomography files for complete planning

(6) Creating a surgical guide

(7) Fully guided dental implant placement

(8) Prosthesis fabrication

After the patient's consent with this option, the first three stages were performed. The models were cast, and the radiopaque mould was made of polymer and base wax to record the occlusion height. At last, a layer of the radiopaque basis of the mould was visible. Then, the models of the upper and lower jaws were scanned separately and together with a mould to create an occlusal file for further virtual wax-up. Also, the mould and the mould with the models of the mandible were also scanned separately. The last two scans are needed for comparison with CBCT. Thus, five scans were obtained.

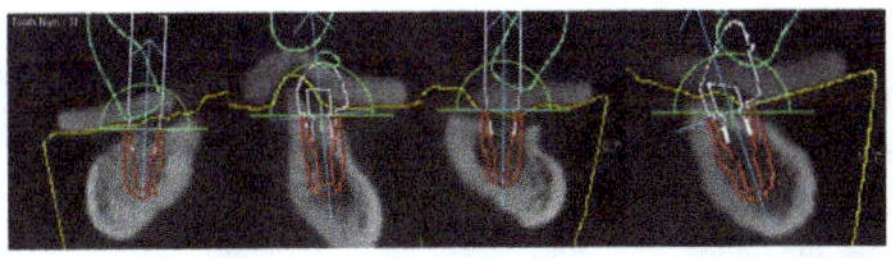

FIGURE 3: The CBCT scan. Coronal mandibular view. Four implants were placed in the 3.2, 3.4, 4.1, and 4.3 teeth regions. Distal implants are tilted at 29 degrees.

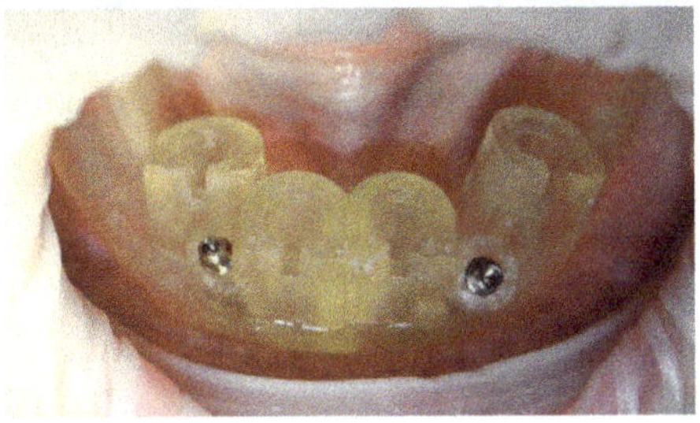

FIGURE 4: Fixed surgical guide.

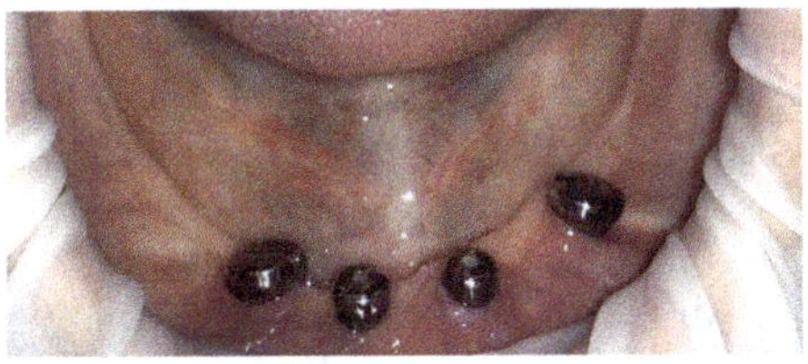

FIGURE 5: Healing abutments in situ.

The R2Gate (Megagen, South Korea) software made a comparison of computed tomography data presented in the ∗.dcm and scans in the ∗.stl. The correlation between mandibular scan and its CBCT scan was matched with the help of the radiopaque mould in the CBCT scan and the 3D scans of this mould.

Further, the available bone in the anterior mandible was assessed. The location of the mandibular incisal canal in the implant site was noted, and the patient was informed, including possible complications after surgery. Four implants are virtually placed, two of which are positioned tilted at 29 degrees due to the lack of available bone (Figure 3).

The final correlation between the implants and the virtual wax-up made it possible to produce a splinted prosthesis, since the scan abutments were relatively parallel to each other.

Next, the design of the surgical guide was developed and printed with a print thickness of 50 microns. Separately, a protocol of recommended drilling was developed for obtaining favorable primary implant stability. It was based on the size of the platform, apex, and type of bone density based on the classification by Lekholm and Zarb [12]. Additionally, a silicone index was made for fixing the guide with the opposite jaw at the time of the pin placement for guide

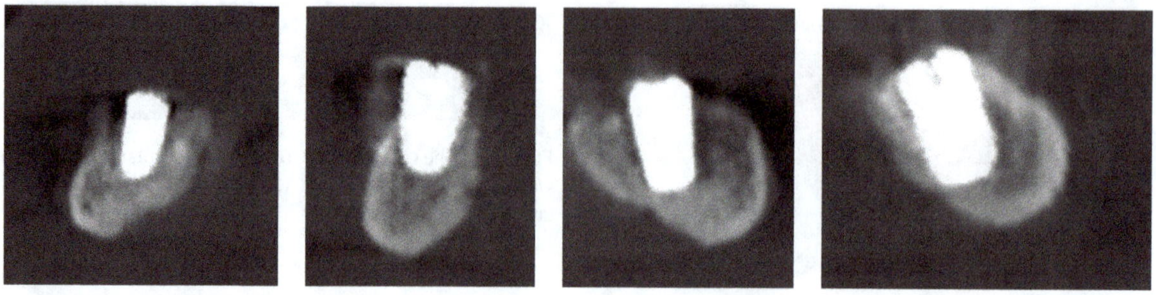

Figure 6: CBCT scan with implants in situ.

stabilization. Before the surgery, the patient was prescribed an antibiotic (lincomycin 500 mg).

3. Surgery Protocol

The general condition is satisfactory; there were no complaints. Antiseptic was performed on the oral cavity with a solution of chlorhexidine digluconate 0.05%, then the local anesthesia was carried out. A surgical guide is placed on the lower jaw, then a silicone index is positioned; after that, the patient squeezed the jaws to fix the position of the guide. Fixing pins were placed and the silicone index was removed (Figure 4).

The first drilling with a special mucotomy-type transgingival drill was performed with the guide to remove the soft tissue. As surgical guides limit irrigation during the drilling, sequential drilling was carried out at a drilling speed of 350 rpm, according to the previously developed protocol. The drills had a cylinder in the apical section with a diameter that was equal to the walls of the guide. The drill's free movement was excluded due to the sequential drilling from a short drill to the required height. Four implants (4.1 region—$4 * 7\,mm$, 3.2 region—$4 * 7\,mm$, 4.3 region—$4 * 7\,mm$ with 29-degree angulation, 3.4 region—$3.5 * 7\,mm$ with 29-degree angulation; AnyOne, Megagen, South Korea) were placed through the guide using a special implant driver for precise height adjustment.

The final torque on the implants was $40\,N * cm$. However, due to the fact that a number of implants were placed in the lower incisal canal, it was decided to install only the healing abutments (Figure 5). Closure was not necessary due to the work with the mucotome.

An antiseptic with chlorhexidine digluconate 0.05% was performed. The radiographic control was provided (Figure 6). Prescriptions including antibiotic prophylaxis were given (lincomycin 500 mg, 1 capsule bis in die for 5 days), and antihistamine and nonsteroidal anti-inflammatory drugs were also prescribed. The existing prosthesis is rebased according to the healing abutments.

The general condition was satisfactory in the next follow-ups; the postoperative region was without inflammatory changes.

A new removable maxillary prosthesis was agreed upon with the patient. Due to pronounced financial constraints, she had to deny the usual prosthesis on multiunit abutments. As implants were placed with a surgical guide, and when planning they were all derived as parallel as possible, transfer checks on titanium bases without a hexagon were previously manufactured. Despite the angulation of the implants, after the try-in of on-transfer checks in the oral cavity, a decision was made about the possibility of manufacturing an all-zirconium prosthesis on these titanium bases. The durability of this design provides contact with a removable denture of the maxilla, so there is no overpressure (Figure 7).

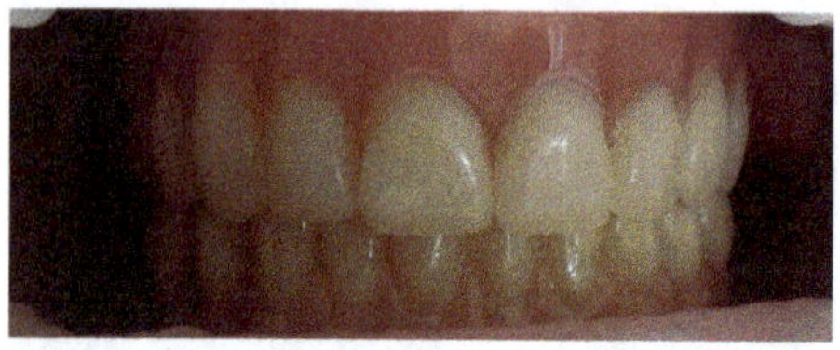

Figure 7: Removable maxillary- and implant-supported mandibular prosthesis in situ.

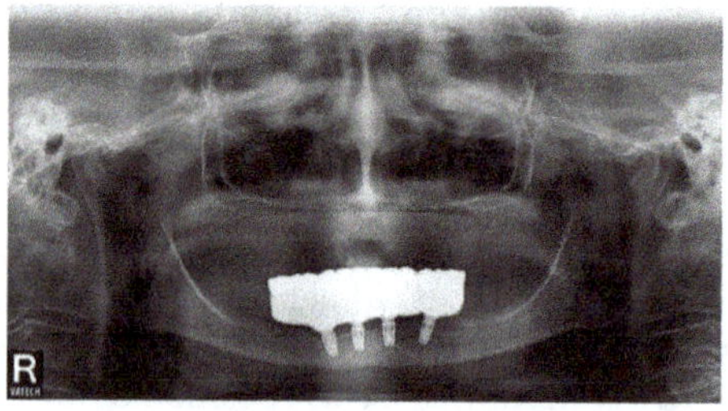

Figure 8: Panoramic view. Radiographic follow-up a year after surgery.

The whole zirconium frame was virtually designed after the determination and analysis of all the nuances on the previously obtained STL file with the position of the scan abutments and CAM fabrication.

The patient follows the recommendations for hygiene and undergoes follow-ups every six months (Figure 8).

4. Discussion and Conclusions

This case report shows the compilation of using short implants in an old patient with fully guided surgery. Short implants have proven their effectiveness with both immediate and delayed loads [4]. In patients with a complex clinical view and the impossibility of restoring bone volume, the use of short implants is a good alternative [1, 4]. The use of short dental implants decreases the need for complicated surgical bone augmentation procedures, which reduces complications, costs, treatment time, and morbidity [14]. Also, the treatment plan with short implants can also be used in age-related patients [13].

There are three types of patterns used for edentulous arches: those designed for freehand drilling, those designed for semiguided controlled directional drilling, and those designed for fully guided controlled directional drilling. Fully guided surgical templates are used when precise control of angulation, location in the arch, and apicocoronal depth are critical to the success of the definitive prosthesis [15]. Fully guided surgery has been proven to be a reliable and accurate method that reduces the damage to the alveolar nerve, sinus perforation, fenestration, etc. [16]. This guide provided not only precise implant placement but also flapless surgery whose advantage is the minimal surgical procedure that supports the preservation of the blood circulation in the soft tissues, which may affect the soft-tissue architecture and reduce bone loss [17, 18].

All these factors combined into a single implant treatment provided the successful implant placement in an old patient without complications. Though the possibilities of short implants are limited, they require further study from the point of view of long-term survival in difficult clinical situations in such patients with such methods described in this article.

Consent

Written consent was signed by the patient for every procedure.

Acknowledgments

The publication has been prepared with support of the International Study Center Dental Guru.

References

[1] M.-S. Howe, W. Keys, and D. Richards, "Long-term (10-year) dental implant survival: a systematic review and sensitivity meta-analysis," *Journal of Dentistry*, vol. 84, no. 9, 21 pages, 2019.

[2] J. A. Griggs, "Dental implants," *Dental Clinics of North America*, vol. 61, no. 4, pp. 857–871, 2017.

[3] H. Birdi, J. Schulte, A. Kovacs, M. Weed, and S.-K. Chuang, "Crown-to-implant ratios of short-length implants," *The Journal of Oral Implantology*, vol. 36, pp. 425–433, 2010.

[4] S. Al-Johany, "Survival rates of short dental implants (≤ 6.5 mm) placed in posterior edentulous ridges and factors affecting their survival after a 12-month follow-up period: a systematic review," *The International Journal of Oral & Maxillofacial Implants*, vol. 34, no. 3, pp. 605–621, 2019.

[5] P. A. Fugazzotto, "Shorter implants in clinical practice: rationale and treatment results," *The International Journal of Oral & Maxillofacial Implants*, vol. 23, pp. 487–496, 2008.

[6] S. R. Schwartz, "Short implants: are they a viable option in implant dentistry?," *Dental Clinics*, vol. 59, pp. 317–328, 2015.

[7] M. Schimmel, M. Srinivasan, G. J. McKenna, and F. Müller, "Effect of advanced age and/or systemic medical conditions on dental implant survival: a systematic review and meta-analysis," *Clinical Oral Implants Research*, vol. 29, pp. 311–330, 2018.

[8] L. J. Heitz-Mayfield, M. Aaboe, M. Araujo et al., "Group 4 ITI consensus report: risks and biologic complications associated with implant dentistry," *Clinical Oral Implants Research*, vol. 29, pp. 351–358, 2018.

[9] R. J. De Groot, M. A. E. M. Oomens, T. Forouzanfar, and E. A. J. M. Schulten, "Bone augmentation followed by implant surgery in the edentulous mandible: a systematic review," *Journal of Oral Rehabilitation*, vol. 45, no. 4, pp. 334–343, 2018.

[10] V. Pohl, D. S. Thoma, K. Sporniak-Tutak et al., "Short dental implants (6 mm) *versus* long dental implants (11–15 mm) in combination with sinus floor elevation procedures: 3-year results from a multicentre, randomized, controlled clinical trial," *Journal of Clinical Periodontology*, vol. 44, no. 4, pp. 438–445, 2017.

[11] A. Lanis, O. Alvarez del Canto, P. Barriga, W. D. Polido, and D. Morton, "Computer-guided implant surgery and full-arch immediate loading with prefabricated—metal framework—-provisional prosthesis created from a 3D printed model," *Journal of Esthetic and Restorative Dentistry*, vol. 31, no. 3, pp. 199–208, 2019.

[12] U. Lekholm and G. A. Zarb, "Patient selection and preparation," in *Tissue integrated prostheses: osseointegration in clinical dentistry*, P. I. Branemark, G. A. Zarb, and T. Albrektsson, Eds., pp. 199–209, Quintessence Publishing Company, Chicago, 1985.

[13] B.-T. N. Grant, F. X. Pancko, and R. A. Kraut, "Outcomes of placing short dental implants in the posterior mandible: a retrospective study of 124 cases," *Journal of Oral and Maxillofacial Surgery*, vol. 67, no. 4, pp. 713–717, 2009.

[14] F. Edher and C. T. Nguyen, "Short dental implants: a scoping review of the literature for patients with head and neck cancer," *The Journal of Prosthetic Dentistry*, vol. 119, no. 5, pp. 736–742, 2018.

[15] P. K. Moy, A. Pozzi, and J. Beumer III, *Fundamentals of Implant Dentistry, Volume II: Surgical Principles*, Quintessence Publishing, USA, 1st edition, 2017.

[16] Y. N. R. Gallardo, I. R. T. da Silva-Olivio, E. Mukai, S. Morimoto, N. Sesma, and L. Cordaro, "Accuracy comparison of guided surgery for dental implants according to the tissue of support: a systematic review and meta-analysis," *Clinical Oral Implants Research*, vol. 28, no. 5, pp. 602–612, 2016.

[17] A. G. Sclar, "Guidelines for flapless surgery," *Journal of Oral and Maxillofacial Surgery*, vol. 65, pp. 20–32, 2007.

[18] J. Cosyn, N. Hooghe, and H. De Bruyn, "A systematic review on the frequency of advanced recession following single immediate implant treatment," *Journal of Clinical Periodontology*, vol. 39, pp. 582–589, 2012.

6

Osteoid Osteoma of the Maxilla Presenting as Dental Implant Pain

R. Al Sadhan,[1] A. Alosaimi,[2] R. Al Shagroud,[1] M. U. Zaman,[1] and M. S. Allahyani[3]

[1]*Department of Oral Medicine and Diagnostic Sciences, College of Dentistry, King Saud University, Riyadh, Saudi Arabia*
[2]*Dental University Hospital, King Saud University Medical City, King Saud University, Riyadh, Saudi Arabia*
[3]*Department of Oral and Maxillofacial Surgery, Al Noor Hospital, Makkah, Saudi Arabia*

Correspondence should be addressed to R. Al Sadhan; rsadhan@ksu.edu.sa

Academic Editor: Anastasios Markopoulos

Osteoid osteoma (OO) is a benign osteogenic lesion, regularly noticed in young individuals. A solitary lesion most frequently appears in long bones but is extremely rare in jawbones. Pain is a distinguishing characteristic of this lesion. Herein, we report a rare case of an OO in the right maxilla of a 37-year-old male presenting as pain associated with dental implants. Clinical and radiographic features were indicative of a benign neoplasia of boney origin. An excisional biopsy and histological examination of the lesion confirmed the diagnosis of osteoid osteoma. Surgical excision was followed by immediate relief of most of the pain. His follow-up visits were documented; complete relief of symptoms with no complications was observed during the postoperative period. There was no evidence of recurrence at a two-year follow-up. Osteoid osteoma of the maxilla may present as pain related to dental implants, and careful radiographic assessment of the entire jawbone should be considered if diagnosis of dental implant pain is unclear.

1. Introduction

Solitary osteoid osteoma (OO) is a rare benign osteogenic tumor of unknown etiology. First described in 1930 by Bergstrand and later classified by Jaffe in1935 [1], it was characterized as an offbeat clinical entity [2]. Walia et al. defined OO as "a small, oval, or roundish tumor-like nidus composed of osteoid and trabeculae of newly formed bone deposited within a substratum of highly vascularized osteogenic connective tissue" [3, 4]. It is characterized by its small size and severe, predominantly nocturnal, localized pain which is frequently relieved by the use of nonsteroidal anti-inflammatory drugs (NSAIDs). The pain may occur with both initial and recurrent disease [5]. Even though the true nature of this lesion is still unknown, different reports suggest it usually occurs in young adults under 30 years of age [6]. An OO is smaller in size than an osteoblastoma, with a central nidus that is usually less than 1 cm in diameter. The osteoid osteoma is more common than osteoblastoma and elucidates approximately 10% to 12% of all primary bone tumors [7–9]. This type of lesion accounts for 3% of all primary bone tumors and 10% of benign bone tumors. It tends to arise more in the long bones of the lower extremities than the long bones of the upper extremities. It may also involve the axial skeleton. According to Dorfman and Czerniak, it barely involves the craniofacial bones [7]. OO most commonly exhibits a prediction for long bones. It rarely occurs within the jaws, with the mandible more commonly affected than the maxilla [10, 11]. Multiple osteomas of the jawbones are seen in Gardner syndrome [12].

Since the original descriptions of osteoid osteoma were first published, 31 examples of isolated osteoid osteoma arising in the jawbones have been reported in the English-language literature until September 2019 [2, 4, 10, 13–40]. OO is seen in less than 1% of jawbones [2]. But it has hardly been described in the jaws [6]. Knowing the proper diagnosis and treatment plan are essential for clinicians because of the specialty and rareness of this tumor.

Hence, to acquaint our awareness in the concerned field, such case reports should be discussed. However, its occurrence in the anterior wall of the maxillary sinus wall just below the infraorbital rim is a rare entity. Here, we presented a rare case report of OO of the maxilla in a 37-year-old patient presenting as pain associated with dental implants.

This case report highlights that osteoid osteoma of the maxilla may present as pain related to dental implants and careful radiographic assessment of the entire jawbone should be considered if diagnosis of dental implant pain is unclear.

2. Case Report

A 37-year-old male patient was seen at the Oral and Maxillofacial Clinic of the Dental University Hospital, King Saud University, Riyadh, Saudi Arabia. He was complaining of localized severe pain in the right maxilla. No swelling or tenderness was noted clinically. The patient had previously undergone the replacement of missing maxillary premolars and molars on the same side with dental implants, and thus, implant-related complication was suspected although the implants were loaded and functional with intact periodontium.

3. Radiographic Examination

A panoramic radiograph (Figure 1) and CT examination (Figure 2) were requested to assess the area, and the images showed a severe marginal alveolar bone loss in the area of the missing upper right posterior teeth and inferior extension of the maxillary sinus floor. The two previously placed dental implants in the area of the missing maxillary right premolars and molars were covered with a very thin surrounding residual alveolar ridge, and localized thickening of the adjacent maxillary sinus lining was noted. Maxillary sinus mucositis of odontogenic origin was initially suspected to be the cause of the patient's pain. But this finding was not fully consistent with the chief complaint of the patient who described his localized pain by pointing at his face just below his right orbital rim and reported that he had severe nocturnal pain at this spot. When the patient signs and symptoms were correlated with the CT examination, a small (3.5 mm in diameter), well-defined, corticated, spherical radiolucency in the superior anterior wall of the right maxillary sinus wall just below the infraorbital rim and medial to the infraorbital foramen was noted. The lesion caused minimal expansion of the boney boundaries especially anteriorly and posteriorly. The CT numbers (HU) indicated that the content is similar to soft tissue. The radiographic observation of a small, well-defined, corticated, unilocular, minimally expansile radiolucency that appears to have originated inside the bone was suggestive of a benign neoplasia of boney origin. The primary radiographic differential diagnosis for small benign neoplasia of the bone that causes pain is osteoid osteoma. Based on the case history, clinical findings, and radiographic presentation, an excisional biopsy of the lesion was planned.

4. Surgical Technique

On the day of the surgery, the patient was brought to the operating theater where the surgical intervention under general anesthesia in a sterile manner was done; the lesion was approached via a transcutaneous incision of the right lower eyelid (midlid incision) after protecting the right eye by employing temporary suture tarsorrhaphy. Sharp and blunt dissection was done exposing the inferior orbital rim adequately. A small bony swelling was located on the facial aspect of the medial portion of the right inferior orbital rim just medial to the right infraorbital nerve and foramen with no violation of the foramen. The lesion was a nodule-like bony mass with central crater-like defect, brownish-red, and gritty. It measured about 3 to 4 mm in dimension and was distinct from the surrounding normal bone (Figure 3(a)). The lesion was excised completely by using a straight surgical bur and chisels. The right infraorbital nerve was protected and not violated (Figure 3(b)). The residual bony defect was reconstructed by using 1 mm thick titanium mesh (Figure 4). The surgical site was irrigated thoroughly with normal saline; the surgical wound was sutured back in layers by using absorbable suture and the lid skin by 6/0 proline suture.

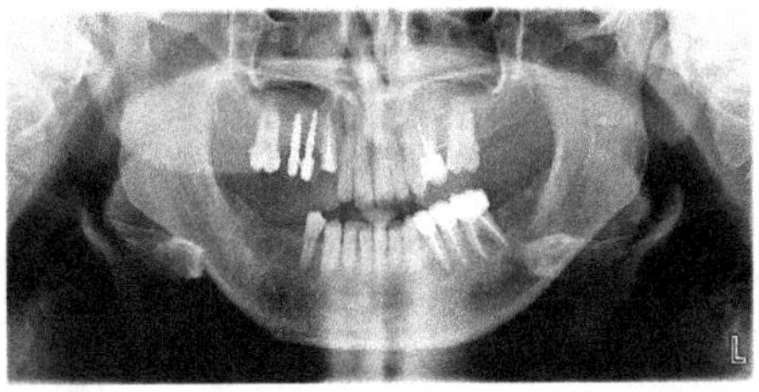

Figure 1: Initial panoramic radiograph.

5. Microscopic Findings

The histopathologic examination of the excised specimen (Figure 5) revealed a well-circumscribed, round, hemorrhagic benign bone-forming tumor surrounded by a thick ring of the mature bone. The tumor was composed of haphazard, irregular trabeculae of woven bone rimmed by osteoblast and embedded in a loose fibrous stroma. The stroma contains dilated blood vessels and occasional hemorrhage. Few scattered osteoclasts are seen often on the surface of the trabeculae. Endothelial cell marker antibodies CD31 and CD34 were used to highlight the wall of the blood vessels (Figure 6). Histopathologically, osteoblastoma and osteoid osteoma can look very similar, and the distension depends on the size of the lesion. Therefore, the clinical, radiographic, and histopathological correlations make us favor osteoid osteoma as a final diagnosis.

6. Postoperative Patient Course

From day one postoperatively, the patient felt a great improvement in the pain intensity which became mild pain and discomfort (about 3 to 4 out of 10) according to his visual analog scale. His follow-up visits were documented regarding his pain perception including the nocturnal pain, which revealed that he is almost in pain-free status. His surgical site after two years healed nicely without noticeable scarring.

7. Discussion

Osteoid osteomas are benign skeletal tumors that are portrayed by an intracortical nidus with a variable amount of calcification, sclerosis, and bone marrow edema [1]. Jaffe

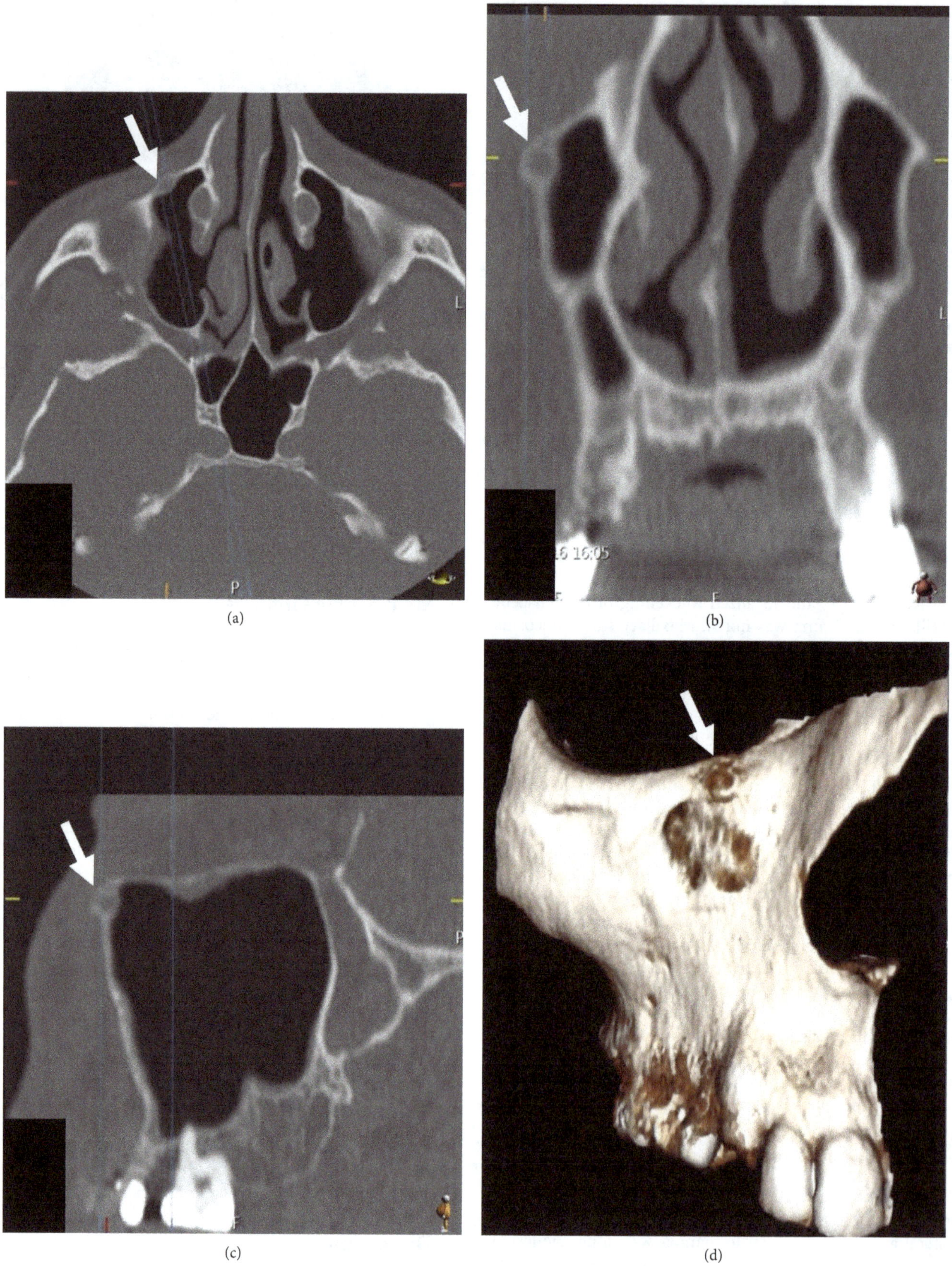

Figure 2: CT examination of the right maxilla in the bone window: (a) axial section, (b) corrected sagittal section, (c) coronal section, and (d) surface rendering; white arrows showing a small, well-defined, corticated, spherical, radiolucency in the superioanterior wall of the right maxillary sinus wall just below the infraorbital rim and medial to the infraorbital foramen.

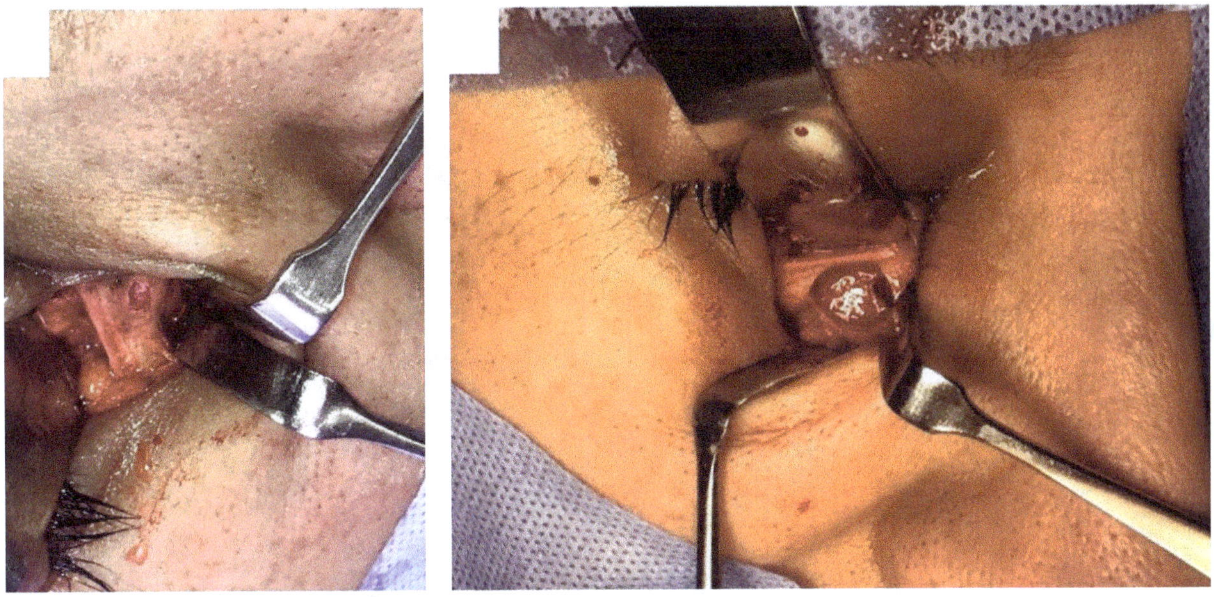

(a) (b)

Figure 3: Intraoperative photographs showing (a) the lesion on the right inferior orbital rim and medial to infraorbital foramen and (b) after complete removal of the lesion with preserving inferior orbital rim.

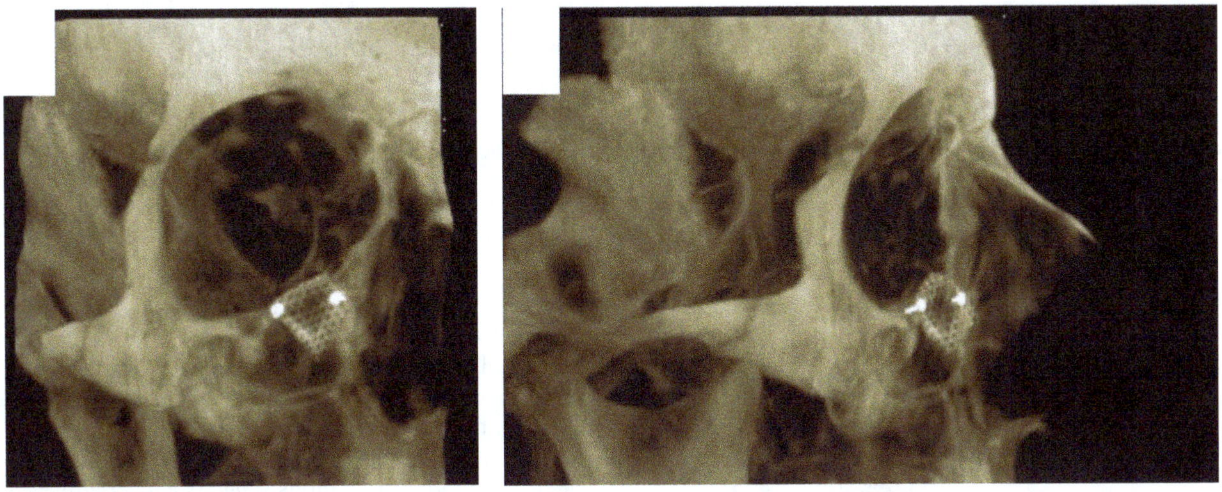

(a) (b)

Figure 4: Thick-slice CT sections in the maximum intensity projection (MIP) in (a) frontal and (b) lateral views showing the reconstruction mesh in place.

described OO as a benign neoplasm with an inflammatory process and considered it a variant of osteoblastoma [1], occurring usually in young adults, with pain as a dominant feature. The pathogenesis of osteoid osteoma has remained controversial. Some authors consider it a neoplasm while some believe it is mainly an inflammatory process. The precise nature is still unclear [14]. Some authors consider it a slow-growing dormant neoplasm or an inflammatory reaction or aftereffect of an unusual healing process [41]. Regarding the nature and genesis of OO, numerous theories have been proposed [1]. The growth of OO is limited, and the lesion size is generally less than 2 cm. A solitary type of this tumor is extremely rare in the head and neck region but relatively common in long bones of the lower limbs [29]. OO typically involves the tibia, femur, fibula, humerus, and vertebral arch [42]. Jaw involvement is rare, with the lingual surface and lower border of the body of the mandible being the most common sites [42]. Its occurrence in the maxillary sinus wall just below the infraorbital rim is rarer.

Clinically, osteoid osteomas are characterized by dull, throbbing, intermittent, local, and nocturnal pain relieved with nonsteroidal anti-inflammatory drugs such as aspirin and are associated with slight local swelling [36]. For decoding the reason for pain, diverse theories were mentioned. Jaffe outlined pain seen in osteoid osteoma as being attributable to the arteriolar blood supply of the lesion [1]. In the current

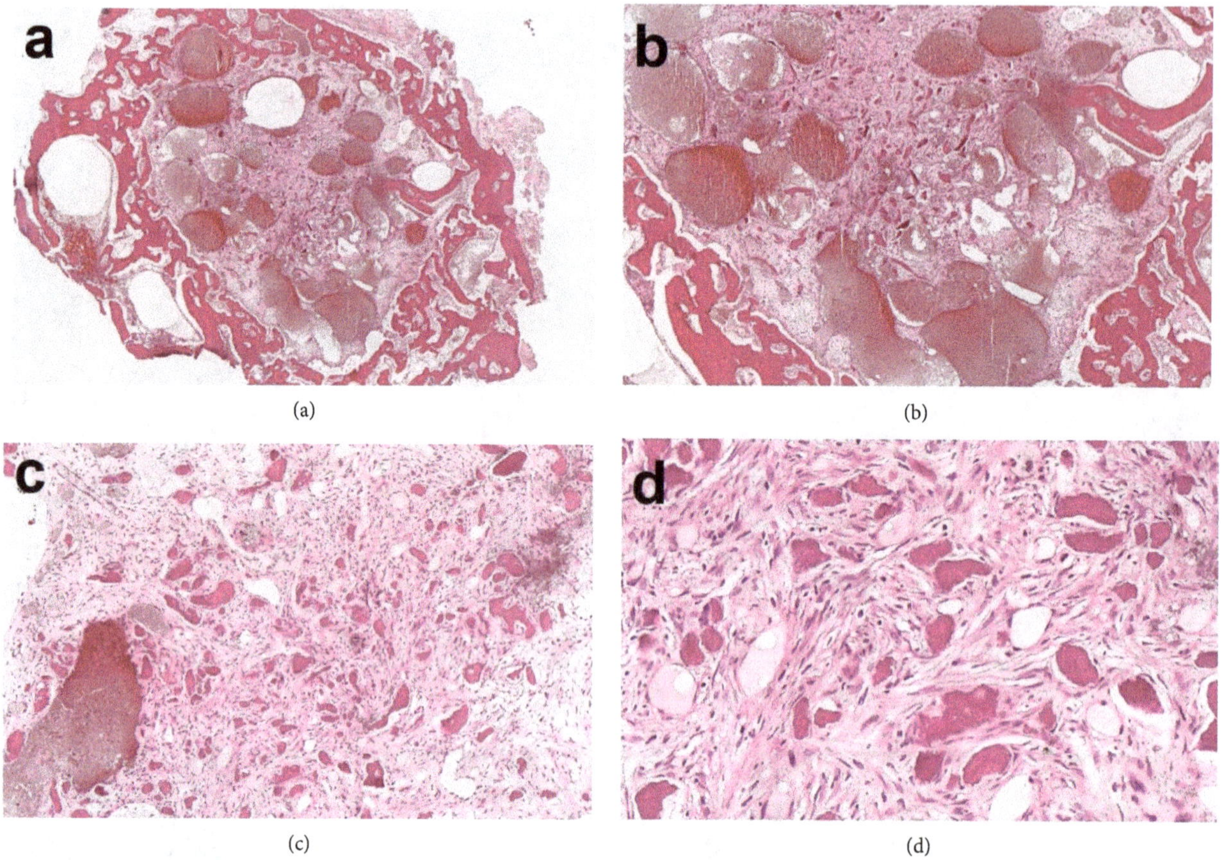

FIGURE 5: H&E-stained histopathologic slides of the excised specimen showing (a) a well-circumscribed and highly vascular tumor surrounded by a thick ring of mature bone. (b) The tumor composed of dilated blood vessels, area of hemorrhage, and numerous scattered irregular calcifications embedded in a fibrous stroma. (c) Cellular fibrous connective tissue containing irregular bony trabeculae. Area of hemorrhage is present. (d) The bony trabeculae are acellular, and the stroma contains plumped osteoblasts with ample cytoplasm and hyperchromatic nuclei.

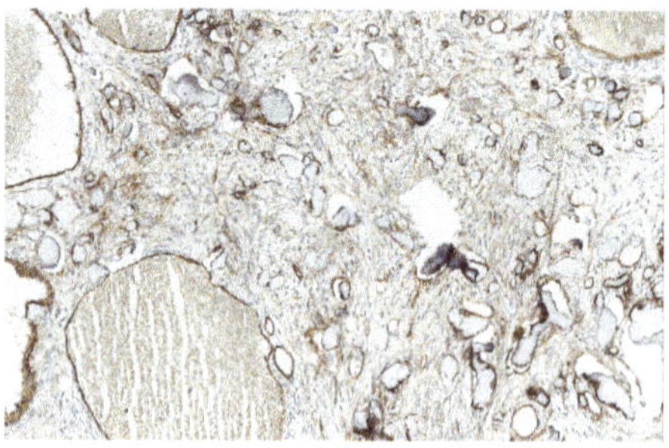

FIGURE 6: CD34 immunoreactivity in the endothelial lining of the blood vessels.

case, the pain was severe in nature, subsiding significantly after the surgery. It is seen to be more common in males compared to females with a ratio of 2 : 1, commonly affecting in the second and third decades of life, and is rarely seen in individuals over 30 years of age [42, 43]. However, the patient reported was a male who was 37 years.

Radiographically, OO is a small, radiolucent intracortical nidus, less than 1 cm in diameter, surrounded by a large, dense sclerotic zone of cortical thickening [44]. Jaffe pointed out that the radiographic features of osteoid osteoma were most important in the ultimate diagnosis of the lesion. He mentioned that the nidus was more radiolucent than radiopaque and that it was surrounded by a reactive radiopacity that extended a variable distance from the nidus [42]. The radiolucent nidus is an ominous sign of a fully mature OO whereas the radiopaque nidus suggests a less mature lesion. Radiolucency with central calcification, located in the cortical bone with surrounding sclerotic bone, is the characteristic feature of osteoid osteoma [3]. The present case was observed in the maxillary anterior region, which is quite uncommon comparing with previously cited cases [2, 4, 10, 13–40]. However, in dentistry, such cases could be underdiagnosed since such a small lesion can be missed on a panoramic radiograph because of the complex anatomic site of the jaws, and CT or CBCT is a useful imaging modality for this diagnosis [3, 30].

The histopathological examination of OO differs according to the site and age of the lesion. Huvos illustrated three specific evolutionary stages of modification of OO. Originally, dense osteoblasts are seen proliferating actively in a highly vascularized stroma followed by deposition of the osteoid matrix between the osteoblasts in the intermediate phase. In the mature stage, the osteoid is transformed into well-calcified, compact trabeculae of atypical bone, which is neither typically woven nor lamellar [2]. Sometimes OO showed possible histological patterns of a neoplastic lesion in the later stages of development [3]. An inflammatory lesion illustrated pain as its constant feature [14]. The cases previously published involving the jaws were abstracted as a type of nidus, more brittle in nature, composed of osteoid tissue predominantly. Describing the microscopic study, Chaudhary and Kulkarni mentioned that a broken nidus may be misguided as granulation tissue and the older lesion might show atypical bone modeled from sheets of osteoid trabeculae [42].

Previously reported cases mentioned several lesions as a differential diagnosis of OO, such as ossifying fibroma, peripheral osteoma, osteoblastoma, osteosarcoma, and fibroosseous lesions. Ossifying fibroma and peripheral osteoma are usually asymptomatic, increase in size, lack nidus, and cause resorption and displacement of teeth [45]. Ossifying fibroma (OF) may have similar radiographic features, presenting as circumscribed well-demarcated bone swellings but lack the presence of a central nidus. OF is typically asymptomatic; therefore, if nocturnal pain is a presenting feature, it can also aid differentiation between these two lesions [43]. Because of clinical, radiographic, and histologic similarities between osteoid osteoma and osteoblastoma, it is very difficult to achieve a differential radiographic diagnosis between them. Also, OO is more painful than osteoblastoma, but this criterion can be subjective, and thus, the patient must provide a clear history of pain [35]. Aspirin and other nonsteroidal anti-inflammatory drugs are very useful in pain associated with OO, but not for an osteoblastoma [45]. Diagnosis of OO is made when the presence of a radiopaque nidus surrounded by sclerotic new bone formation is noted [35]. OOs are defined by their limited growth and size of less than 2 cm in diameter, distinguishing them from osteoblastoma which is usually greater than 2 cm in size, with most 3–10 cm [43]. Osteosarcoma can be excluded based on the clinical behavior of the lesion, which would present as a more rapidly growing painful swelling as well as different histopathological presentation. Fibrous dysplasia can be differentiated from OO radiographically, as fibrous dysplasia is poorly defined with a "ground-glass" appearance. Histologically, fibrous dysplasia shows features typical of any fibrous osseous lesion, with the replacement of normal bone by a variably cellular stroma within which abnormal bone is noted; however, unlike OO, fibrous dysplasia shows little or no osteoblastic rimming [43].

In the present case, the diagnosis of osteoid osteoma was made considering the reported symptom of gradually increasing pain (with which the patient presented to the emergency dental clinic), the CT radiographic appearance, and the histopathologic examination of the specimen.

Studies suggested complete excision should be the treatment of choice with intact removal of the nidus. Recurrence of the lesion depends upon the complete removal of the lesion. To date, no history of malignant transformation of OO has been reported [3, 42]. Albeit some reports of spontaneous remission of osteoid osteoma, complete excision of the osteoid osteoma nidus is the ultimate treatment of choice as it brings immediate relief of pain and completely cures the patient [10].

Wexell et al. recently reported a 7-year follow-up of a 37-year-old woman with Gardner syndrome who had multiple osteomas in both jaws with dental implant treatment with no complication. However, in that case, the patient had known long standing preexisting nonpainful multiple osteomas as part of the Gardner syndrome [46].

8. Conclusion

Herein, we reported a case of osteoid osteoma that occurred in the right maxilla of an adult male patient. The correct diagnosis was achieved by considering clinical, radiographic, and pathological features. To avoid confusion with similar bony pathosis, the treating physician should have a clear concept and keen observation skill. Osteoid osteoma is a benign bone lesion that occurs very rarely in the jawbones. Due to the rarity of this lesion, it is essential to report these cases to increase awareness among dental surgeons worldwide. Osteoid osteoma of the maxilla may present as pain related to dental implants and careful radiographic assessment by CT or CBCT of the entire jawbone should be considered if diagnosis of dental implant pain is unclear.

References

[1] H. Jaffe, "A benign osteoblastic tumor composed of osteoid and atypical bone," *Archives of Surgery*, vol. 31, pp. 701–728, 1935.

[2] S. Karandikar, G. Thakur, M. K. S. Tijare, and K. Agrawal, "Osteoid osteoma of mandible," *BMJ Case Reports*, vol. 2011, no. dec05 1, 2011.

[3] C. Walia, P. Devi, V. B. Thimmarasa, and S. Jayadev, "Osteoid osteoma of the mandible: a rare entity," *Journal of Indian Academy of Oral Medicine and Radiology*, vol. 22, no. 3, pp. 162–164, 2010.

[4] B. S. Manjunatha and D. Nagarajappa, "Osteoid osteoma," *Indian Journal of Dental Research*, vol. 20, no. 4, pp. 514-515, 2009.

[5] J. H. Healy and B. Ghelman, "Osteoid osteoma and osteoblastoma current concepts and recent advances," *Clinical Orthopaedics and Related Research*, vol. 204, pp. 76–85, 1986.

[6] R. Rajendran, B. Sivapathasundaram Shafer, and L. Hine, *Shafer's Textbook of Oral Pathology*, Elsevier, India, 5th edition, 2006.

[7] H. D. Dorfman and B. Czerniak, *Bone tumors*, Mosby, St Louis, 1998.

[8] K. K. Unni, *Dahlin's bone tumors. General aspects and data on 11,087 cases*, Lippincott-Raven, Philadelphia, 1996.

[9] F. J. Frassica, R. L. Waltrip, P. D. Sponseller, L. D. Ma, and E. F. McCarthy, "Clinicopathologic features and treatment of osteoid osteoma and osteoblastoma in children and adolescents," *The Orthopedic Clinics of North America*, vol. 27, no. 3, pp. 559–574, 1996.

[10] B. Rahsepar, A. Nikgoo, and S. A. Fatemitabar, "Osteoid osteoma of subcondylar region: case report and review of the literature," *Journal of Oral and Maxillofacial Surgery*, vol. 67, no. 4, pp. 888–893, 2009.

[11] E. O. Kirwan, P. A. Hutton, J. L. Pozo, and A. O. Ransford, "Osteoid osteoma and benign osteoblastoma of the spine. Clinical presentation and treatment," *Journal of Bone and Joint Surgery*, vol. 66, pp. 21–26, 1984.

[12] E. J. Gardner and R. C. Richards, "Multiple cutaneous and subcutaneous lesions occurring simultaneously with hereditary polyposis and osteomatosis," *American Journal of Human Genetics*, vol. 5, p. 139, 1953.

[13] M. A. Ruston, "An osteoid-osteoma of the mandibular alveolus," *Oral Surgery, Oral Medicine, Oral Pathology, Oral Radiology, and Endodontics*, vol. 4, no. 1, pp. 86–88, 1951.

[14] E. L. Foss, M. B. Dockerty, and C. A. Good, "Osteoid osteoma of the mandible; report of a case," *Cancer*, vol. 8, no. 3, pp. 592–594, 1955.

[15] A. R. Nelson, "Osteoid osteoma of maxilla," *Archives of Surgery*, vol. 70, no. 3, pp. 459–461, 1955.

[16] J. C. Stoopack, "Sialolith and osteoid osteoma," *Oral Surgery, Oral Medicine, Oral Pathology, Oral Radiology, and Endodontics*, vol. 11, no. 11, pp. 1220–1225, 1958.

[17] P. O. Lind and K. Hillerström, "Osteoid-osteoma in the mandibular condyle:Case report and survey of the literature," *Acta Oto-Laryngologica*, vol. 57, pp. 467–474, 1964.

[18] B. S. Hillman and H. G. Birck, "Osteoid osteoma of the maxilla in a four-year-old patient," *Laryngoscope*, vol. 75, no. 12, pp. 1872–1876, 1965.

[19] G. W. Greene Jr., J. R. Natiella, and P. N. Spring Jr., "Osteoid osteoma of the jaws," *Oral Surgery, Oral Medicine, Oral Pathology, Oral Radiology, and Endodontics*, vol. 26, no. 3, pp. 342–351, 1968.

[20] I. Brynolf, "Osteoid osteoma and fibrous dysplasia in the periapical region of maxillary incisors," *Oral Surgery, Oral Medicine, Oral Pathology, Oral Radiology, and Endodontics*, vol. 28, no. 2, pp. 243–248, 1969.

[21] O. P. Gupta, R. K. Jain, M. K. Agarwal, S. Khanna, and A. Shrivastava, "Osteoid osteoma of the mandible," *Ear, Nose, & Throat Journal*, vol. 64, pp. 206–208, 1985.

[22] M. A. Zulian, S. K. Vincent, and W. R. Hiatt, "Osteoid osteoma of the mandibular ramus," *Journal of Oral and Maxillofacial Surgery*, vol. 45, no. 8, pp. 712–714, 1987.

[23] S. Tochihara, T. Sato, H. Yamamoto, K. Asada, and K. Ishibashi, "Osteoid osteoma in mandibular condyle," *International Journal of Oral and Maxillofacial Surgery*, vol. 30, no. 5, pp. 455–457, 2001.

[24] C. Yang and W. L. Qiu, "Osteoid osteoma of the eminence of the temporomandibular joint," *The British Journal of Oral & Maxillofacial Surgery*, vol. 39, no. 5, pp. 404–406, 2001.

[25] M. Ida, T. Kurabayashi, Y. Takahashi, M. Takagi, and T. Sasaki, "Osteoid osteoma in the mandible," *Dento Maxillo Facial Radiology*, vol. 31, no. 6, pp. 385–387, 2002.

[26] C. J. Liu, K. W. Chang, K. M. Chang, and C. Y. Cheng, "A variant of osteoid osteoma of the mandible: report of a case," *Journal of Oral and Maxillofacial Surgery*, vol. 60, no. 2, pp. 219–221, 2002.

[27] C. Badauy, V. Carrard, P. Rados, and F. M. Sant'ana, "Radiopaque mass of the posterior mandible with lingual expansion," *Journal of Oral and Maxillofacial Surgery*, vol. 65, no. 12, pp. 2498–2502, 2007.

[28] B. C. Do Egito Vasconcelos, G. G. Porto, and R. V. Bessa-Nogueira, "Rare benign tumors of the mandibular condyle: report of 2 cases and literature review," *Journal of Oral and Maxillofacial Surgery*, vol. 65, no. 9, pp. 1830–1835, 2007.

[29] I. Mohammed, N. A. Jannan, and A. Elrmali, "Osteoid osteoma associated with the teeth: unusual presentation," *International Journal of Oral and Maxillofacial Surgery*, vol. 42, no. 2, pp. 298–302, 2013.

[30] S. Y. An, H. I. Shin, K. S. Choi, J. W. Park, Y. G. Kim, and E. Benavides, "Unusual osteoid osteoma of the mandible: report of case and review of the literature," *Oral Surgery, Oral Medicine, Oral Pathology, Oral Radiology*, vol. 116, pp. 134–140, 2013.

[31] P. Gadre, D. Singh, K. Gadre, and I. Khan, "Piezosurgery for excision of large osteoid osteoma," *The Journal of Craniofacial Surgery*, vol. 27, no. 7, pp. e701–e702, 2016.

[32] P. Infante-Cossio, A. Restoy-Lozano, F. Espin-Galvez, and L. M. Gonzalez-Perez, "Mandibular osteoid osteoma," *The Journal of Emergency Medicine*, vol. 52, no. 3, pp. e83–e84, 2017.

[33] S. Richardson, R. V. Khandeparker, and K. Sharma, "A large osteoid osteoma of the mandibular condyle causing conductive hearing loss: a case report and review of literature," *Journal of the Korean Association of Oral and Maxillofacial Surgeons*, vol. 43, no. 2, pp. 106–114, 2017.

[34] J. T. Deferm, S. C. A. Steens, D. Vriens, E. M. Bekers, S. I. Kalaykova, and W. A. Borstlap, "Chronic temporomandibular joint pain: two cases of osteoid osteoma and a review of the literature," *International Journal of Oral and Maxillofacial Surgery*, vol. 46, no. 9, pp. 1130–1137, 2017.

[35] A. Singh and M. C. Solomon, "Osteoid osteoma of the mandible: a case report with review of the literature," *Journal of Dental Sciences*, vol. 12, no. 2, pp. 185–189, 2017.

[36] T. Khaitan, P. Ramaswamy, U. Ginjupally, and A. Kabiraj, "A bizarre presentation of osteoid osteoma of maxilla," *Iranian Journal of Pathology*, vol. 11, no. 5, pp. 431–434, 2016.

[37] M. Bajpai and N. Pardhe, "Osteoid osteoma of jaw in a 54-year male," *Journal of the College of Physicians and Surgeons–Pakistan*, vol. 28, no. 6, p. 498, 2018.

[38] L. Matthies, T. Rolvien, T. J. Pakusa et al., "Osteoid osteoma of the mandible-clinical and histological findings," *Anticancer Research*, vol. 39, no. 1, pp. 291–296, 2018.

[39] S. A. Issa, H. A. Abdulnabi, and A. S. H. Alshewered, "Intra-articular osteoid osteoma of tempromandibular joint: a case report," *International Journal of Surgery Case Reports*, vol. 62, pp. 9–13, 2019.

[40] I. A. Díaz-Rengifo, A. J. Díaz-Caballero, K. R. Oro, and Y. Y. Hernández-Arenas, "Painless osteoid osteoma in the maxilla of an elderly female patient," *Journal of Oral and Maxillofacial Pathology*, vol. 23, no. 2, pp. 280–283, 2019.

[41] E. H. Lee, M. Shafi, and J. H. Hui, "Osteoid osteoma: a current review," *Journal of Pediatric Orthopedics*, vol. 26, pp. 965–970, 2006.

[42] M. Chaudhary and M. Kulkarni, "Osteoid osteoma of mandible," *Journal of Oral and Maxillofacial Pathology*, vol. 11, no. 2, pp. 52–55, 2007.

[43] D. M. Fletcher, K. Unni, and F. Mertens, *Pathology and Genetics: Tumours of Soft Tissue and Bone*, IARC Press, Lyon, 2002.

[44] L. Schulman and H. D. Dorfman, "Nerve fibers in osteoid osteoma," *The Journal of Bone & Joint Surgery*, vol. 52, no. 7, pp. 1351–1356, 1970.

[45] M. S. Greenburg and M. Gick, *Burket's Oral Medicine Diagnosis and Treatment*, BC Decker, Ontario, Canada, 11th edition, 2003.

[46] C. L. Wexell, S. Bergenblock, and A. Kovács, "A case report on gardner syndrome with dental implant treatment and a long-term follow-up," *Journal of Oral and Maxillofacial Surgery*, vol. 77, no. 8, pp. 1617–1627, 2019.

7

Laser Therapy for Infected Sites and Immediate Dental Implants in the Esthetic Zone: A Case Report and Review of Literature

Rolando Crippa,[1] Riccardo Aiuto,[2] Mario Dioguardi,[3] María Peñarrocha-Diago,[2] Miguel Peñarrocha-Diago,[2] and Francesca Angiero[4]

[1]*Department of Oral Pathology, Italian Stomatological Institute, Milan, Italy*
[2]*Department of Oral Surgery, University of Valencia, València, Spain*
[3]*Department of Clinical and Experimental Medicine, University of Foggia, Italy*
[4]*Department of Medical Sciences and Diagnostic Integrated, S. Martino Hospital, University of Genoa, Genova, Italy*

Correspondence should be addressed to Riccardo Aiuto; riccardo.aiuto@unimi.it

Academic Editor: Kevin Seymour

Placement of postextraction dental implants has become a common practice. Here, we reviewed current literature, along with clinical procedures, outcomes, and incidence of complications, associated with immediate implants in infected postextraction sites. The YSGG (yttrium, scandium, gallium, and garnet) laser can significantly reduce the bacterial concentration after extracting a compromised tooth. We treated a 40-year-old woman with a compromised tooth in the esthetic zone, presenting clinical and radiological signs of infection, particularly a periapical periodontitis. The tooth was extracted after administering local anesthesia using Optocain® (mepivacaine and adrenalin 1 : 100,000), following which the site was treated with an ErCr : YSGG (erbium, chromium-doped yttrium, scandium, gallium, and garnet) 2780 nm laser device (Biolase iPlus®). The implant (Straumann® fixture) was inserted with minimum 35 N torque, 1 mm below the most apical bone peak. Bio-Oss® and resorbable membrane were applied to improve bone healing. The use of ErCr : YSGG laser has ensured success of implant therapy performed on an infected site. There were no complications such as peri-implantitis or loss of peri-implant bone. The implant achieved good primary stability, immediate placement into an infected site did not increase complications, and the 5-year follow-up confirmed the treatment success.

1. Introduction

Placement of postextraction dental implants has become a common practice, due to its numerous advantages, such as it facilitated maintenance of the horizontal and vertical dimensions of the osseous tissues [1], reduced treatment times, enhanced patient comfort, and good esthetic results. The immediate implant placement technique was first described by Lazzara in 1989 [2]. However, only a small number of studies report the clinical outcomes of immediate implants inserted in postextraction sockets.

One of the primary indications to this technique is the need to replace endodontically compromised teeth in cases when periapical surgery is inadvisable [3]. In such cases, it is imperative to note that certain local and systemic factors may contraindicate placement of the dental implant [4]. Recent studies have demonstrated that the presence of a periradicular infection may not compromise immediate implant placement, provided that the site is adequately decontaminated with a disinfection protocol [5]. The YSGG laser can significantly reduce the bacterial concentration present in the socket of an extracted tooth [6].

A number of studies have reported high success rates for immediately placed, in some cases immediately loaded, implants that are inserted in infected or inflamed postextraction sites [7]. However, to ensure the success of this technique, it is imperative to establish certain preoperative and postoperative measures, such as meticulous cleansing, alveolar debridement, administration of antibiotics, and postoperative 0.12% chlorhexidine mouth rinses [8].

Recent studies have reported that laser technology is capable of eliminating bacteria more effectively than chemical products. Kusek suggests that the hydroacoustic phenomenon, which combines bactericidal effects with the ability to reach anatomically complex regions, is the principal factor that ensures complete disinfection [6]. The article reviews the studies concerning the immediate implant technique after laser disinfection and presents a clinical case to illustrate the main steps for correct management of the procedure and the 5-year follow-up.

2. Case Report

We encountered the case of a 40-year-old woman with a compromised upper left lateral incisor presenting with clinical and radiological signs of an infection, particularly periapical periodontitis (Figures 1 and 2). The tooth had been unsuccessfully treated with apicectomy. The patient was in good general health and had a good oral hygiene and was motivated to begin the treatment. We decided to proceed with a postextraction dental implant, considering the conditions and the area of high esthetic value.

Optocain® (mepivacaine 1 : 100.000) was used as local anesthetic, and tooth 2.2 was extracted as atraumatically as possible. The full thickness flap was carried out by a crestal incision with vertical releases. The postextraction site was treated with the ErCr : YSGG 2780 nm laser device Waterlase iPlus® (Biolase) with handpiece gold having two modes of operation, namely, the soft tissue and hard tissue modes (Figure 3). Configuration for the soft tissue mode includes tip MC-3, length 9 mm, air 20%, and water 40%; alternatively, the configuration for the hard tissue mode includes tip MZ-8, length 9 mm, air 40%, water 60%, 3.5 W, and 60 Hz. The site was debrided and decontaminated after extraction using the same laser device (2.0 W, 15 Hz, 40% air, 60% water, and 100 mL H_2O/min in hard tissue mode) while mounting a MZ-6 tip and 9 mm in length. Debridement time depended on the amount of pathological tissue and bone volume, whereas decontamination lasted from 60 to 90 seconds per socket, ensuring no physical contact between the tip and the tissues. Straumann® fixtures were selected for the implant surgery. The implant (1 T.E. ø 3.3 mm RN, SLA®; 10 mm, Roxolid®) was inserted with a minimum 35 N torque and 1 mm below the most apical bone peak. Bio-Oss® and GUIDOR matrix barrier (DeOre Materials®) were used to improve bone healing (Figures 4 and 5). The suture was placed with particular care to obtain primary closure over the implant. The suturing material used was PTFE Omnia 3/0, 19 mm 3/8. We postoperatively administered amoxicillin (1 gr ×2/day for 6 days) and chlorhexidine gluconate 0.20% twice daily for 15-20 days. The temporary prosthetic phase before loading was managed with a Maryland bridge. The implant was loaded after 4 months, and a clinical check 2 years later demonstrates satisfactory esthetic outcomes (Figure 6). Radiographic checkups were scheduled on the 1st, 4th, 8th, and 12th months in the first year (Figure 7).

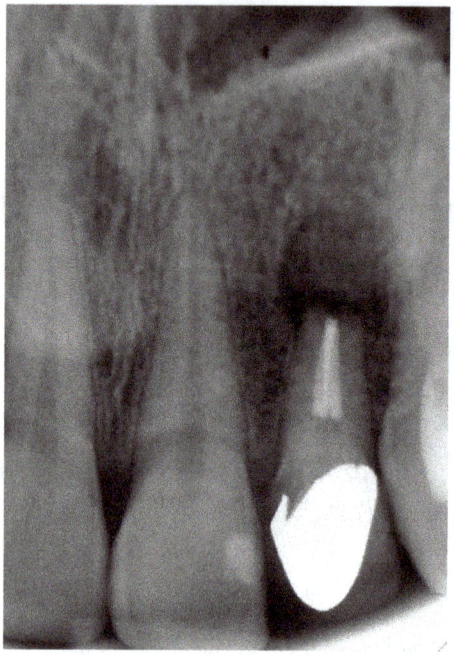

Figure 1: Preoperative X-ray.

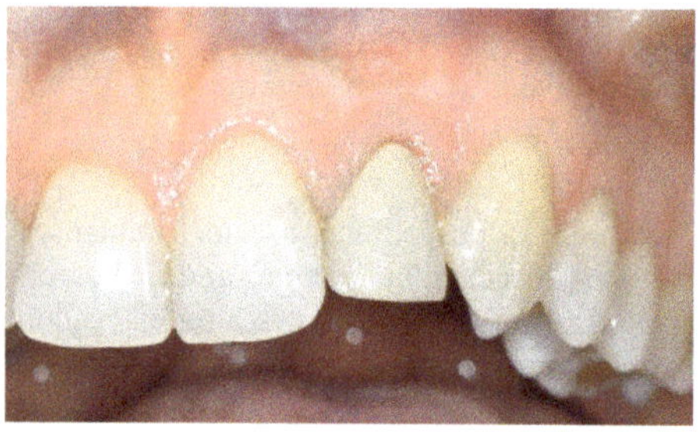

Figure 2: Preoperative clinical condition.

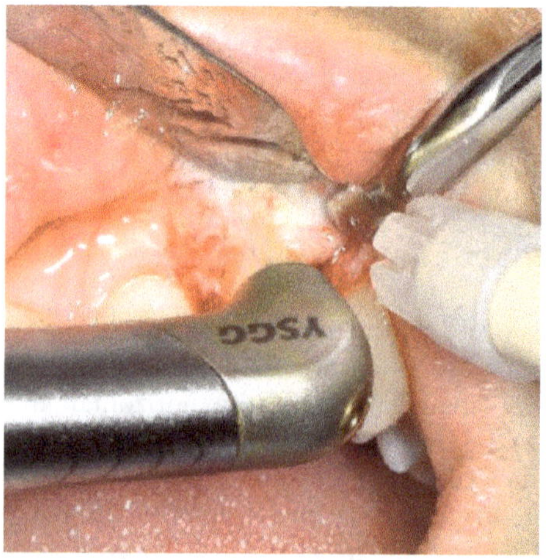

Figure 3: Phases of surgery.

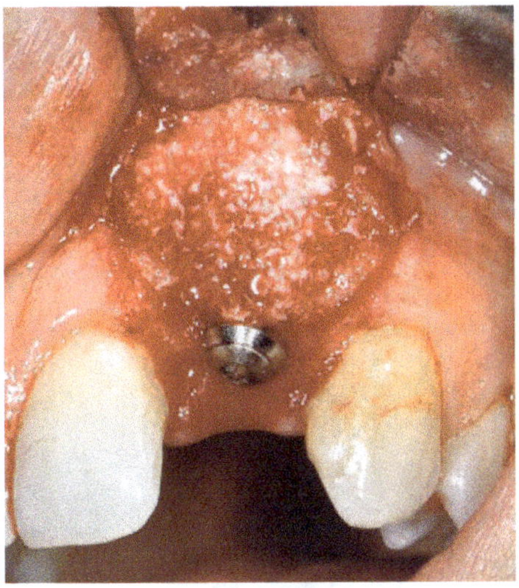

FIGURE 4: Tissue regeneration.

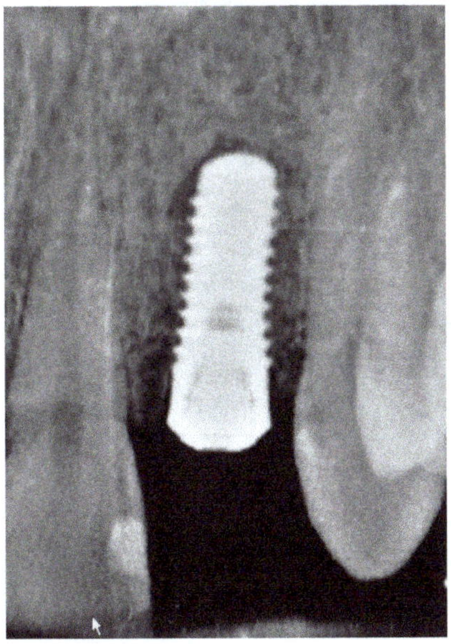

FIGURE 5: Postoperative X-ray.

3. Discussion

We did not observe any complications, such as implant loss, peri-implantitis, or loss of the peri-implant bone. The implant achieved a good primary stability (>35 N/cm) and indicated that immediate placement into infected sites does not lead to more number complications than the traditional technique. This is evidenced by the 5-year follow-up (Figure 8) and research performed to analyze the scientific literature. The PICO assessment worksheet was used to define the topic and plan the search strategy, before commencing the review [9]. We searched for the studies including those limited to the period from January 1, 1980, to June 30, 2019. Furthermore, we used a specific set of keywords such as "immediate implant placement" AND "laser", "dental implants" AND "laser" AND "postextrac-

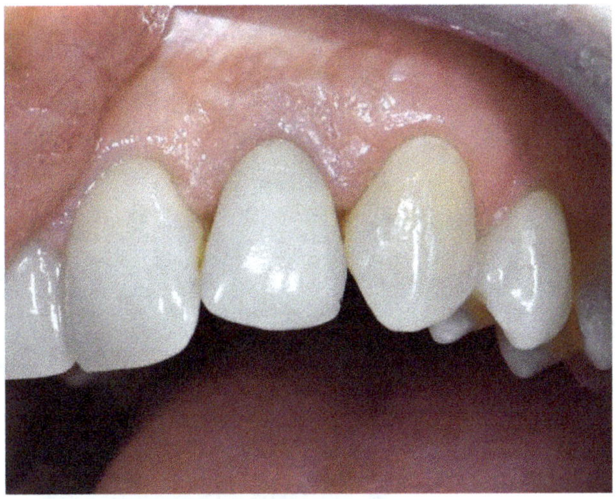

FIGURE 6: Clinical conditions after 2 years.

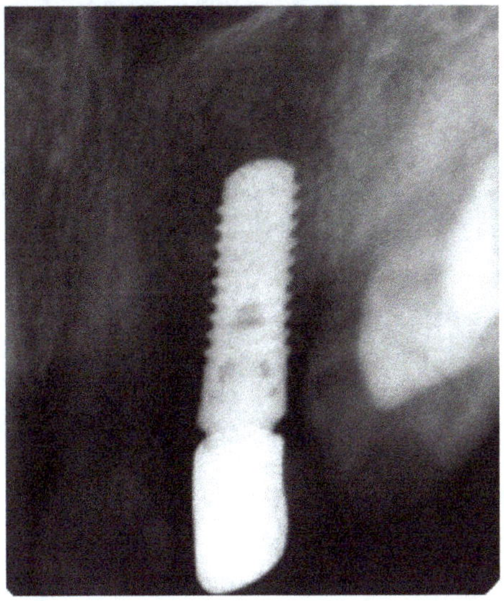

FIGURE 7: 1-year follow-up.

tion". The search was restricted to the study subjects due to the use of Boolean connectives. We used the PubMed (Medline) search engine and the NCBI database. All types of studies published in dental journals were considered.

Although the postextraction implant placement technique has been widely validated, little has been reported concerning the applications of laser decontamination of the infected sites for immediate implant placement. A search through the published studies produced only four clinical articles that combined laser treatment and immediate implant therapy (Table 1). Kusek presented 10 cases of immediate implant placement subjected to the ErCr : YSGG laser disinfection therapy and affirmed that these cases would have taken 3 times longer to heal if treated through traditional methods. Using this technique would therefore enable both the patient and dentist to benefit from a reduced treatment time [6].

Montoya-Salazar et al. also reported a similar study: they analyzed 36 immediate implants replacing teeth lost due to chronic periapical lesions, with a history of endodontic

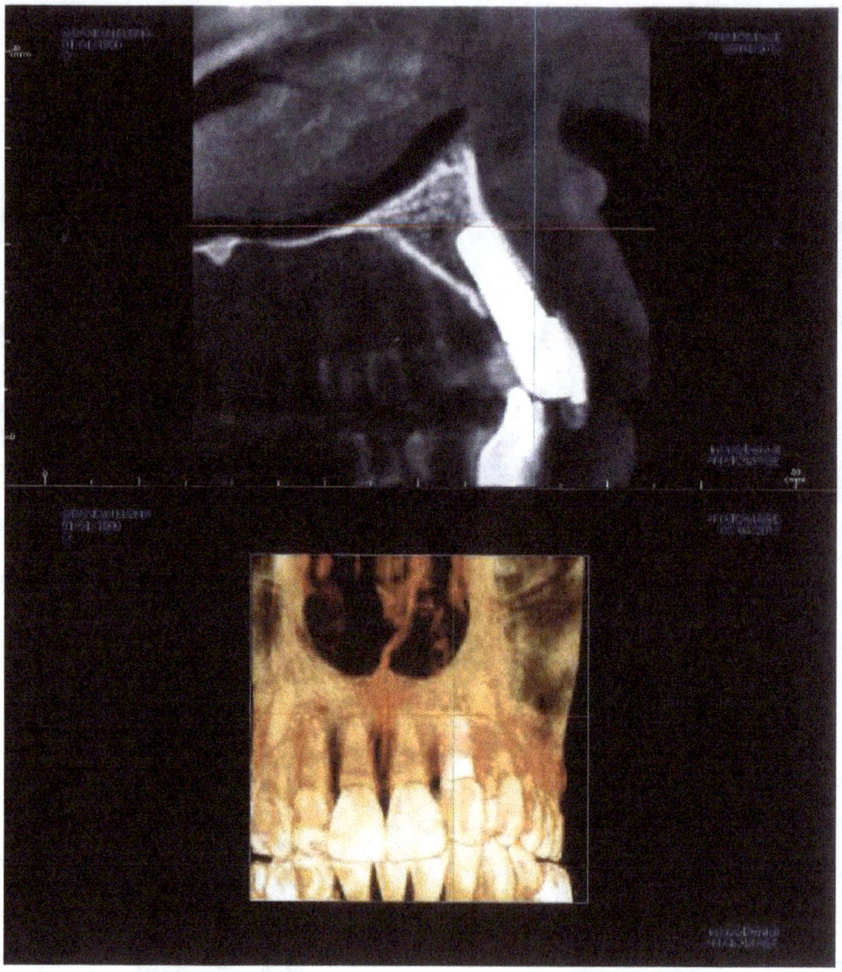

Figure 8: 5-year follow-up.

Table 1: Articles about laser treatment and immediate implant therapy.

Author	Study design	Infected sites	Laser	Implants (no.)	Follow-up	Survival rate
Kusek	Case series	Yes	ErCr : YSGG	10	1 year	10/10
Montoya-Salazar et al.	Prospective	Yes	ErCr : YSGG	18	3 years	17/18
Crippa et al.	Case series	Yes	ErCr : YSGG	94	6 months/4 years	89/94
Choi et al.	Case series	No	Nd : YAG	6	9 months	6/6

failure, and concluded that this therapy may be considered safe option to restore fresh infected postextraction sockets, provided that a strict debridement protocol was respected. Their protocol comprised curettage, cleansing with 90% hydrogen peroxide, irradiation with ErCr : YSGG laser, and chlorhexidine rinses, together with guided bone regeneration under antibiotic cover [7].

Crippa et al. described a series of 94 postextraction implants with a follow-up from 6 months to 4 years and a success rate of 94.6% (89/94) [10].

Additionally, Choi et al. described the advantages of using the laser for ridge conservation. However, that study was not pertinent to infected sites. The authors affirmed that using the Nd : YAG laser energy with 650 μs pulse duration consistently supported rapid clot formation and graft containment at immediate implant and ridge preservation sites [11].

An important systematic review of the literature on immediate implants in infected sites was carried out by Waasdorp et al., but it does not include studies on the effects of laser decontamination [12].

Success after 5 years of follow-ups, the case described in this work reflects what the other authors observed in previous studies. According to the current scientific evidence, provided the presence of adequate primary stability, the implant immediate placement into infected sites would not present with increased rate of complications. However, according to the studies reviewed, it is imperative to conduct an RCT study on this objective, while following appropriate clinical protocol.

The effectiveness of the YSGG laser in disinfecting the surgical site depends on the photoacoustic effect of laser radiation, which attacks bacterial colonies [13, 14]. This effect has been extensively studied in vitro, through experiments that have demonstrated its validity [15, 16]. An important factor is the power setting of the laser: the power must be adjusted to ensure optimum disinfection of the site without risking collateral tissue damage [17]. Moreover, the operator's experience with this technique also plays a fundamental role. Using the laser device for implant surgery may also be advantageous in reducing intraoperative bleeding, therefore keeping the operative field clear [18].

4. Conclusion

Immediate implant placement in infected or inflamed post-extraction sites, after laser decontamination, does not seem to increase the risk of failure, as demonstrated by this case and other previously published reports. The technique also offers interesting advantages of treating esthetic areas with postextraction implants. It is necessary to follow a certain set of protocols and procedures to prevent peri-implantitis and infective complications. However, further studies will undoubtedly be needed to fully elucidate the importance and mechanism underlying the technique.

References

[1] S. W. Chang, S. Y. Shin, J. R. Hong et al., "Immediate implant placement into infected and noninfected extraction sockets: a pilot study," *Oral Surgery, Oral Medicine, Oral Pathology, Oral Radiology, and Endodontics*, vol. 107, no. 2, article S1079210408004320, pp. 197–203, 2009.

[2] R. J. Lazzara, "Immediate implant placement into extraction sites: surgical and restorative advantages," *International Journal of Periodontics and Restorative Dentistry*, vol. 9, no. 5, pp. 332–343, 1989.

[3] P. Diz, C. Scully, and M. Sanz, "Dental implants in the medically compromised patient," *Journal of Dentistry*, vol. 41, no. 3, pp. 195–206, 2013.

[4] J. A. H. Lindeboom, Y. Tjiook, and F. H. M. Kroon, "Immediate placement of implants in periapical infected sites: a prospective randomized study in 50 patients," *Oral Surgery, Oral Medicine, Oral Pathology, Oral Radiology, and Endodontics*, vol. 101, no. 6, pp. 705–710, 2006.

[5] D. W. Siegenthaler, R. E. Jung, C. Holderegger, M. Roos, and C. H. F. Hämmerle, "Replacement of teeth exhibiting periapical pathology by immediate implants: a prospective, controlled clinical trial," *Clinical Oral Implants Research*, vol. 18, no. 6, pp. 727–737, 2007.

[6] E. R. Kusek, "Immediate implant placement into infected sites: bacterial studies of the Hydroacoustic effects of the YSGG laser," *Journal of oral implantology*, vol. 37, no. sp1, pp. 205–211, 2011.

[7] V. Montoya-Salazar, R. Castillo-Oyagüe, C. Torres-Sánchez, C. D. Lynch, J. L. Gutiérrez-Pérez, and D. Torres-Lagares, "Outcome of single immediate implants placed in post-extraction infected and non-infected sites, restored with cemented crowns: a 3-year prospective study," *Journal of Dentistry*, vol. 42, no. 6, pp. 645–652, 2014.

[8] S. Marconcini, A. Barone, F. Gelpi, F. Briguglio, and U. Covani, "Immediate implant placement in infected sites: a case series," *Journal of Periodontology*, vol. 84, no. 2, pp. 196–202, 2013.

[9] S. A. Miller and J. L. Forrest, "Enhancing your practice through evidence-based decision making: PICO, learning how to ask good questions," *Journal of Evidence-Based Dental Practice*, vol. 1, no. 2, article S1532338201700243, pp. 136–141, 2001.

[10] R. Crippa, R. Aiuto, M. Guardincerri, M. Peñarrocha Diago, and F. Angiero, "Effect of laser radiation on infected sites for the immediate placement of dental implants," *Photobiomodulation, photomedicine, and laser surgery*, 2019.

[11] A. Y. Choi, C. M. Reddy, R. T. McGary et al., "Adjunctive Nd:YAG laser irradiation for ridge preservation and immediate implant procedures: a consecutive case series," *Clinical advances in periodontics*, vol. 9, no. 3, pp. 125–134, 2019.

[12] J. A. Waasdorp, C. I. Evian, and M. Mandracchia, "Immediate placement of implants into infected sites: a systematic review of the literature," *Journal of Periodontology*, vol. 81, no. 6, pp. 801–808, 2010.

[13] M. E. Licata, A. Albanese, G. Campisi, D. M. Geraci, R. Russo, and G. Gallina, "Effectiveness of a new method of disinfecting the root canal, using Er, Cr:YSGG laser to kill Enterococcus faecalis in an infected tooth model," *Lasers in medical science*, vol. 30, no. 2, article 1410, pp. 707–712, 2015.

[14] U. Schoop, W. Kluger, A. Moritz, N. Nedjelik, A. Georgopoulos, and W. Sperr, "Bactericidal effect of different laser systems in the deep layers of dentin," *Lasers in Surgery and Medicine*, vol. 35, no. 2, pp. 111–116, 2004.

[15] A. Moritz, O. Doertbudak, N. Gutknecht, K. Goharkhay, U. Schoop, and W. Sperr, "Nd: YAG laser irradiation of infected root canals in combination with microbiological examinations," *The Journal of the American Dental Association*, vol. 128, no. 11, pp. 1525–1530, 1997.

[16] W. Gordon, V. A. Atabakhsh, F. Meza et al., "The antimicrobial efficacy of the erbium, chromium:yttrium-scandium-gallium-garnet laser with radial emitting tips on root canal dentin walls infected with Enterococcus faecalis," *Journal of the American Dental Association*, vol. 138, no. 7, pp. 992–1002, 2007.

[17] L. Zhu, M. Tolba, D. Arola, M. Salloum, and F. Meza, "Evaluation of effectiveness of Er,Cr:YSGG laser for root canal disinfection: theoretical simulation of temperature elevations in root dentin," *Journal of Biomechanical Engineering*, vol. 131, no. 7, article 071004, 2009.

[18] R. Crespi, P. Capparè, and E. Gherlone, "Fresh-socket implants in periapical infected sites in humans," *Journal of Periodontology*, vol. 81, no. 3, pp. 378–383, 2010.

8

Optimised Implant Selection using Digital Volume Tomography (DVT) Osteodensitometry

Manfred Nilius[1,2] and Jörg Winterhoff[1]

[1]*Niliusklinik, Londoner Bogen 6, D-44269 Dortmund, Germany*
[2]*Universitätsklinikum, Carl Gustav Carus, Technische Universität Dresden, Fakultät für Zahn, Mund-und Kieferheilkunde, Dresden, Germany*

Correspondence should be addressed to Manfred Nilius; manfrednilius@niliusklinik.de

Academic Editor: Sukumaran Anil

Purpose. The density of the jaw bone has an inhomogeneous distribution and, even within partial volumes, varies more or less strongly from the size of typical implants. Consequently, the primary stability of implants using conventional techniques can only ever be determined postimplantation. The aim of the present case report is to present digital volume tomography (DVT) osteodensitometry as a procedure for assessing the primary stability preimplantation and to evaluate its benefits. *Methods.* An orthopantomogram (OPT) and vertical sections, including bone density measurement, were obtained from a DVT in the course of preimplantological diagnosis. Conventional implant planning and densitometric simulation were performed on this basis. *Results.* Densitometric simulation enabled assessment of the bone density at the interface to the implant body preimplantation. This procedure provides not only an overall value (averaged density) but also allocation of bone areas with different densities to the adjacent areas on the implant surface. This then allows the implant with the best possible macroscopic geometry and optimum position to be selected, with the aim of maximising primary stability. In the present case, the maximum torques during insertion confirmed the densitometric values recorded in advance. *Conclusion.* DVT osteodensitometry enables selection of an implant optimised to bone density distribution. At the same time, the point at which loading occurs can already be defined at the planning stage, thanks to the predictable primary stability. A standard integration of DVT osteodensitometry in the algorithms of implant planning software thus seems desirable.

1. Introduction

There are a variety of technologies using Cone Beam-Computer Tomography (CB-CT) scan and CAD/CAM to measure implant stability: cutting resistance analysis (CRA), reverse torque test (RTT), resonance frequency analysis (RFA), and impact hammer method [1].

The standard methods in implantology—torque measurement during insertion [2, 3] and implant stability quotient (ISQ) [4–6] for evaluating the primary stability—have proven successful in implant planning. They have the disadvantage, however, of providing the required information only after insertion is complete. But reliable assessment of bone quality for evaluating the possible moment of loading already at the planning stage would be useful for the clinician, so that the timing of the treatment sequence is predictable and can be communicated in a patient-oriented manner.

The use of DVT osteodensitometry opens up the possibility of a predictive method [7–11]. With the aid of DVT, not only the bone density can be evaluated, but also the expected bone contact with the implant can be shown—differentiated according to areas of different quality/thickness. This allows the expected primary stability already to be predicted in preoperative diagnosis. The dental surgeon can decide individually in advance, whether prosthetic immediate loading is possible or whether a delayed restoration is to be preferred, to reduce the risk of implant failure in the early stage. Bone condensing or augmentative measures can also be evaluated in this way [7, 8].

The following case shows an example of a densitometrically planned implantation from the planning stage to prosthetic rehabilitation and to the 3-year follow-up.

2. Case Presentation

A 55-year-old female patient presented with the request for a fixed restoration in the left mandible. She was in good general condition and had no systemic preexisting diseases. The periodontal indices were inconspicuous. There was a slight narrowness in the lower jaw front. Previous patient's dental history was an abutment loss of tooth 36 with shortening of the existing bridge to the distal of the crowned tooth 34. In this area, there was evidence of a completely healed region with moderate atrophy of the alveolar ridge (Figure 1).

Following comprehensive patient history, diagnosis, and consultation, the patient decided in favour of an implant-borne restoration in the form of all-ceramic crowns. Likewise, the insufficient crowns on 33 and 34, which were on teeth worth preserving, should also be replaced.

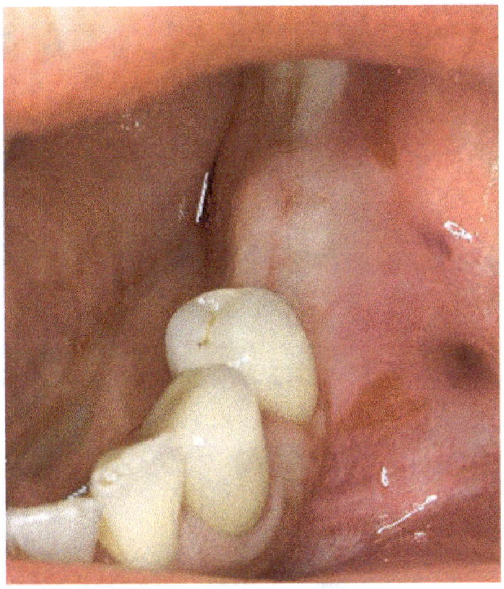

FIGURE 1: The initial clinical situation.

2.1. Preimplantological Diagnosis and Planning. The aim of preimplantological diagnosis was to ensure the best possible selection of implants for the local bone with regard to the expected primary stability and thus the planning of the time of loading.

Intraoral scans (3Shape Trios 3 Basic Pod, Software: 3Shape Implant Studio Version 20.1.1, Copenhagen/Denmark) of the initial situation were taken and a DVT created (CB-CT: KaVo 3D-eXam ConeBeam XG; software: eXam-VisionQ, version 1.9.3.13, both by Kaltenbach & Voigt Dental GmbH, Biberach/Riss, Germany). From these, a level-optimised OPT and a vertical section in the region of implants to be placed were also generated using Hounsfield unit measurement (Figures 2(a)–2(c)).

After importing the DVT data, including Hounsfield values, in an implant planning software (Implant Studio, 3Shape, Copenhagen), the densitometric-supported planning for the guided surgery process was completed (Figure 3).

In addition to the usual determination of implant position, length, and diameter, a densitometric-based simulation could also be created using this data/software combination. This provides visualisation of which parts of the implant body come into contact with areas of different bone density.

Apart from limited and restricted flexible parameters, such as implant length and diameter due to anatomical conditions, this additional information now allows the macrostructure of the implant body to be evaluated in relation to its effect on the (primary) stability in the bone site and selected accordingly.

For this, it was also an advantage to have an implant system available that provides various implant bodies with the same instrumentarium and the same prosthetic interface (SIC invent, Basel, Switzerland). The system selected in the present case allows selection between three different types of implant body (SICace, SICmax, SICtapered, Figures 4(a)–4(c)) using the same drill instrumentarium and protocol.

We performed densitometric simulation for the different implant bodies of the system and ultimately decided in favour of the conical implant (SICtapered), as there was mainly soft bone present towards the buccal side at the implant position (Figures 5 and 6). The defined compression effect of the conical implant seemed the sensible option to us in this case (Figure 6).

Immediate loading was excluded due to the predominantly D3/D4 bone density, and unloaded healing was planned. According to planning, the guided surgery template was fabricated in the dental laboratory using the implant software, and the drill protocol to be used was printed and provided for treatment.

2.2. Implantation and Prosthetic Restoration. Treatment was performed using electronically controlled intraosseous anaesthesia (Quicksleeper 5, Dental HiTec, Gronau, Germany) with approximately 0.8 ml Ultracain DS-Forte osteocentral in the implant insertion region [12]. This avoided the use of block anaesthesia and associated risk, while also reducing the volume of local anaesthetic. Thanks to the planning reliability of the DVT-based guided surgery technique, a flapless procedure could be performed to ensure minimum traumatisation of the surrounding hard and soft tissue. Preparation of the implant site was guided, i.e., using the template with the corresponding instrumentarium (SIC Guided Surgery, SIC invent, Basel). Preparation and implant insertion proceeded without any complications, and the implants were inserted using maximum torques of 14 Ncm (35) and 30 Ncm (36) (Figures 7 and 8). This corresponded to the expected values from the densitometry of minimum compression of the spongiosa, without a final peak through the crestal compact bone, and supported the planning of unloaded healing.

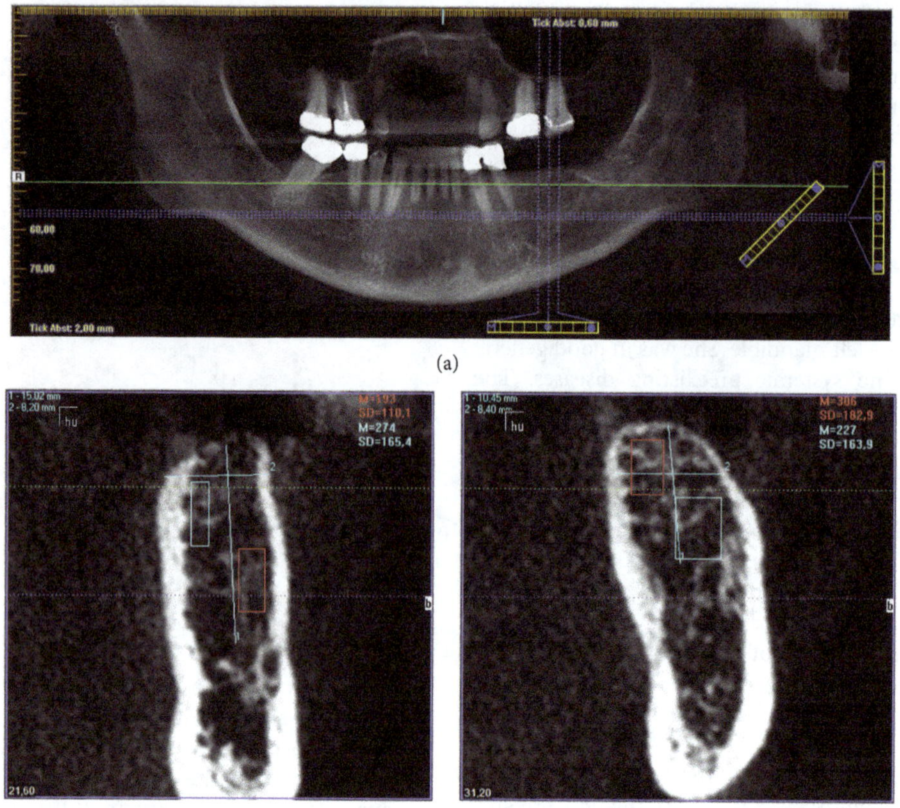

(a)

(b) (c)

FIGURE 2: An OPT and a vertical section in the region of the implants to be inserted were derived from the DVT.

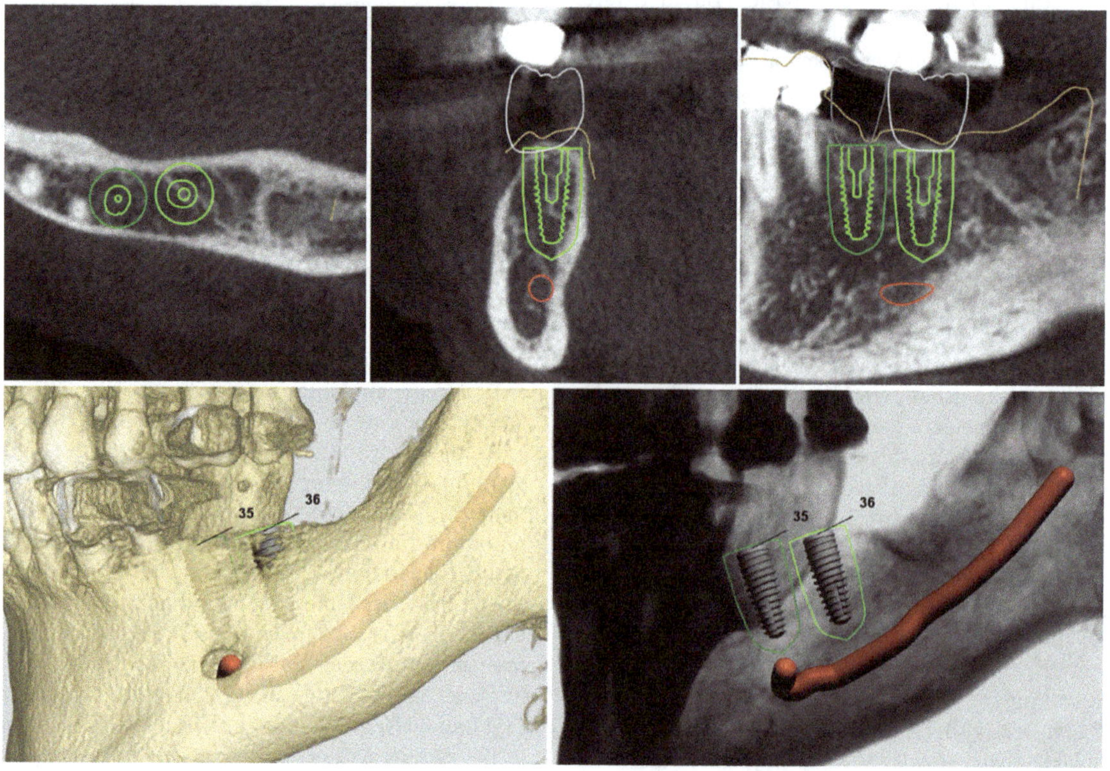

FIGURE 3: Screenshot from the guided surgery planning.

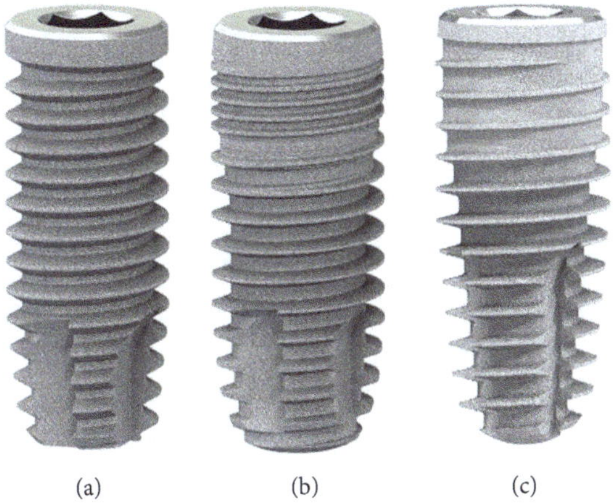

FIGURE 4: (a) SICace (cylindrical). (b) SICmax (mainly cylindrical). (c) SICtapered (conical).

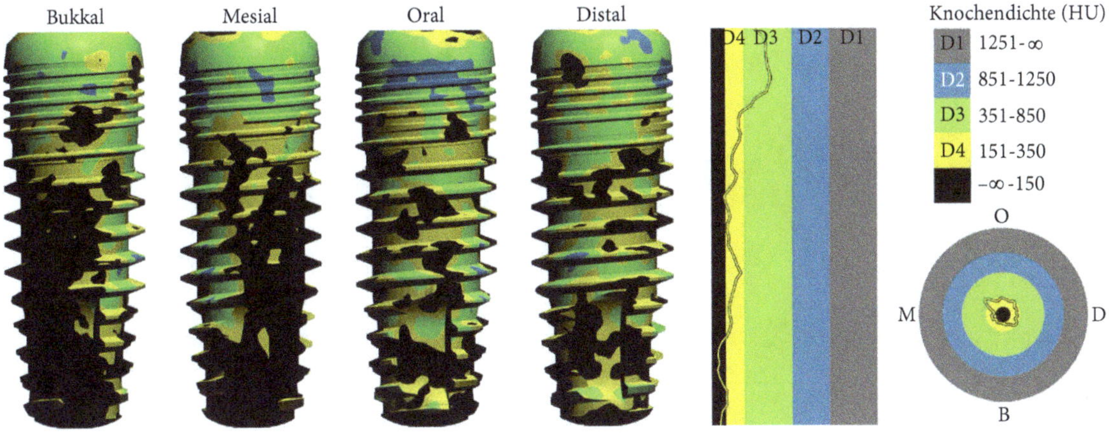

FIGURE 5: Example: simulation with mainly cylindrical implant (SICmax).

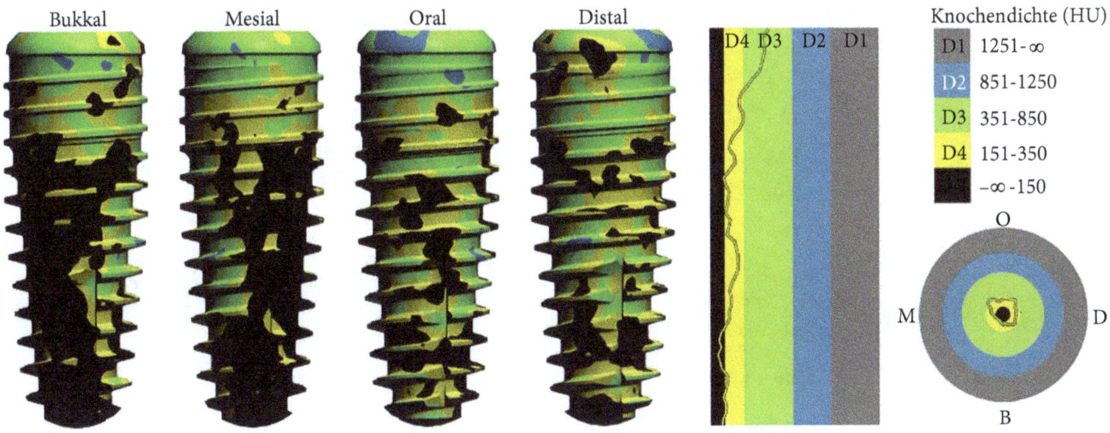

FIGURE 6: Simulation with conical implant (SICtapered).

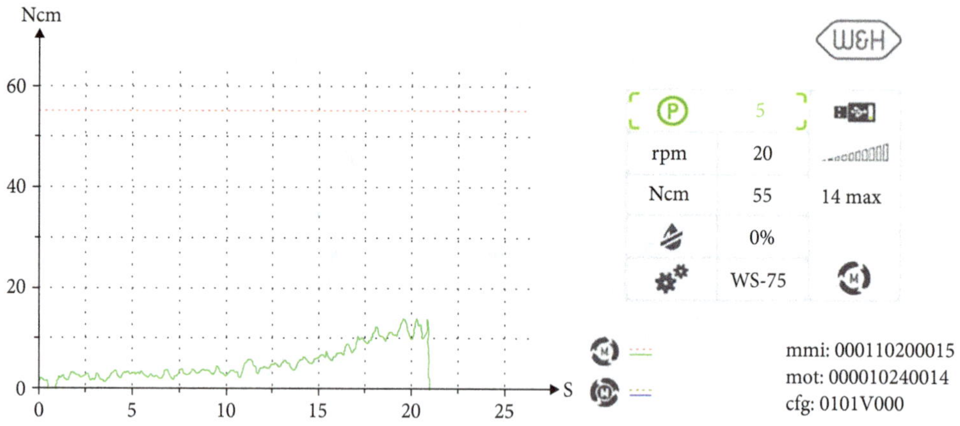

FIGURE 7: Insertion torque curve 35.

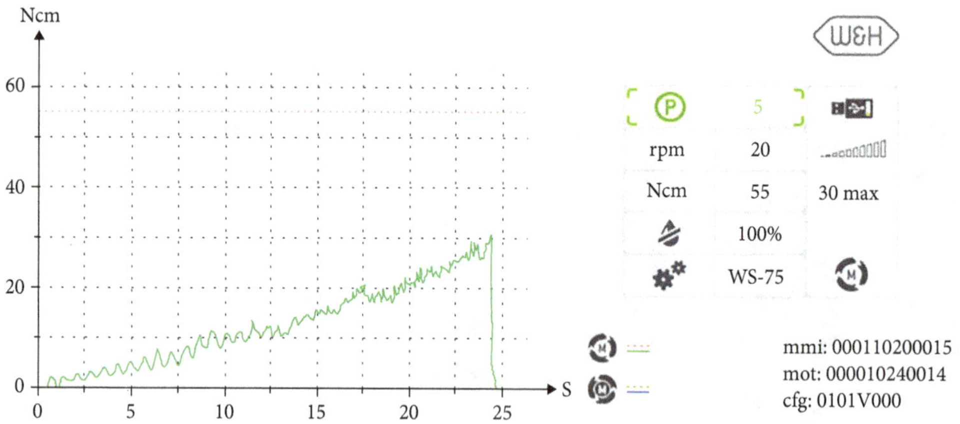

FIGURE 8: Insertion torque curve 36.

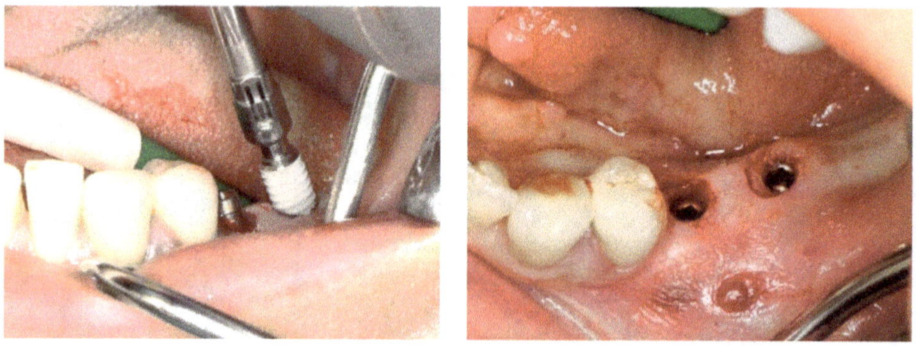

(a) (b)

FIGURE 9: The implants were inserted in regions 35 and 36.

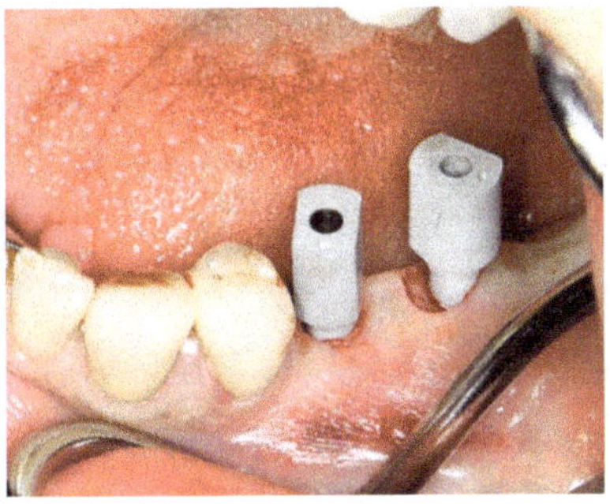

FIGURE 10: Digital impression posts (SIC Scan Adapter for CAD/CAM abutments and milling blanks) with buccal alignment of the point for the immediate postoperative scan.

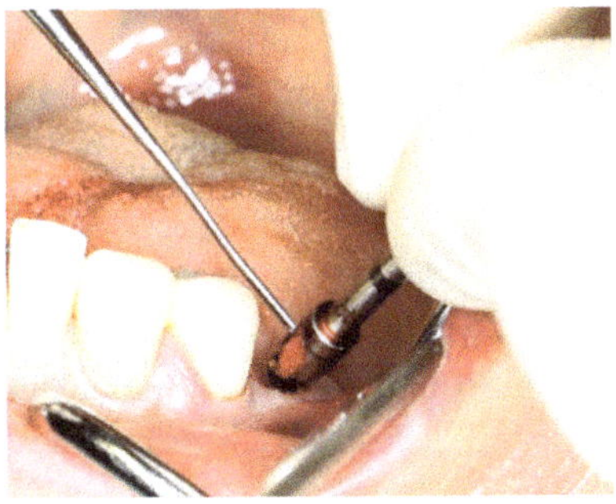

FIGURE 11: Subcrestal relocation of local bone (bone chips from the crestal cutter, SIC Crestal Cutter) on the implant shoulder following insertion of the implant cover screw.

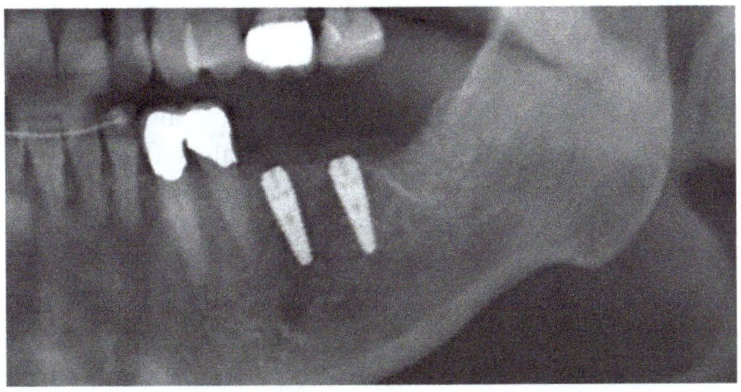

FIGURE 12: X-ray check after insertion.

The intraoral scan for the long-term temporary restoration (LTT) was taken immediately after insertion (Figures 9(a), 9(b), and 10).

Filling of small bone defects in the cervical areas of the implant using intraoperatively harvested host bone chips and closure using sutures (Profimed 3/0, medipac, Kilkis, Greece) completed the treatment (Figures 11 and 12).

The patient explicitly expressed her satisfaction with the treatment procedure at the check-up on the following day and reported discreet initial wound pain.

Based on the intraoral scan from the day of treatment and the DVT data, which was matched in the implant planning

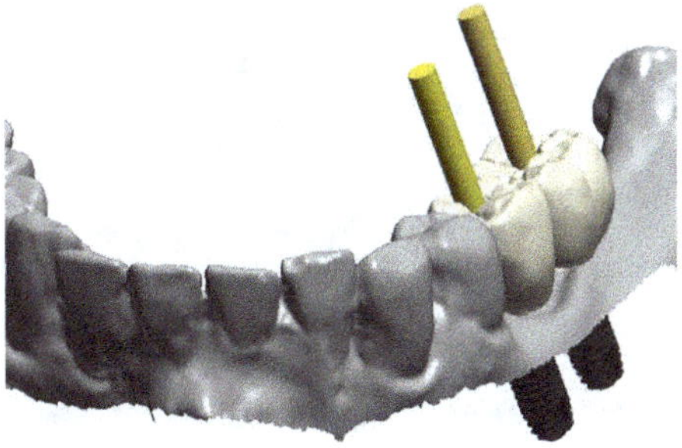

FIGURE 13: Verification of the implant axes (yellow pins) for implants 35 and 36 and comparison with the prosthetic digital crown planning.

software, the LTT was then digitally planned in the form of two single crowns (Figure 13). The temporary restorations were fabricated using a multilayer polymethylmethacrylate (PMMA) composite milling blank (Copra Temp Symphony A2-PMMA-Blank, Whitepeaks, dental solutions GmbH) on titanium- (Ti-) bonding bases (SIC bonding bases CAD/CAM) with the final ZrO_2 abutments (DD cube ONE, white, Dental Direkt, Spenge, Germany), which are also custom milled.

Ti bases with PMMA, with the required transgingival emergence profile for contouring the soft tissue, were fabricated as gingival formers following implant exposure and fitted five months after insertion. Both implants proved to be optimally osseointegrated and exhibited ISQ values of 72 and 75 (Penguin RFA Instrument Kit, P-I Brånemark, Askim, Sweden/SIC invent, Basel). X-ray images and sound on percussion affirmed the clinical findings.

Due to the accompanying aligner treatment (Invisalign, Align Technology, Tempe, Arizona, USA) desired during the course of treatment, the temporary restoration was only fitted two months later (Figure 14). The customised final ZrO_2 abutments on Ti bonding bases (DD cube ONE, white, Dental Direkt, Spenge) were finally screwed in position using the recommended torque of 20 Ncm for fitting. The insufficient crowns on teeth 33 and 34, which were due to be renewed, were removed, and the teeth built up at the same appointment. The opportunity was also used to take an X-ray (Figure 15).

After final preparation of teeth 33 and 34, a renewed intraoral mandibular scan was created for fabricating the final restoration following completion of the aligner treatment. In addition to the prepared teeth 33 and 34, the scan also included the 35 and 36 abutments.

The final crowns were designed virtually in the dental laboratory in the CAD process (Figure 16) and then milled from ZrO_2 (DD cube ONE, white, Dental Direkt, Spenge) and characterised (MiYO, Jensen, Metzingen, Germany).

After a total treatment time of approximately 18 months, including aligner treatment, the final restoration of the support zone could be completed using crowns on the teeth and implants 33, 34, 35, and 36 (Figures 17(a)–17(c)). The crowns were fitted using dual-curing luting composite (Variolink Esthetic DC neutral, Ivoclar Vivadent, Schaan, Liechtenstein). The patient was highly satisfied with the aesthetics and function.

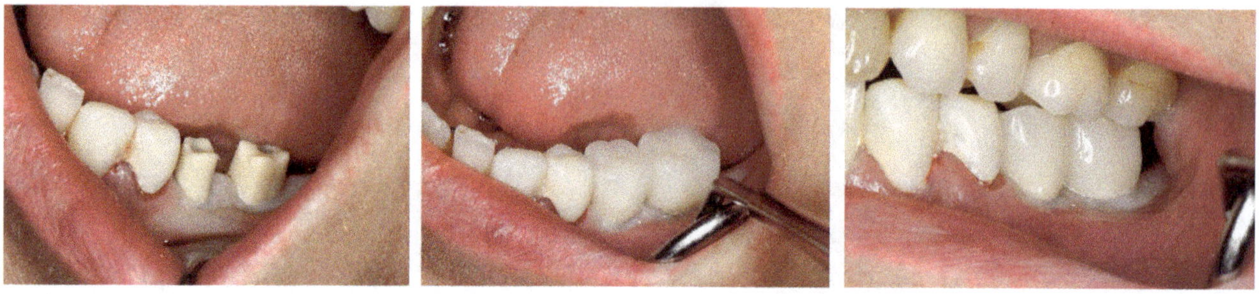

Figure 14: Fitting the long-term temporary restorations.

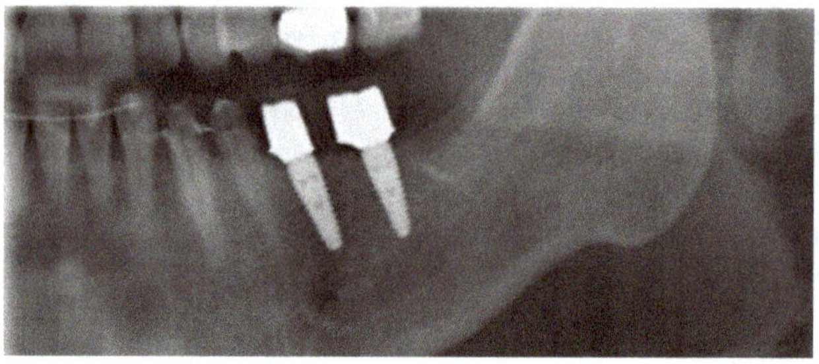

Figure 15: X-ray check during LTT fitting.

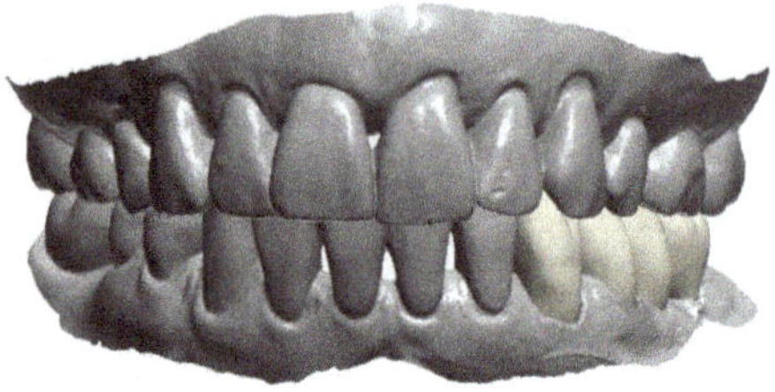

Figure 16: The design of the final crowns in the CAD process.

A final X-ray check was also taken at the same appointment (Figure 18).

The patient still comes regularly for a check-up. The latest check OPG three years after implant insertion shows an unchanged stable bone level (Figure 19). The clinical functionality and soft tissue situation are also unchanged, and the patient is highly satisfied with them.

3. Discussion

The present case demonstrates how implant planning and treatment using modern digital methods for diagnosis, planning, and fabrication lead to treatment reliability and predictable results. DVT-based planning, with osteodensitometry analysis and insertion simulation, plays a decisive role in this. It allows case-by-case selection and optimum positioning of the implants. In this way, it is possible for the first time, using objective data and their imaging, to be able to evaluate osseointegration conditions already at the planning stage and to make the correct decision for the time at which to load the implants.

Any changes to the planning, such as the required aligner treatment after beginning treatment in the present case, could be implemented in the digital workflow without problem based on the intraoral scan. Flapless technique can be used when the minimal keratinized tissue height of 2 mm has remained [13].

Any prosthetic adjustments to the masticatory function due to the long-term temporary restorations could also be undertaken. The selected approach proved flexible, including with the decision for a specific type of implant body (cylindrical, mainly cylindrical or conical). The decision can still even be made at the moment of insertion after preparation is complete. In contrast to parallel forms, the tapered form selected in the present case still allows compression of the bone to be varied by slightly adjusting the insertion depth to create better primary stability [14].

The next stage in the ongoing development of implantological planning software could consequently be in the inclusion of DVT-based osteodensitometry in the algorithm. The programme would then make far-reaching suggestions for implant positions, insertion (conventional or flapless), and suitable type of implant body. This could possibly be further optimised using artificial intelligence—just like the suggestions of the planning software.

It is self-evident that treatment decisions are ultimately made by the implantologists, if necessary following a consultation meeting together with the patient. It would seem preferable that this can be explained even more clearly regarding possible treatment options using imaging of the further advanced software. "Implantology must become simpler"! If this dogma is followed, we expect in future informed patients who, following a visit to an implantological centre, are highly motivated and look forward to their implantological rehabilitation, thanks to appropriate explanation and reliably predicted treatment schedule.

Note: some photographs in this case were unspecifically, for clarification of an example of a treatment procedure, already published in the magazine *EDI Journal* within the framework of a study into the reliability of a certain implant design (SICtapered) [15].

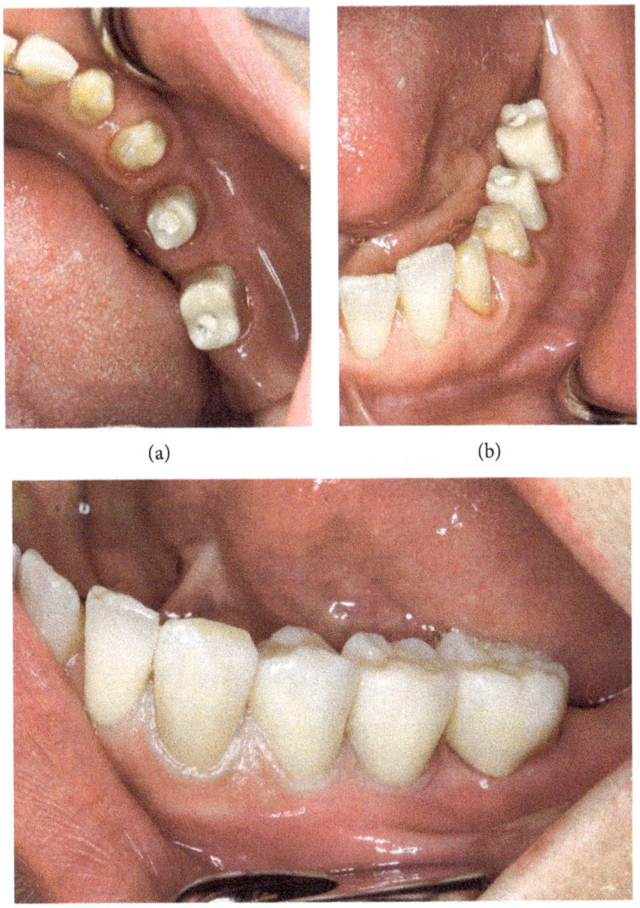

(a) (b)

(c)

FIGURE 17: Fitting of the final crowns using dual-curing cement.

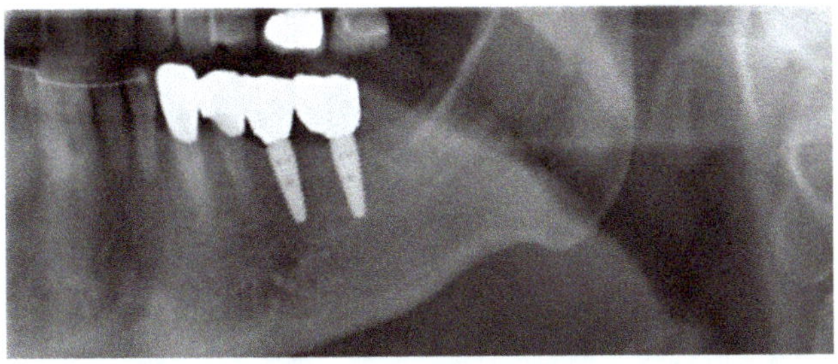

FIGURE 18: X-ray check at the crown fitting.

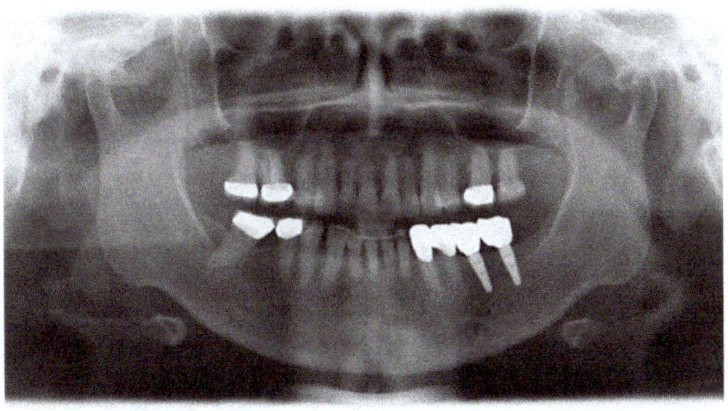

FIGURE 19: X-ray check 3 years after implant insertion.

Consent

The patient gave written consent for publication.

References

[1] J. Matys, K. Świder, R. Flieger, and M. Dominiak, "Assessment of the primary stability of root analog zirconia implants designed using cone beam computed tomography software by means of the Periotest® device: an ex vivo study. A preliminary report," *Advances in Clinical and Experimental*

MedicineClinical and Experimental Medicine, vol. 26, no. 5, pp. 803–809, 2017.

[2] M. Wada, T. Suganami, M. Sogo, and Y. Maeda, "Can we predict the insertion torque using the bone density around the implant?," *International Journal of Oral and Maxillofacial Surgery*, vol. 45, no. 2, pp. 221–225, 2016.

[3] L. R. Walker, G. A. Morris, and P. J. Novotny, "Implant insertional torque values predict outcomes," *Journal of oral and maxillofacial surgery*, vol. 69, no. 5, pp. 1344–1349, 2011.

[4] H. Huang, G. Wu, and E. Hunziker, "The clinical significance of implant stability quotient (ISQ) measurements: a literature review," *Journal of Oral Biology and Craniofacial Research*, vol. 10, no. 4, pp. 629–638, 2020.

[5] Y. H. Park, U.-W. Jung, C. S. Kim, S.-H. Choi, K.-S. Cho, and J.-S. Lee, "Resonance frequency analysis of tapered implants placed at maxillary posterior sites after lateral sinus augmentation: a 1.5-year follow-up prospective study," *Implant Dentistry*, vol. 28, no. 1, pp. 62–67, 2019.

[6] N. Sargolzaie, S. Samizade, H. Arab, H. Ghanbari, L. Khodadadifard, and A. Khajavi, "The evaluation of implant stability measured by resonance frequency analysis in different bone types," *Journal of the Korean Association of Oral and Maxillofacial Surgeons*, vol. 45, no. 1, pp. 29–33, 2019.

[7] A. Troedhan, D. Skiba, M. Ziad, and M. Wainwright, "Can CBCT-bone-densitometry predict implant stability in augmented sinus-sites ? Results of a randomized clinical trial," *Clinical Oral Implants Research*, vol. 30, no. S19, pp. 10–10, 2019.

[8] A. Troedhan, "Klinische anwendung der DVT-basierten knochendensitometrie," *Implantologie Journal*, vol. 24, no. 12, pp. 26–32, 2020.

[9] D. Schulz and U.-J. Rother, "Die osteodensitometrie mittels DVT," *Implantologie Journal*, vol. 14, no. 5, pp. 34–40, 2010.

[10] I. Turkyilmaz, C. Tumer, E. N. Ozbek, and T. F. Tözüm, "Relations between the bone density values from computerized tomography, and implant stability parameters: a clinical study of 230 regular platform implants," *Journal of Clinical Periodontology*, vol. 34, no. 8, pp. 716–722, 2007.

[11] S. Haghanifar, A. Yousefi, E. Moudi et al., "Accuracy of densitometry of two cone beam computed tomography equipment in comparison with computed tomography," *Elektron Physician*, vol. 9, no. 5, pp. 4384–4390, 2017.

[12] M. Nilius, C. Mueller, M. H. Nilius, D. Haim, H. Leonhardt, and G. Lauer, "Intraosseous anesthesia in symptomatic irreversible pulpitis: impact of bone thickness on perception and duration of pain," *Journal of Dental Anesthesia and Pain Medicine*, vol. 20, no. 6, pp. 367–375, 2020.

[13] J. Matys and M. Dominiak, "Assessment of pain when uncovering implants with Er: YAG laser or scalpel for second stage surgery," *Advances in Clinical and Experimental Medicine Clinical and Experimental Medicine*, vol. 25, no. 6, pp. 1179–1184, 2016.

[14] F. Javed and G. E. Romanos, "The role of primary stability for successful immediate loading of dental implants. A literature review," *Journal of Dentistry*, vol. 38, no. 8, pp. 612–620, 2010.

[15] M. Nilius, J. Winterhoff, and G. Lauer, "Performance of a novel implant design," *EDI Journal*, vol. 17, no. 2, pp. 64–76, 2021.

9

Rare Case of Dental Implantation in the Segment with Residual Filling Material in the Mandibular Canal

Yury Georgievich Sedov,[1] Kamil Nail'evich Khabiev,[2] Zulfiya Iltuzurovna Yarulina,[3] Vasiliy Stanislavovich Tarasuk,[2] Anatoliy Mikhailovich Avanesov,[1] Nikolay Ivanovich Sergeev,[4] Vitaliy Georgievich Pantsulaya,[2] and Irina Gennad'evna Sedova[2]

[1]*Department of General and Clinical Dentistry, RUDN University, Medical Institute, Moscow, Russia*
[2]*Private Dental Practice, Moscow, Russia*
[3]*Department of Orthopedic Dentistry, Kazan State Medical University of the Ministry of Health of Russia, Kazan, Russia*
[4]*Scientific Centre of Roentgenoradiology and Russian National Research Medical University, n.a. N.I. Pirogov, Moscow, Russia*

Correspondence should be addressed to Yury Georgievich Sedov; sedov_yug@pfur.ru

Academic Editor: Kevin Seymour

Dental implantation is the most popular method of restoring lost teeth. There are risk factors for dental implantation. These risk factors include the localization of residual filling material in the lumen of the mandibular canal in the selected jaw segment for implantation. A rare clinical case of dental implant placement with preservation of the safety zone relative to the residual siler in the mandibular canal is presented. A surgical guide was used for precise positioning. The treatment protocol was carried out without an immediate loading stage to monitor the possible development of symptoms.

1. Introduction

Dental implantation is the most popular method of lost teeth restoration [1, 2]. The complications of dental implants vary in the range of 5-10% [3, 4]. An important component of this method of treatment is the planning stage and, in particular, the use of radiological examination methods [5, 6]. To date, we recommend the use of cone-beam computed tomography, which allows the doctor to determine if there is enough bone volume for implant placement and the type of architectonic bone and also to take into account the location of important anatomical structures. On the lower jaw, such a structure includes the mandibular channel. Its diameter is 2-3 mm on average, and it is important for the clinician to know that in 80% of cases, the vessels are located in the upper part of the channel, and the nerve is located below them [7, 8]. Another anatomical feature is that the lower alveolar nerve is the third branch of the trigeminal nerve; it means that it is a large formation and has polyphasticity, which together increases its regenerative abilities [9].

Existing recommendations dictate that in order to avoid nerve damage, it is recommended to observe a safety zone of 2 mm from the apex of the implant to the upper border of the mandibular channel [10]. However, if there is a violation of the integrity of the channel, there are currently no clear official clinical recommendations on how to rehabilitate such a patient. The situation may get worse if you need to install a dental implant and there is already a residual filling material in the interesting area, which is also visualized in the mandibular channel. According to the Seddona classification, there are three types of nerve damage: neuropraxia, axonotmesis, and neurotmesis. If the last two are characterized by structural damage to the nerve, then neuropraxia is a compression or stretching of the nerve [11]. Localization of the siler in the channel usually results in neuropraxia, and it is assumed that sensitivity can be restored if there is no

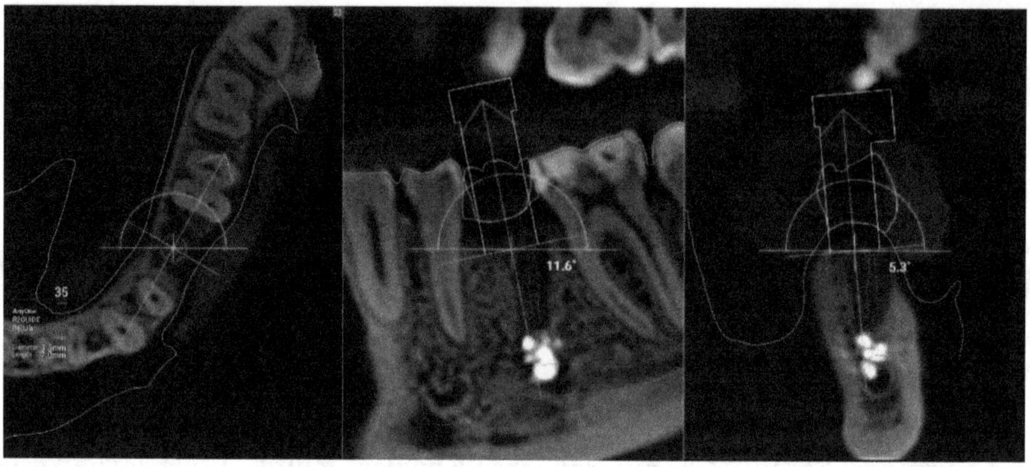

Figure 1: CBCT. The implant is installed virtually in the area of the missing 3.5 tooth. Fragments of filling material are visualized in the lumen of the mandibular canal.

structural damage to the epinephrium and, as a result, toxic effects on the axons [9].

In connection with aforesaid, the question arises whether it is possible to perform dental implantation in patients with available data on the localization of the filling material in the mandibular channel in the same jaw segment. As a demonstration and subsequent discussion, we want to cite a clinical case.

2. Clinical Case

The patient, 29 years old, went to the clinic to make a fixed structure in the area of the missing 3.5 tooth. The tooth was removed due to complications from apical periodontitis. During the consultation, the patient made panoramic zoning of the jaws, which showed a foreign body in this jaw segment projected into the mandibular channel. When collecting anamnesis, the patient denied any symptoms associated with damage to the inferior lunatic nerve. In view of the complexity of the situation and a more detailed analysis of the possibility of implantation, the patient was made cone-beam computed tomography with a special X-ray contrast positioner, so that in the future it will be possible to make a navigation guide. Analysis of the tomogram showed the presence of a foreign body, which was visualized as a heterogeneous, high-contrast round shadow with a clear, irregular contour of 4 × 3.4 mm in size, partially localized in the lumen of the mandibular channel, classified as a sealer. The foreign body was surrounded by bone tissue on all sides except the mandibular canal. The absence of symptoms is explained by the preservation of the integrity of the nerve sheath. In view of the complexity of the situation, it was finally agreed to conduct a dental implant with a navigation guide R2Gate to preserve the security zone between the apex of the implant and the top edge sealer, to avoid possibility of displacement in the channel. The entire planning protocol was conducted in digital mode (Figure 1).

Then, it was necessary to choose an implantation system. The best option in this case was the use of a so-called "supercortical" implant, which has a taper and a microthread on the neck. This makes it possible to achieve good primary stability in medium-density bone tissue and to ensure that the implant does not move deeper than planned [12].

Then, using 3D printing, a surgical guide was made for the full drilling protocol.

The operation algorithm included anesthesia, positioning of the surgical guide on adjacent teeth, and a complete protocol for drilling through the guide with the installation of a dental implant. The drilling speed did not exceed 300 rpm. The torc when fixing the implant was 35 N/cm. The ISQ Index was equal to 69 units of CI. Since the use of a "supercortical" implant virtually eliminated the loss of stability at the obtained torc and ISQ values, a gum shaper with a diameter of 5.5 mm and a height of 5 mm was immediately installed. It is important to note that due to the complexity of the situation, it was decided to install a gingival cuff shaper for the observation period and not to carry out immediate loading, despite the design of the implant. The postoperative image showed the optimal location of the implant with the preservation of the safety zone between the apex and the sealer border (Figure 2).

During the three months of follow-up, the patient made no complaints. Before the prosthetics stage, the frequency-resonance analysis indicators demonstrated the onset of osteointegration. Prosthetics was performed with an all-zirconium crown on a titanium base with transocclusal fixation. Two months after fixation of the permanent crown, a CT scan was performed to assess the position of the implant after loading. According to CBCT, the distance from the implant apex to the upper border of the sealer is 0.72 mm. The peri-implant bone structure was normal. The patient did not complain (Figure 3).

3. Discussion

Injury to the lower alveolar nerve is a serious mistake in dental treatment. As a rule, this occurs after endodontic treatment and dental implantation [13]. The recommendations of most experts suggest surgical intervention for 72 hours in the presence of pain symptoms and determination of the

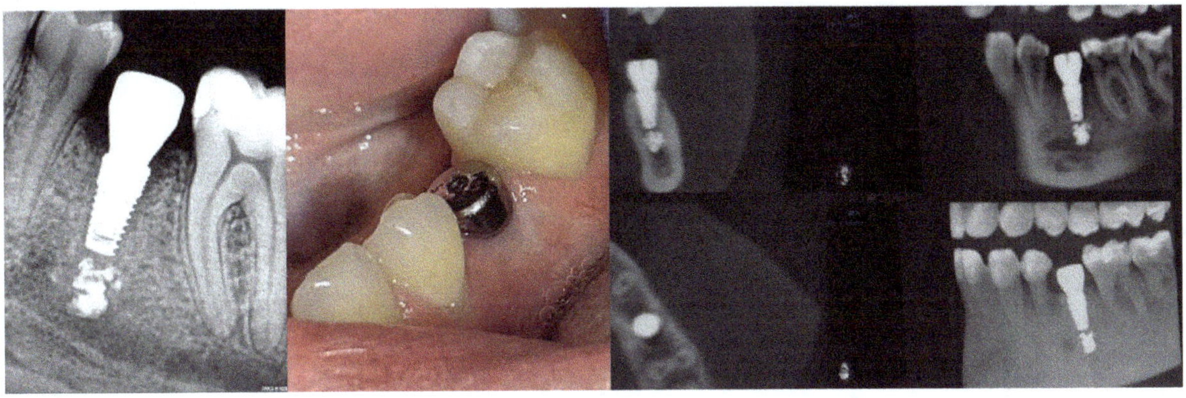

FIGURE 2: Intraoral X-ray. Condition in the oral cavity with the installation of the gum shaper. CBCT 1 month after implant placement.

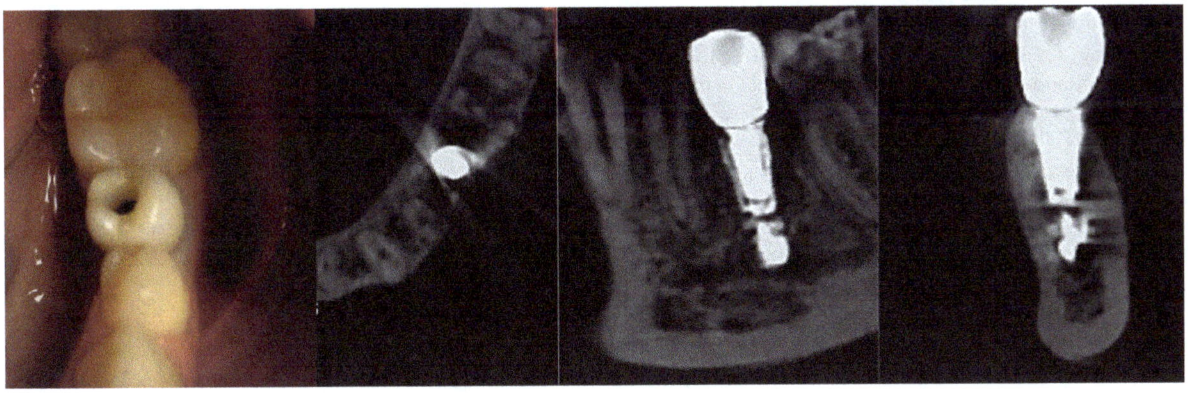

FIGURE 3: Fixing a permanent structure. CBCT. After the final restoration, the implant is also located in compliance with the safety zone.

mandibular channel damage on X-ray. In the absence of symptoms or its weak variations, the patient is undergoing dynamic observation or conservative therapy [14]. Filling material without damage to the nerve sheath may not cause clinical symptoms, while radiographs determined it in the lumen of the mandibular canal [9].

Based on our clinical case, it follows that restoration of the lost tooth in patients with diagnosed involvement of the mandibular canal due to dental treatment is possible. However, a preliminary assessment is required that combines the absence or presence of complaints with a CT scan analysis. If symptoms are present and damage to the integrity of the canal is visualized on the X-ray image, it is necessary to treat such a patient in the maxillofacial department. If the tomogram shows the presence of a foreign body in the lumen of the canal, but there are no symptoms, it is necessary to determine the identity of this foreign body and plan dental implantation. In our opinion, if the sealer is visualized, it is better not to carry out immediate loading even with adequate primary stability. This is due to the fact that before the onset of osseointegration, there may be excessive external pressure that can displace the implant, and this will aggravate the impact of the sealer on the n.h. channel. The safety zone was chosen from the apex of the implant to the sealer in 1 mm, because the distance to the channel exceeded 2 mm and even the tip of the cutter could not damage the integrity of this structure. Drilling speed up to 300 rpm helped to enhance the tactile sensation of the attending physician in the drilling process and reduce the risk of overheating the bone bed due to lack of irrigation due to the use of a surgical guide. The latter was the determining factor for controlling the location of the implant according to the virtual planning protocol.

4. Conclusion

The use of modern digital technologies allows for the transfer of this data intraoperatively. Even complex cases involving the mandibular canal due to iatrogenic treatment are not a contraindication to dental implantation but should be solved in each case individually from the analysis of symptoms and X-ray examination data. Also, it is recommended that the load on the implant is at the onset of osseointegration.

Additional Points

Materials and Tools Used. The materials and tools used are implantation system Impro (ImproManagement, Germany), R2gate program (Megagen), and device for determining the stability of ISQ Penguin.

Acknowledgments

The publication has been prepared with support of the International Study Center Dental Guru.

References

[1] M.-S. Howe, W. Keys, and D. Richards, "Long-term (10-year) dental implant survival: a systematic review and sensitivity meta-analysis," *Journal of Dentistry*, vol. 84, no. 9, pp. 9–21, 2019.

[2] J. A. Griggs, "Dental implants," *Dental Clinics of North America*, vol. 61, no. 4, pp. 857–871, 2017.

[3] T. Jemt, "A retro-prospective effectiveness study on 3448 implant operations at one referral clinic: a multifactorial analysis. Part II: clinical factors associated to peri-implantitis surgery and late implant failures," *Clinical Implant Dentistry and Related Research*, vol. 19, no. 6, pp. 972–979, 2017.

[4] C. K. Rösing, T. Fiorini, A. N. Haas, F. W. M. G. Muniz, R. V. Oppermann, and C. Susin, "The impact of maintenance on peri-implant health," *Brazilian Oral Research*, vol. 33, article e074, suppl 1, 2019eCollection 2019.

[5] A. M. Avanesov, Y. G. Sedov, and O. S. Mordanov, "Morphology of mandibular lingual concavities," *Stomatologiya*, vol. 98, no. 5, pp. 113–117, 2019.

[6] D. W. Beals, V. Parashar, J. R. Francis, G. M. Agostini, and A. Gill, "CBCT in advanced dental education: a survey of U.S. postdoctoral periodontics programs," *Journal of Dental Education*, vol. 84, no. 3, pp. 301–307, 2020.

[7] K. C. Vidya, J. Pathi, S. Rout, A. Sethi, and N. C. Sangamesh, "Inferior alveolar nerve canal position in relation to mandibular molars: a cone-beam computed tomography study," *National Journal of Maxillofacial Surgery*, vol. 10, no. 2, pp. 168–174, 2019.

[8] H.-J. Kim, H. Kang, Y.-S. Seo, D. K. Kim, and S.-K. Yu, "Anatomic evaluation of the retromolar canal by histologic and radiologic analyses," *Archives of Oral Biology*, vol. 81, pp. 192–197, 2017.

[9] M. A. Pogrel, "Nerve damage in dentistry," *General Dentistry*, vol. 65, no. 2, pp. 34–41, 2017.

[10] E. Sener, E. Onem, G. C. Akar et al., "Anatomical landmarks of mandibular interforaminal region related to dental implant placement with 3D CBCT: comparison between edentulous and dental mandibles," *Surgical and Radiologic Anatomy*, vol. 40, no. 6, pp. 615–623, 2018.

[11] R. A. Meyers, "Prevention and management of nerve problems in implant dentistry," *Journal of Oral Implantology*, vol. 25, no. 2, pp. 127–129, 1999.

[12] K. N. Khabiev, "The choice of implant system depending on the tasks," *New Dent*, vol. 1, no. 237, pp. 68–70, 2019.

[13] T. Koivisto, D. Chiona, L. L. Milroy, S. B. McClanahan, M. Ahmad, and W. R. Bowles, "Mandibular canal location: cone-beam computed tomography examination," *Journal of Endodontia*, vol. 42, no. 7, pp. 1018–1021, 2016.

[14] R. Castro, M. Guivarc'h, J. M. Foletti, J. H. Catherine, C. Chossegros, and L. Guyot, "Endodontic-related inferior alveolar nerve injuries: a review and a therapeutic flow chart," *Journal of Stomatology, Oral and Maxillofacial Surgery*, vol. 119, no. 5, pp. 412–418, 2018.

10

Implant-Supported Rehabilitation using GBR Combined with Bone Graft on a Reconstructed Maxilla with the Fibula Free Flap

S. Di Carlo, V. Valentini, E. Grasso, F. De Angelis, L. Piccoli, A. Quarato, S. Jamshir, and E. Brauner

Dipartimento Scienze Odontostomatologiche e Maxillo Facciali, Università degli Studi di Roma La Sapienza Facoltà di Medicina e Odontoiatria, Rome, Italy

Correspondence should be addressed to A. Quarato; aleq_91@hotmail.it

Academic Editor: Jose López-López

Alveolar ridge augmentation procedures allow restoring jaw defects due to teeth extractions, periodontal diseases, trauma, or outcomes from a previous surgery. This case report describes a patient suffering from Fibrous Dysplasia of the right upper maxilla surgically reconstructed by fibula free flap. In 2003, four dental implants were placed in the 1.2, 1.3, 1.5, and 1.6 areas. Twelve years later, the onset of peri-implantitis led to the failure of osseointegration with consequent thinning of the fibula flap. To avoid the risk of fracture and to restore the bone volumes necessary for a new implant-prosthetic rehabilitation, we used heterologous biomaterials in combination with a non-reabsorbable membrane, according to the Guided Bone Regeneration (GBR) technique. GBR was performed using the Equimatrix® natural bone mineral matrix, Cytoplast™ Ti-150, a non-reabsorbable titanium-reinforced membrane, and four fastening screws to pin the membrane. After six months, the membrane was removed and two Zimmer® implants 3.7×13 mm were placed in the 1.1 and 1.2 areas. A fixed implant-supported prosthesis with a custom-milled titanium bar screwed to the implants was made. Computed tomography (CT) six months after GBR showed a good bone regeneration of 1.5 cm mesiodistal (MD), 1.8 cm buccopalatal (BP), and 2.8 cm in height. The main difficulty of this clinical case concerns the low predictability of success of GBR on a maxillary reconstructed area with a free fibula flap: there is no previous evidence in the literature. Clinical and radiographic exams nowadays show that there is no macroscopic bone reabsorption; however, further research is needed to obtain more information.

1. Introduction

Oral implant rehabilitation in patients formerly subjected to partial or total resection of the facial bones is increasingly common [1].

A successful implant rehabilitation requires adequate bone volume which is essential to house the implant and provide esthetics and function [2].

The reconstruction of maxillomandibular defects has undergone considerable progress due to the development of microsurgical techniques. Using vascularized free flaps, nowadays it is possible to reconstruct complex defects providing both soft and bone tissues. The aim of modern surgery is not only the aesthetic outcome of reconstruction but also, and above all, the functional restoration of the stomatognathic apparatus. Aesthetic and functional achievements together enhance the patient's quality of life [3].

The particularity of this case consists in the association of the GBR technique using a bone grafting material and a nonabsorbable membrane on a hemimaxillary reconstruction with the fibula free flap.

2. Materials and Methods

A 27-year-old female was referred to the Department of Oral and Maxillofacial Sciences to rehabilitate the upper right quadrant. Her medical history was positive for Fibrous Dysplasia (FD) of the right side of the maxillofacial bones.

Fibrous Dysplasia is a disorder characterized by the replacement of normal bone and marrow with fibrous tissue, resulting in the formation of bone that is weak and prone to expansion. Therefore, most complications result from fracture, deformity, functional impairment, and pain [4].

The patient reported the appearance of a facial swelling at the age of nine.

Due to the increased size of the swelling, in 2001 she underwent right-sided maxillomalar reconstruction for osteodysplastic obliteration of the facial bones.

She was operated at the Maxillofacial Surgery Unit of the hospital Policlinico "Umberto I" in Rome. During surgery, the right half of the maxillary bone was removed, and it was submitted to definitive histological examination, which confirmed the initial diagnosis of Fibrous Dysplasia. A fibula free flap was shaped to reconstruct the alveolar ridge, the orbital margin, the zygomatic knob, and the orbital lateral pillar. The bone, revascularized by Termino-Terminal anastomosis (T-T), was fixed with 6 different plates (2 right-angled plates in the left jaw, 1 X-plate in the frontal process of the jaw, and 3 miniplates in the frontoorbital suture and temporozigomatic suture).

In 2003, the fibula flap was remodelled and 4 dental implants were inserted. The implant abutments were placed during the 12th postoperative month, and the implantation of a resin cement-retained temporary prosthesis was performed. The patient was not finally fit with a permanent prosthesis due to her own negligence.

In 2007, she underwent another surgery for peri-implant inflammatory gingiva removal. After the removal of the inflamed alveolar mucosa at the 1.2-1.5 level, a graft of palatal mucosa was executed. A pink resin for the improvement of the flange prosthetic was, however, added.

Eight years later, the patient came to our attention. Clinical examination showed the presence of gingival hypertrophy and peri-implantitis (Figure 1(a)). Peri-implantitis had caused the loss of one of the four dental implants, accompanied by a substantial bone resorption.

Our treatment plan was, firstly, to carefully reestablish oral hygiene especially to ablate peri-implant oral mucosa and to allow tissue to heal; therefore, we put the patient into a periodontal maintenance program. The next step was to remove the severely compromised 1.2 implant, carry out a bone graft, and undertake rehabilitation with a tooth-implant-supported fixed partial denture (FPD) including the 2.1 element to ensure better aesthetics and stability of the prosthesis. In preparation for GBR, a temporary prosthesis which did not lean on the graft to avoid inevitable bone reabsorption was performed.

After orthopanthomography (OPT) and computer tomography (CT) X-ray analysis, and considering the amount of bone resorption, we opted for the GBR technique. The bone defect was calculated on the basis of three-dimensional (3D) computational analysis of the CT imaging and measured 1.9 cm MD, 1.8 cm BP, and 2.8 cm in height (Figure 1(b)).

The patient received a prophylactic preoperative dose of an oral antibiotic (2 g amoxicillin/clavulanic acid 1 hour before surgery), and a mouth rinse with 15 mL of 0.2% chlorhexidine solution was used before surgery for 1 minute. After administration of local anesthesia, induced with mepivacaine 2% + epinephrine 1 : 100,000 (2% carbocaine) to ensure deeper pain control and contain bleeding, the compromised implant 1.2 was removed. Then, a ridge incision was performed, and bone tissue was exposed (Figure 1(c)). Multiple cortical perforations, which created openings for osteopromotion, were then made to stimulate blood and cell migration from the bone marrow spaces to the regeneration area. A nonresorbable titanium-reinforced membrane (Cytoplast Ti-150) was positioned to create a barrier effect against epithelium cells and to maintain the grafted space. The membrane was pinned by three buccal osteosynthesis screws (distal, central, and mesial); then, a graft material was positioned in the defective area. We used Equimatrix (0.2-1.0 mm) natural bone mineral matrix, an equine-derived natural bone graft substitute with a complex, porous network that closely resembles natural human bone. After positioning the graft material which was left protruding from the crest, another palatal (distal) screw was used for fixing the membrane (Figures 1(c)–1(e)). A tension-free suture was performed to allow healing by first intention and to prevent membrane exposure, a complication that may occur in bone regeneration.

3. Results

After a healing period of 6 months, newly formed bone beneath the membrane was obtained (Figures 1(f) and 1(g)). Another surgical procedure was required to remove the nonresorbable membrane with the osteosynthesis screws and to place the implants. A CT Dentascan with a radiological template inserted in the oral cavity was performed. Computed tomography (CT) six months after GBR showed a bone regeneration of 1.5 cm mesiodistal, 1.8 cm buccopalatal, and 2.8 cm in height (Figure 1(h)). With the aid of this procedure, it was decided to place two Zimmer Trabecular Metal™ implants (Ø 3.7 mm, L 13.0 mm) in the maxillary canine and central incisive area. The clinical situation after removal of the membrane showed a compact and non-reabsorbed graft. The implant insertion torque was greater than 32 Newtons, and implant stability had a value greater than 60 ISQ. Measurements were made by the Osstell® system. They confirmed good bone quality and a good bone-implant interface. Primary intention healing had been obtained: periosteal incisions were performed to make the flap passive and it was sutured using Donati stiches with an absorbable suture to close the flap and simple sutures with a nonabsorbable suture on the occlusal margin. After the procedure, the patient was told to continue the antibiotic therapy for 6 days (1 g every 8 h), to use a 0.2% chlorhexidine mouthwash 3 times a day for two weeks, and to take an anti-inflammatory drug as needed. After 6 months during which the membrane had not been exposed, implant uncovering was performed, and healing screws were inserted (Figure 1(i)).

After 3 months, the soft tissue had healed completely and prosthetic rehabilitation for implant-supported fixed dentures was begun. The primary structure is a custom-milled titanium bar screwed onto the dental implants. The secondary structure has a series of geometrical elements shaped

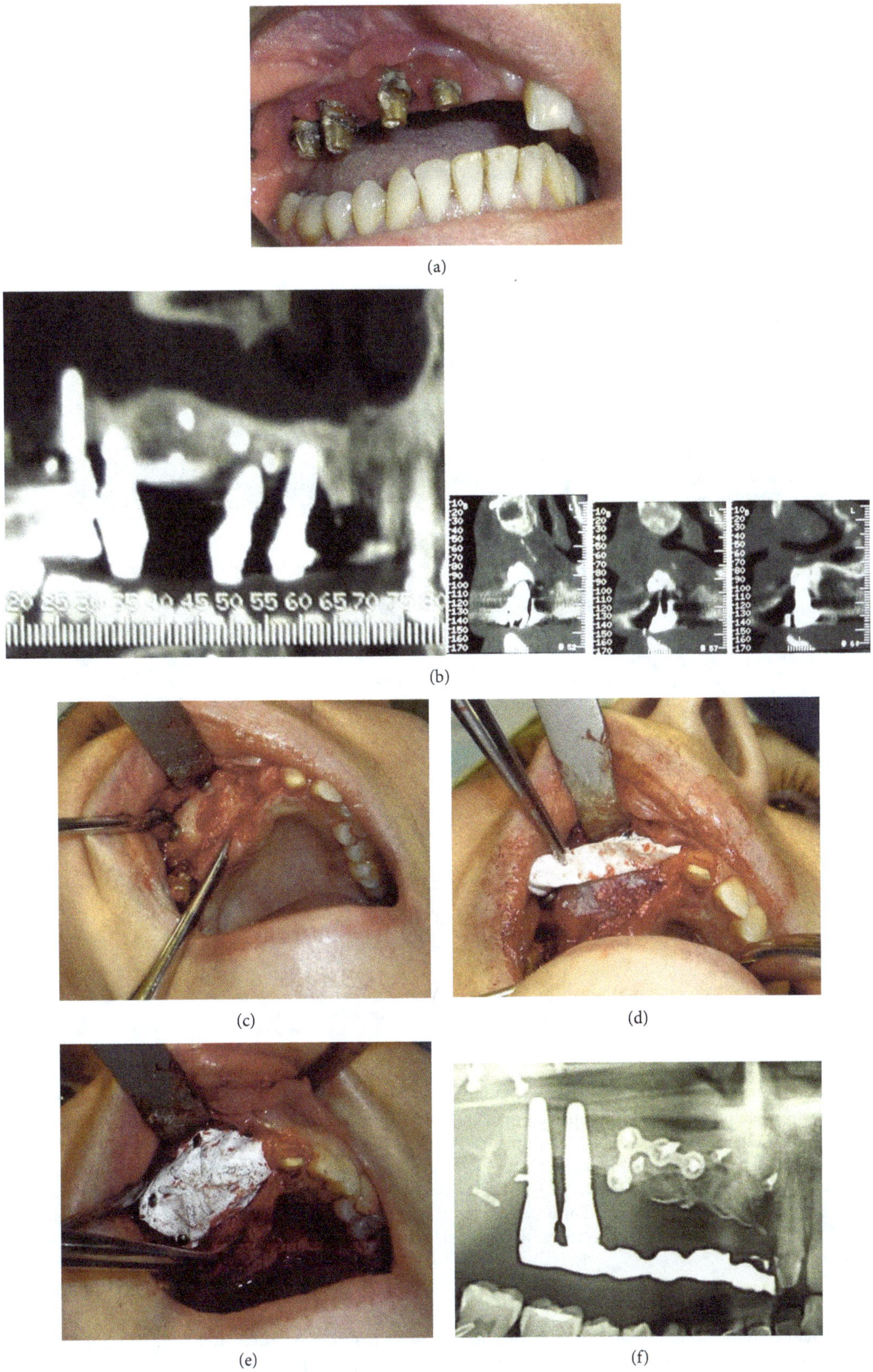

Figure 1: Continued.

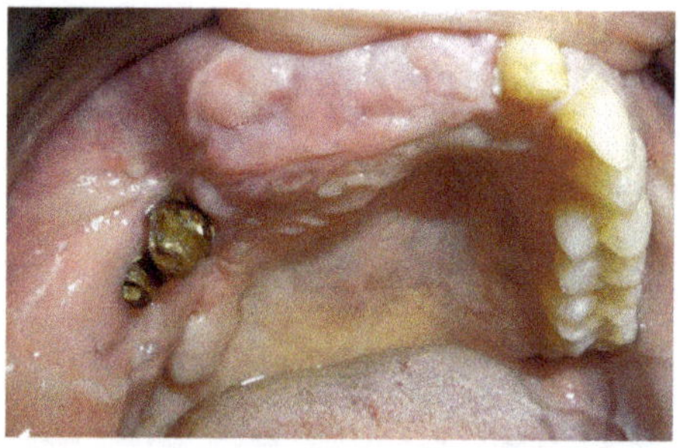

(g)

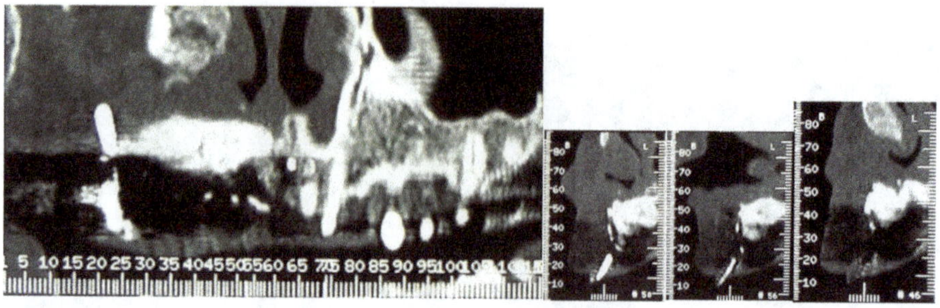

(h)

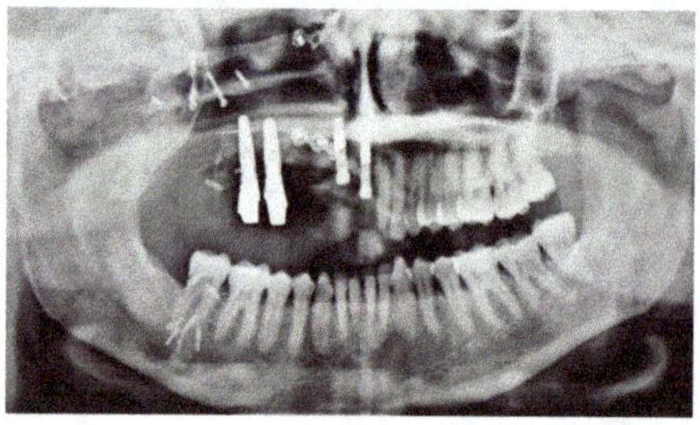

(i)

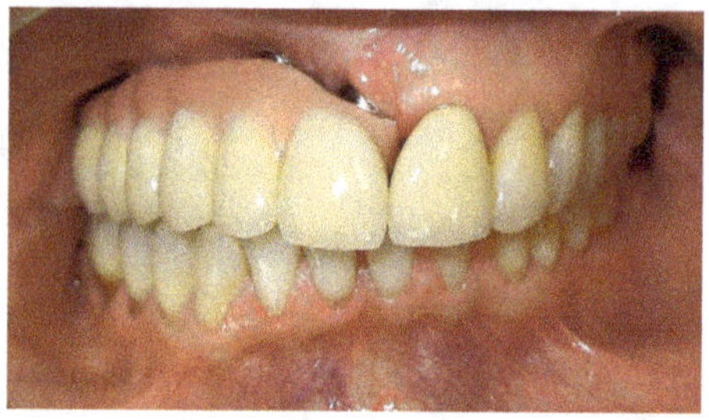

(j)

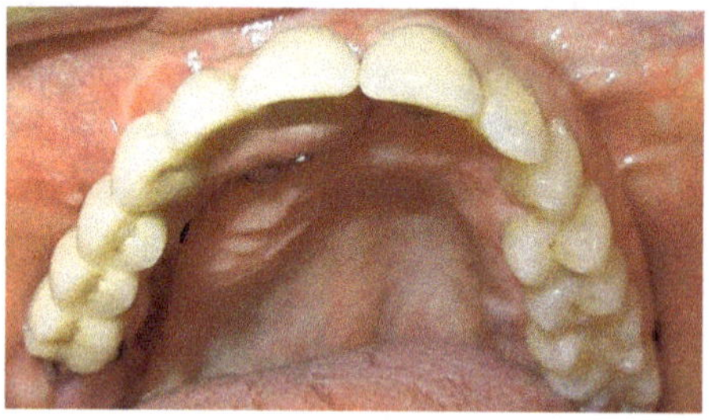

(k)

FIGURE 1: (a) Clinical image shows peri-implantitis, hypertrophy, and severe gingival inflammation. (b) Computerized tomography scan. Preoperative view showing insufficient bone in the apicocoronal and buccolingual dimension to place implants according to the prosthetic needs. (c) Clinical image showing bone defect. (d) Clinical image prior to fixing the membrane on the palatal side showing the graft that completely covers the defect. (e) Clinical image with the membrane completely in place. (f) Panoramic radiograph post-GBR. (g) Clinical image shows tissue healing at three months. (h) Computerized tomography scan. Postoperative view showing robust bone regeneration in the area corresponding to the radiopaque marks on the surgical stent. (i) Panoramic radiograph postimplant surgery. (j) Clinical view of the implant-supported fixed prosthesis. Frontal view. (k) Clinical view of the implant-supported fixed prosthesis. Maxillary occlusal view.

inversely to the grooves of the primary structure and consists of a metal covered with porcelain for the teeth and composite for the pink gum (Figures 1(j) and 1(k)).

The occlusal plane presented alteration. In fact, since the patient had been affected by Fibrous Dysplasia during developmental age, mesiodistal lower plane growth was present. Therefore, onlays made using an indirect method were inserted on the 4.4, 4.5, 4.6, and 4.7 elements to restore the occlusal plane.

4. Discussion

Facial reconstructive surgery has seen great progress over the last century, improving the quality of life for patients following ablative surgery, by restoring both function and aesthetic outcome. Microvascular flap employment and the development of implantology have largely helped to achieve these goals [5–7].

With regard to the flaps employed, the fibula is one of the most versatile options. The use of the fibula microvascular flap for maxillomandibular reconstruction and especially for dental rehabilitation has the following major advantages: its length makes it possible to use up to 25 cm of bone for the reconstruction and it provides the chance of shaping it; its extraordinary periosteal vascularization gives the possibility of performing multiple osteotomies; and it has lower morbidity in the donor area [3, 8].

The bone structure of the fibula is very similar to the mandible, where cortical bone dominates. This structural similarity allows a good osteintegration of dental implants, the same as for the mandible [9–11]. Therefore, in this clinical case the problem was not only to achieve regeneration and to insert implants but also to consider the type of autologous bone already grafted. Surgery regarded the upper jaw but was the same as that for the mandible. Furthermore, the absence of baseline bone implicated a risk a pathological fracture in that area. Then, we had to pay close attention to the risk of fractures.

Various methods have been developed to increase bone volume and augment new tissue growth [12–15]: (1) distraction osteogenesis, which describes the surgical induction of a fracture and the subsequent gradual separation of the two bone ends to create spontaneous bone regeneration between the two fragments; (2) osteoinduction, which employs appropriate growth factors and/or stem/osteoprogenitor cells to encourage new bone formation; (3) osteoconduction, in which a grafting material serves as a scaffold for new bone formation; and (4) guided bone regeneration (GBR), which provides spaces using barrier membranes that subsequently become filled with new bone [16, 17].

Among these different regenerative techniques, GBR seemed to us the best option because it was necessary to fill a predominantly vertical bone defect [18, 19]; therefore, the stiffness of the nonresorbable titanium membrane was used to support the soft tissues and thus allow the formation of new bone [20, 21]. To ensure successful GBR, four principles need to be met: exclusion of epithelium and connective tissue, space maintenance, stability of the fibrin clot, and primary wound closure.

This case goes to show that by following the operative protocol scrupulously and respecting its principles, it is possible to obtain good bone regeneration even in complex cases [22].

The main difficulty of the present clinical case concerned the low predictability of success of GBR on a maxillary reconstructed area with a free fibula flap. There is no evidence to support the claims made in the literature. To maximize success in similar advanced clinical cases, a scrupulous surgical protocol must be followed. Furthermore, it is important for the dentist to approach these patients knowing the kind of surgery they received because this aspect will influence rehabilitative choices [23–26]. The amount of regeneration we achieved was 1.5 cm MD, 1.8 cm BP, and 2.8 cm in height. Follow-up controls of patients must be performed every 3-4 months for monitoring and reevaluation. Clinical and radiographic findings (bone sounding and intraoral X-ray images) suggested that there was no significant bone resorption. The patient was satisfied with the prosthesis both esthetically and functionally and reported significant improvements in oral function and psychosocial activities. However, further research in this area and long-term monitoring are needed to obtain more information.

Authors' Contributions

Di Carlo S is the implanto-prosthetic department head who coordinated our work. Valentini V is the maxillofacial surgeon who performed the fibula free flap in the first surgery on the patient. Grasso E and De Angelis F helped us document the case report and write the work. Piccoli L, Jamshir S, and Quarato A were involved in the prosthetic rehabilitation after the surgeries. Brauner E is the surgeon who performed GBR (Guided Bone Regeneration) surgery and dental implant insertion and supervised my work on the patient's prosthesis. Piccoli L initially was not included in authors' list because of an oversight by the corresponding author, and I would like to put him on the list because he worked together with all the other authors. There are no other clinicians or students involved in the treatment of the case report's patient.

References

[1] Y. Mittal, G. Jindal, and S. Garg, "Bone manipulation procedures in dental implants," *Indian Journal of Dentistry*, vol. 7, no. 2, pp. 86–94, 2016.

[2] T. Albrektsson, P. I. Brånemark, H. A. Hansson, and J. Lindström, "Osseointegrated titanium implants: requirements for ensuring a long-lasting, direct bone-to-implant anchorage in man," *Acta Orthopaedica Scandinavica*, vol. 52, no. 2, pp. 155–170, 1981.

[3] J. L. Cebrian-Carretero, J. Guinales-Diaz de Cevallos, J. A. Sobrino, T. Yu, and M. Burgueno-Garcia, "Predictable dental rehabilitation in maxillomandibular reconstruction with free flaps. The role of implant guided surgery," *Medicina Oral Patología Oral y Cirugia Bucal*, vol. 19, no. 6, pp. e605–e611, 2014.

[4] A. M. Boyce, P. Florenzano, L. F. de Castro, and M. T. Collins, "Fibrous dysplasia/McCune-Albright syndrome," in *GeneReviews*, M. P. Adam, H. H. Ardinger, R. A. Pagon, S. E. Wallace, L. J. H. Bean, K. Stephens, and A. Amemiya, Eds., University of Washington, Seattle, WA, USA, 2018.

[5] M. L. Urken, D. Buchbinder, P. D. Costantino et al., "Oromandibular reconstruction using microvascular composite flaps: report of 210 cases," *Archives of Otolaryngology–Head & Neck Surgery*, vol. 124, no. 1, pp. 46–55, 1998.

[6] D. A. Hidalgo and A. Rekow, "A review of 60 consecutive fibula free flap mandible reconstructions," *Plastic and Reconstructive Surgery*, vol. 96, no. 3, pp. 585–596, 1995.

[7] E. Brauner, V. Valentini, F. De Angelis et al., "Gingival hyperplasia around dental implants in jaws reconstructed with free vascularized flaps: a case report series," *Journal of International Dental and Medical Research*, vol. 11, no. 1, 2018.

[8] V. Pompa, E. Brauner, L. Bresadola, S. di Carlo, V. Valentini, and G. Pompa, "Treatment of facial vascular malformations with embolisation and surgical resection," *European Review for Medical and Pharmacological Sciences*, vol. 13, pp. 407-4137, 2012.

[9] R. Kuprys, V. Varinauskas, A. Gervickas, and R. Stanaityte, "A review of mandibular reconstruction with free microvascularised fibular flap," *Health Sciences*, vol. 22, no. 3, pp. 170-174, 2012.

[10] G. Pompa, E. Brauner, S. Jamshir, F. De Angelis, R. Giardino, and S. Di Carlo, "Quality of life in patients rehabilitated with palatal obturator without reconstruction versus fixed implant-prosthesis after reconstruction of maxillectomy defects," *Journal of International Dental and Medical Research*, vol. 10, no. 1, pp. 1–8, 2017.

[11] E. Brauner, A. Quarato, F. De Angelis et al., "Prosthetic rehabilitation involving the use of implants following a fibula free flap reconstruction in the treatment of Osteosarcoma of the maxilla: a case report," *La Clinica Terapeutica*, vol. 168, no. 6, pp. e392–e396, 2017.

[12] E. Brauner, G. Guarino, S. Jamshir et al., "Evaluation of highly porous dental implants in postablative oral and maxillofacial cancer patients: A prospective pilot clinical case series report," *Implant Dentistry*, vol. 24, no. 5, pp. 631-637, 2015.

[13] M. Chiapasco, M. Zaniboni, and M. Boisco, "Augmentation procedures for the rehabilitation of deficient edentulous ridges with oral implants," *Clinical Oral Implants Research*, vol. 17, no. S2, pp. 136–159, 2006.

[14] M. Chiapasco, P. Casentini, and M. Zaniboni, "Bone augmentation procedures in implant dentistry," *The International Journal of Oral & Maxillofacial Implants*, vol. 24, pp. 237-259, 2009.

[15] V. Valentini, V. Terenzi, A. Cassoni et al., "Giant cell lesion or langerhans' cell histiocytosis of the mandible? A case report," *European Journal of Inflammation*, vol. 10, no. 1, pp. 159-164, 2012.

[16] J. Liu and D. G. Kerns, "Mechanisms of guided bone regeneration: a review," *The Open Dentistry Journal*, vol. 8, no. 1, pp. 56–65, 2014.

[17] H. L. Wang and L. Boyapati, ""PASS" principles for predictable bone regeneration," *Implant Dentistry*, vol. 15, no. 1, pp. 8–17, 2006.

[18] M. Ronda, A. Rebaudi, L. Torelli, and C. Stacchi, "Expanded vs. dense polytetrafluoroethylene membranes in vertical ridge augmentation around dental implants: a prospective randomized controlled clinical trial," *Clinical Oral Implants Research*, vol. 25, no. 7, pp. 859–866, 2014.

[19] E. Brauner, F. de Angelis, S. Jamshir et al., "Aesthetic satisfaction in lip and palate clefts: a comparative study between secondary and tertiary bone grafting," *La Clinica Terapeutica*, vol. 169, no. 2, pp. e62–e66, 2018.

[20] C. H. F. Hammerle and R. E. Jung, "Bone augmentation by means of barrier membranes," *Periodontology 2000*, vol. 33, no. 1, pp. 36–53, 2003.

[21] M. Trobos, A. Juhlin, F. A. Shah, M. Hoffman, H. Sahlin, and C. Dahlin, "In vitro evaluation of barrier function against oral bacteria of dense and expanded polytetrafluoroethylene (PTFE) membranes for guided bone regeneration," *Clinical Implant Dentistry and Related Research*, vol. 20, no. 5, pp. 738–748, 2018.

[22] R. Dimitriou, G. I. Mataliotakis, G. M. Calori, and P. V. Giannoudis, "The role of barrier membranes for guided bone regeneration and restoration of large bone defects: current experimental and clinical evidence," *BMC Medicine*, vol. 10, no. 1, p. 81, 2012.

[23] F. De Felice, M. de Vincentiis, V. Valentini et al., "Management of salivary gland malignant tumor: the Policlinico Umberto I, "Sapienza" University of Rome Head and Neck Unit clinical recommendations," *Critical Reviews in Oncology/Hematology*, vol. 120, pp. 93–97, 2017.

[24] E. Brauner, G. Pompa, A. Quarato et al., "Maxillofacial prosthesis in dentofacial traumas: A retrospective clinical study and introduction of new classification method," *BioMed Research International*, vol. 2017, Article ID 8136878, 8 pages, 2017.

[25] E. Brauner, V. Valentini, S. Jamshir et al., "Retrospective review of 78 rehabilitated head and neck postoncological patients: a new classification method," *Minerva Stomatologica*, vol. 65, no. 1, pp. 17–32, 2016.

[26] E. Brauner, V. Valentini, S. Jamshir et al., "Two clinical cases of prosthetical rehabilitation after a tumor of the upper maxilla," *European Review for Medical and Pharmacological Sciences*, vol. 16, no. 13, pp. 1882–1890, 2012.

Autologous Deciduous Tooth-Derived Material for Alveolar Ridge Preservation: A Clinical and Histological Case Report

Elio Minetti,[1] **Silvio Taschieri**,[1,2,3] **and Stefano Corbella**[1,2,3]

[1]*Department of Biomedical, Surgical, and Dental Science, Università degli Studi di Milano, Milan, Italy*
[2]*IRCCS Istituto Ortopedico Galeazzi, Milan, Italy*
[3]*Federal State Autonomous Educational Institution of Higher Education I.M. Sechenov First Moscow State Medical University of the Ministry of Health of the Russian Federation (Sechenov University), 8-2 Trubetskaya St., 119991 Moscow, Russia*

Correspondence should be addressed to Elio Minetti; elio.minetti@gmail.com

Academic Editor: Giuseppe Alessandro Scardina

The management of the alveolar socket is fundamental to create conditions that would allow the positioning of dental implants in the same site, when required. A number of biomaterials were described in scientific literature to be used for alveolar socket preservation immediately after tooth extraction: autogenous grafts, allograft (of various origin), and synthetic products. Among the autogenous biomaterials, some authors proposed the use of autogenous dentin and/or enamel, retrieved from teeth, adequately managed, and purified. The present case report with two-year follow-up shows one case of alveolar socket preservation by using tooth graft material that was subsequently treated with one implant-supported rehabilitation in the same site. The paper presents clinical and histological outcomes and confirms the feasibility of adopting such autogenous biomaterial in standard procedures.

1. Introduction

The possibility of positioning dental implants in sites that underwent tooth extraction is strictly related on the amount of the available bone volume that results from bone healing and remodeling after tooth removal. Bone remodeling is a continuous, complex process that involves all the bone tissues in the organism and, obviously, could cause the resorption of alveolar bone when one tooth is no longer present [1]. In order to overcome the presence of insufficient available bone volume, a number of surgical procedures were described and validated by scientific literature aimed at increasing the bone volume [2].

As we know from the literature, after tooth extraction, the healing of the alveolar socket happens through the succession of many phases, beginning from the stabilization of the bone clot, the formation of fibrin, and, in the end, the recruitment of osteoblasts that will be responsible for new bone formation [3]. A number of biomaterials and technique were described for alveolar socket volume preservation, with many functions (osteoconduction, osteoinduction, or even stimulation) depending on the characteristics of each material [4]. MacBeth and colleagues in 2017 published one systematic review of the literature and reported that alveolar ridge preservation (ARP) may limit the necessity of further guided bone regeneration (GBR) procedures, reducing the bone changes during the healing period [4]. Such results confirmed what was found in previously published systematic reviews of the literature [5, 6]. However, all the authors concluded that ARP outcomes were extremely heterogeneous, and even though the techniques are effective, they cannot arrest the bone remodeling process and its reduction [7].

Considering studies about histomorphometric analysis, none of the commonly used biomaterials was found to be superior, in terms of new bone formation, as compared to the others [8].

In many clinical situations, the autogenous bone graft has been considered the most effective biomaterial [8, 9]. Human dentin and bone show many similarities in terms of mineralization. In fact, after demineralization, both the

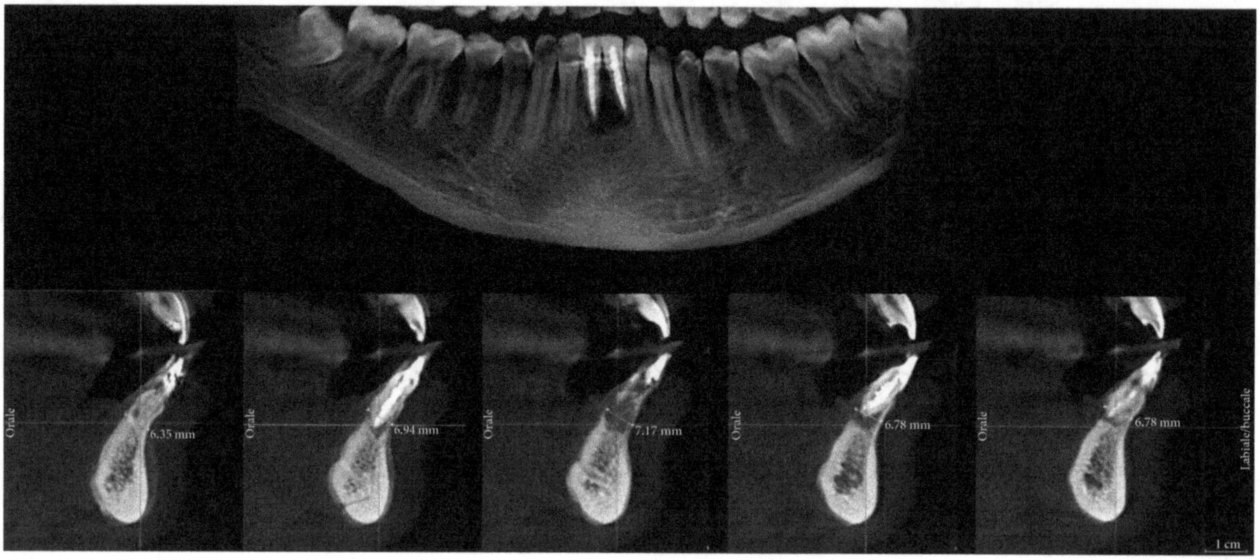

FIGURE 1: Radiographs of preoperative situation.

demineralized dentin matrix (DDM) and demineralized bone matrix (DBM) are predominantly composed of type I collagen (95%) and noncollagenous proteins (NCPs), and, among them, growth factors; for such reason, human DDM is a biological collagenous scaffold containing osteoinductive growth factors that provides an appropriate environment for stimulating new bone formation [10].

In 2015, Park et al. [11] suggested the use of the deciduous tooth as source of graft materials. They made an in vivo study, and the conclusion was that the deciduous teeth had structural and physicochemical characteristics suitable for grafting with appropriate demineralization.

In 2018, Bono et al. [12] described that deciduous teeth could be used as grafting materials in bone augmentation procedures. They also shed light on the effects of demineralization on deciduous teeth material, evaluating whether or not collagen and BMP-2 protein contents were preserved after the chemical treatment. Moreover, they evaluated in vitro the response of osteoblastic cells to exogenous BMP-2 stimulation (at different protein concentrations) with the aim of identifying the minimum BMP-2 concentration able to induce the expression of alkaline phosphatase, the early marker of the osteoblastic phenotype.

The aim of the present report is to present a case of ARP using autogenous deciduous tooth material, presenting both clinical and histologic results.

2. Case Presentation

The subject of the case report was one 26-year-old women, nonsmoker, ASA-1 (following the classification proposed by the American Society of Anesthesiologists), and able to understand the information given about the treatment.

The patient referred pain and mobility in the area of 3.1 and 4.1 (mandibular central incisors). The radiographic (by periapical radiograph and CBCT) and clinical examination revealed that the teeth (both) underwent nonsurgical endodontic treatment that was unsuccessful. It was evident the presence of a large bone loss area in the periapical region with partial preservation of the buccal bone. The teeth were both affected by mobility (more than 2 mm), suppuration, and spontaneous pain (Figure 1).

For this particular case, the treatment alternatives were limited. The operator proposed the removal of both teeth, alveolar ridge preservation, and, after healing, the placement of two dental implants to support one fixed prosthesis. The patient approved the proposed treatment protocol, accepting to use her own deciduous teeth (stored by the patient in plastic box for at least 15 years) as bone grafting material. The decision of using deciduous teeth materials was due to the impossibility of using the extracted teeth for the same purposes. In fact, the amount of potentially available material, after removing the endodontic fillings, would not be sufficient in such clinical situation. The patient signed an informed consent form before surgery.

Before surgery, as standard protocol, the patient received professional oral hygiene with supragingival scaling.

After local anesthesia performed with articaine 4% and epinephrine 1 : 100.000 in the 3.1-4.1 position, the extraction of affected teeth was performed without flap elevation, preserving the buccal bone plate. A piezoelectric device was used to debride the alveolar socket, removing infected tissues [13].

In order to use deciduous teeth as bone substitute material, the following procedure was adopted: (1) the teeth were adequately selected avoiding teeth with caries and cleaned, (2) the teeth were cut in small portions, and (3) they were grinded, demineralized, and sterilized using a specific device (Tooth Transformer®, Milan, Italy), following a standard and automatic procedure.

The so-obtained biomaterial, weighting approximately 1.5 grams (made of both dentin and enamel, in granules with diameter ranging between 0.4 and 0.8 mm), was placed and compacted in the alveolar sockets and the soft tissues were sutured with bioresorbable material (Vicryl 5-0, Ethicon Inc., Johnson & Johnson, Bridgewater, USA).

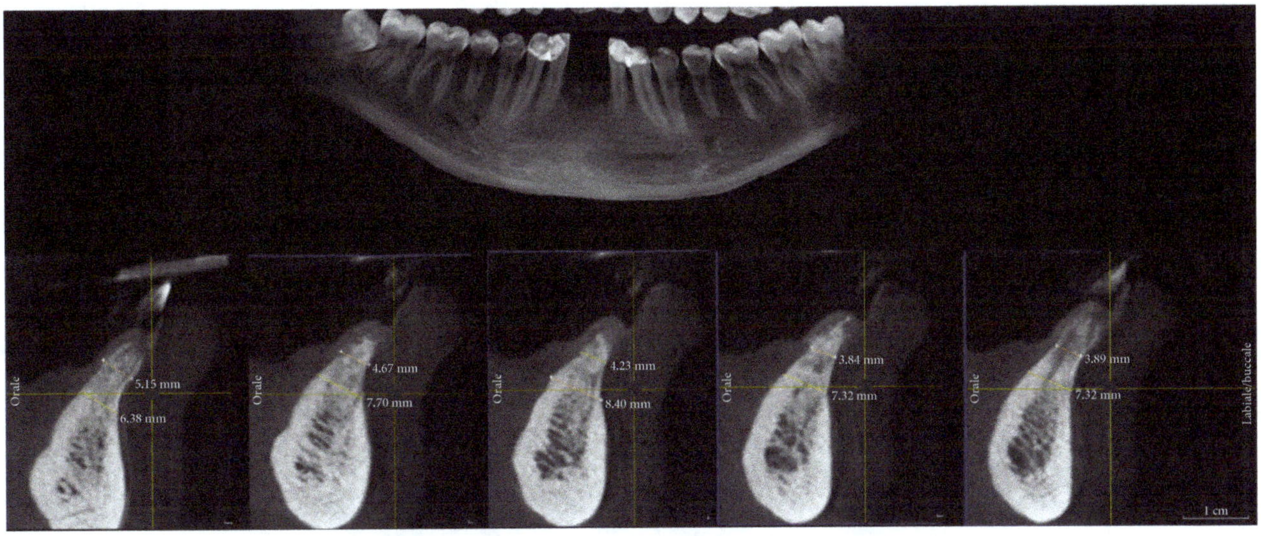

FIGURE 2: Section of CBCT scan, taken after 5 months, showing bone healing after grafting.

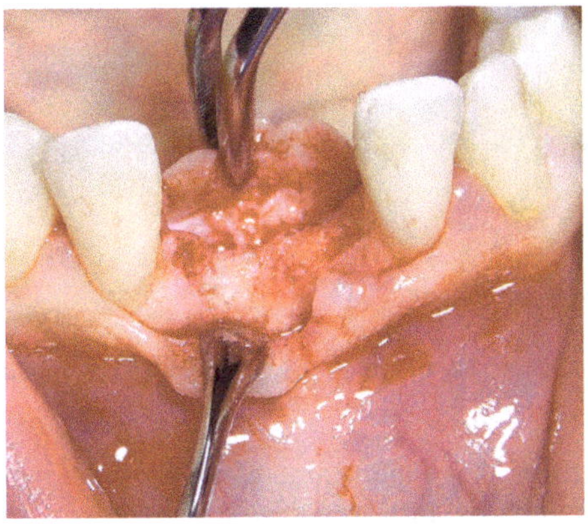

FIGURE 3: Clinical image showing a sufficient amount of bone volume.

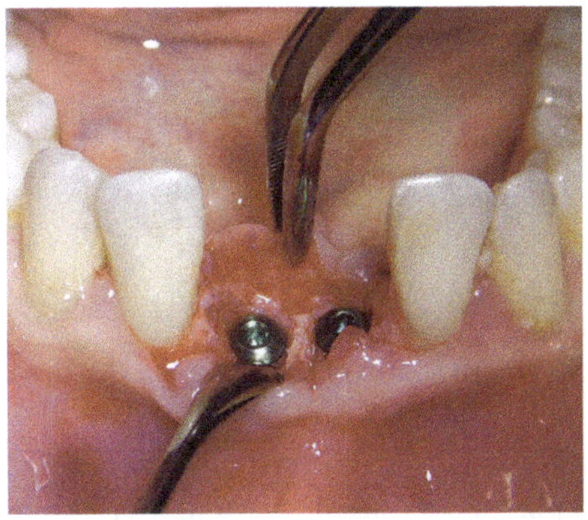

FIGURE 4: Clinical image showing the situation after placement of the two dental implants.

Standard postoperative instructions were provided, prescribing the use of 15 mL 0.2% chlorhexidine mouthwashes twice a day for seven days and nonsteroidal anti-inflammatory drug (ibuprofen 600 mg twice a day for three days).

After five months from the ARP intervention, we performed a CBCT scan to evaluate the healing of the bone and to plan dental implant placement (Figure 2). The radiographic investigation revealed the presence of sufficient available bone to place two 3.5 × 13 mm implants (Visio One ®, CEA Medical Sa, Geneva, Switzerland). After local anesthesia, a full-thickness mucoperiosteal flap was raised in the 3.1-4.1 region, and it was possible to confirm the presence of available bone volume and quality to place two dental implants in that region, without needing further procedures for bone augmentation (Figure 3). While preparing the implant site, using a 3 mm trephine bur, a biopsy of the bone tissues was taken with the aim of analyzing the characteristics of the healed bone in the region of autogenous grafting (Figure 4). The surgical procedure ended after implant placement by suturing the repositioned flap. Healing was uneventful. Second stage surgery was performed after three months, and the metal-ceramic prosthesis was delivered after a total of nine months from the ARP procedure.

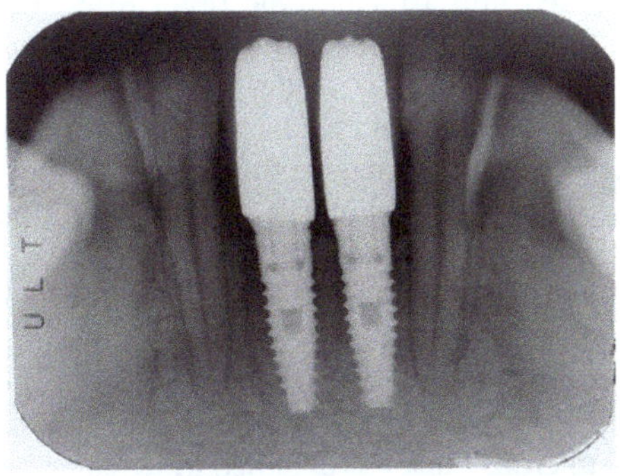

FIGURE 5: Periapical radiograph taken 2 years after prosthetic loading.

The clinical and radiographic follow-up revealed, after two years from loading, the absence of bone resorption process and stability of soft tissues (Figure 5).

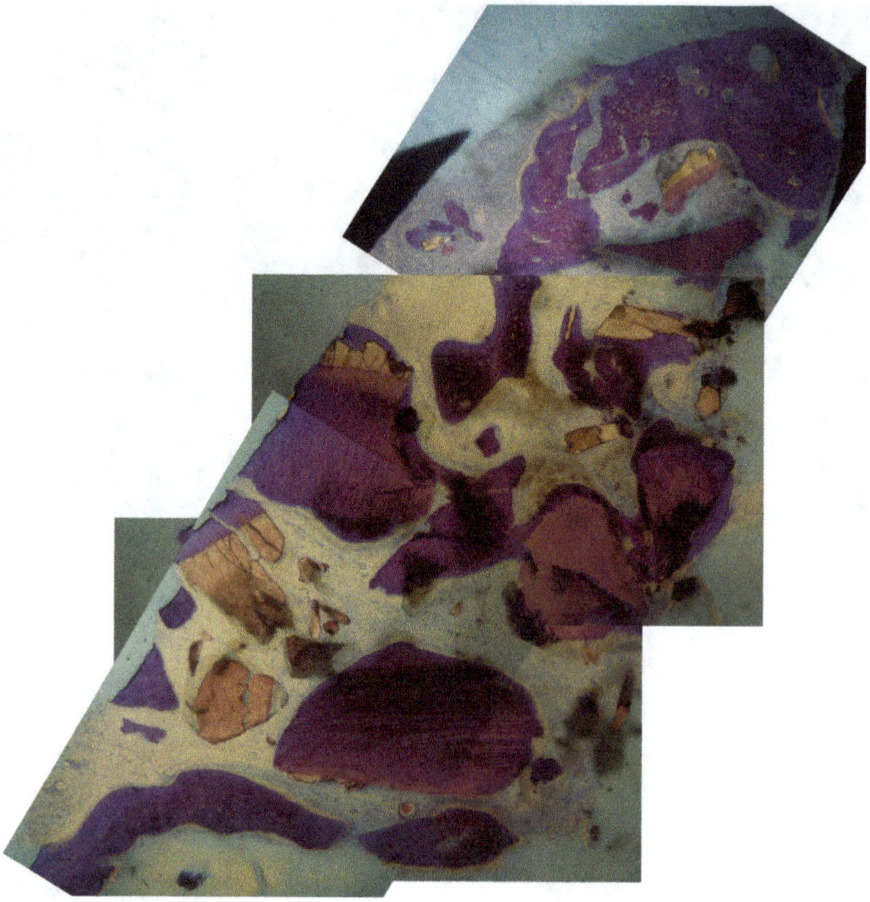

Figure 6: Section used for histologic analysis. In dark violet, the tooth-derived material; in violet, the bone, with Havers' canals.

2.1. Histologic Analysis. The histologic analysis was performed in the laboratory of the Biomaterial Clinical and Histological Research Association in Pescara, Italy.

The samples were dehydrated by a series of solutions with increasing alcohol concentration, up to pure alcohol, and then infiltrated into a methacrylic resin. After light curing of the resin, the sample was processed to obtain nondecalcified sections due to wear, using a disk abrasion system (LS2-Remet, Bologna) and a diamond disk cutting system (Micromet-Remet, Bologna). In the first phase, the inclusion in resin was abraded to eliminate the resin component that covered the sample; the area of the biopsy to be observed was thus brought to the surface. Then, the surface was glued to a showcase with cyanoacrylate-based adhesives. Subsequently, cutting with a high speed and cooling diamond blade was performed. In this way, a slide with a sample of about 200 microns thick was obtained which must be thinned by abrasion. With low abrasive paper, the sample was then abraded on the lapping machine with thickness control that allowed to progressively reduce the sample thickness up to about 40-50 microns. At this point, the slide was polished with polishing papers and colored with basic fuchsin and blue toluidine for the final observation in light and polarized light microscopy.

For histomorphometric measurements, the histological images obtained from the transmitted light microscope were digitized through a digital camera and analyzed by means of the image analysis software IAS 2000.

For each sample we calculated the following: BV% is the percentage of residual bone volume with exclusion of medullary tissues; Graft% is the percentage of the remaining graft, excluding the bone and marrow; and VB% is the percentage of vital bone with exclusion of the medulla and residual graft.

The histologic analysis (Figure 6) revealed 47.22% of BV, 18.68% of graft volume, and 28.55% of VB, indicating a substantial integration of the biomaterial used without signs of inflammation.

3. Discussion

The present case report demonstrated that deciduous teeth could be used as a source of bone substitute material, with good results in terms of histologic integration of the biomaterials and of clinical outcomes, thus allowing an effective ARP procedure.

Healing of the extraction socket has been widely studied by a number of published papers of high quality [3, 14]. One of the most important factors in determining the extent of the bone resorption process is represented by the presence of the buccal bone wall and by its width [14]. The so-called ARP techniques were proposed in order to maintain the bone volume even after tooth extraction and to reduce the need of performing complex and invasive bone augmentation procedures to place dental implants [4].

Over the years, a number of bone substitute materials were described in alveolar socket preservation procedures, but none of them demonstrated significantly better outcomes from the histomorphometric analysis [8].

For this case report, we decided to use such autologous material for several reasons, which represents the main advantages of the presented technique. First is the fact that we have great availability in terms of volume, then the use of completely autogenous material would have been beneficial in order to lower the possibility of adverse immune reactions, the patient refuses receiving biomaterials of animal origin, and finally, the use of the deciduous tooth was completely free of any biological or economic cost. Moreover, on the basis of the results of the research performed by Schmidt-Schultz and Schultz in 2005, we assumed that the characteristics of the teeth were not changed over the storing period, maintaining both the mineral and the nonmineral composition [15]. Therefore, the decision of using deciduous teeth was supported by the fact that they have structural and chemical characteristics that are suitable for grafting, having less enamel than permanent teeth, and, thus, an increased osteoinduction and resorption rate [11].

There are several papers about the use of tooth materials (dentin and enamel) as bone substitutes, acknowledging the advantage of being available after tooth extraction, thus avoiding other surgical procedures to be grafted (as it happens for the block graft from the mandibular ramus, for example) [10, 16, 17].

In 2018, one systematic review of the literature was published by Gual-Vaques et al., with the aim of evaluating autogenous teeth used as bone grafting material before implant placement [10]. The authors examined the existing literature of about 6 papers for a total of 182 dental implants. On the basis of the available data and admitting that the number of papers was insufficient for conclusive considerations, the authors stated that the use of such biomaterial was safe and effective for allowing implant placement in sites requiring bone augmentation [10].

The positive outcomes of the case we treated found support by other studies describing similar cases, even though not using deciduous teeth. The pilot study published by Del Canto-Diaz et al. in 2019 reported the results obtained using autogenous tooth material in nine patients. The outcomes they obtained were promising, since bone volume changes were significantly lower in the test group than in sites left to heal spontaneously [18]. Similar results were found also in more demanding bone regeneration procedures, such as the treatment of furcation defects [19].

To our knowledge, this is the first case described in the literature of regeneration performed in an adult using an autologous deciduous tooth. The present case report validity is limited by the study design itself. More studies (randomized controlled clinical trials) with a larger sample size are needed to confirm the results obtained in a significant number of pilot studies.

Consent

Informed consent was obtained from all individual participants included in the study.

References

[1] J. A. Siddiqui and N. C. Partridge, "Physiological bone remodeling: systemic regulation and growth factor involvement," *Physiology (Bethesda)*, vol. 31, no. 3, pp. 233–245, 2016.

[2] M. Chiapasco, P. Casentini, and M. Zaniboni, "Bone augmentation procedures in implant dentistry," *The International Journal of Oral & Maxillofacial Implants*, vol. 24, Supplement, pp. 237–259, 2009.

[3] T. Berglundh, I. Abrahamsson, J. P. Albouy, and J. Lindhe, "Bone healing at implants with a fluoride-modified surface: an experimental study in dogs," *Clinical Oral Implants Research*, vol. 18, no. 2, pp. 147–152, 2007.

[4] N. MacBeth, A. Trullenque-Eriksson, N. Donos, and N. Mardas, "Hard and soft tissue changes following alveolar ridge preservation: a systematic review," *Clinical Oral Implants Research*, vol. 28, no. 8, pp. 982–1004, 2017.

[5] M. A. Atieh, N. H. M. Alsabeeha, A. G. T. Payne et al., "Interventions for replacing missing teeth: alveolar ridge preservation techniques for dental implant site development," *Cochrane Database of Systematic Reviews*, no. 5, article CD010176, 2015.

[6] N. Mardas, A. Trullenque-Eriksson, N. MacBeth, A. Petrie, and N. Donos, "Does ridge preservation following tooth extraction improve implant treatment outcomes: a systematic review," *Clinical Oral Implants Research*, vol. 26, Supplement 11, pp. 180–201, 2015.

[7] M. Willenbacher, B. Al-Nawas, M. Berres, P. W. Kammerer, and E. Schiegnitz, "The effects of alveolar ridge preservation: a meta-analysis," *Clinical Implant Dentistry and Related Research*, vol. 18, no. 6, pp. 1248–1268, 2016.

[8] S. Corbella, S. Taschieri, L. Francetti, R. Weinstein, and M. del Fabbro, "Histomorphometric results after postextraction socket healing with different biomaterials: a systematic review of the literature and meta-analysis," *The International Journal of Oral & Maxillofacial Implants*, vol. 32, no. 5, pp. 1001–1017, 2017.

[9] S. Corbella, S. Taschieri, R. Weinstein, and M. Del Fabbro, "Histomorphometric outcomes after lateral sinus floor elevation procedure: a systematic review of the literature and meta-analysis," *Clinical Oral Implants Research*, vol. 27, no. 9, pp. 1106–1122, 2016.

[10] P. Gual-Vaques, C. Polis-Yanes, A. Estrugo-Devesa, R. Ayuso-Montero, A. Mari-Roig, and J. Lopez-Lopez, "Autogenous teeth used for bone grafting: a systematic review," *Medicina Oral, Patología Oral y Cirugía Bucal*, vol. 23, no. 1, pp. e112–e119, 2017.

[11] M. Park, Y. J. Mah, D. H. Kim, E. S. Kim, and E. J. Park, "Demineralized deciduous tooth as a source of bone graft material: its biological and physicochemical characteristics," *Oral Surgery, Oral Medicine, Oral Pathology, Oral Radiology*, vol. 120, no. 3, pp. 307–314, 2015.

[12] N. Bono, P. Tarsini, and G. Candiani, "BMP-2 and type I collagen preservation in human deciduous teeth after demineralization," *Journal of Applied Biomaterials & Functional Materials*, vol. 17, no. 2, 2018.

[13] T. Vercellotti, "Technological characteristics and clinical indications of piezoelectric bone surgery," *Minerva Stomatologica*, vol. 53, no. 5, pp. 207–214, 2004.

[14] V. Chappuis, O. Engel, K. Shahim, M. Reyes, C. Katsaros, and D. Buser, "Soft tissue alterations in esthetic postextraction sites: a 3-dimensional analysis," *Journal of Dental Research*, vol. 94, 9_Supplement, pp. 187S–193S, 2015.

[15] T. H. Schmidt-Schultz and M. Schultz, "Intact growth factors are conserved in the extracellular matrix of ancient human bone and teeth: a storehouse for the study of human evolution in health and disease," *Biological Chemistry*, vol. 386, no. 8, pp. 767–776, 2005.

[16] E. Minetti, A. Palermo, F. Ferrante et al., "Autologous tooth graft after endodontical treated used for socket preservation: a multicenter clinical study," *Applied Sciences*, vol. 9, no. 24, article 5396, 2019.

[17] D. Wu, L. Zhou, J. Lin, J. Chen, W. Huang, and Y. Chen, "Immediate implant placement in anterior teeth with grafting material of autogenous tooth bone vs xenogenic bone," *BMC Oral Health*, vol. 19, no. 1, p. 266, 2019.

[18] A. del Canto-Diaz, J. de Elio-Oliveros, M. del Canto-Diaz, M. A. Alobera-Gracia, M. del Canto-Pingarron, and J. M. Martinez-Gonzalez, "Use of autologous tooth-derived graft material in the post-extraction dental socket. Pilot study," *Medicina Oral Patología Oral y Cirugia Bucal*, vol. 24, no. 1, pp. e53–e60, 2018.

[19] P. Upadhyay, V. Blaggana, P. Tripathi, and M. Jindal, "Treatment of furcation involvement using autogenous tooth graft with 1-year follow-up: a case series," *Clinical Advances in Periodontics*, vol. 9, no. 1, pp. 4–8, 2019.

12

Reoperation on an Implant-Supported Restoration in the Maxillary Anterior Region to Correct a Complex Aesthetic Deficit

M. M. Figliuzzi, L. Parentela, A. Forte, and D. Aiello

Health Sciences Department "Magna Graecia", University of Catanzaro, Catanzaro, Italy

Correspondence should be addressed to M. M. Figliuzzi; figliuzzi@unicz.it

Academic Editor: Konstantinos Michalakis

Introduction. In an era in which patients are becoming more and more demanding and in which there are many ways to satisfy their needs, modern implantology must consider the correct management of soft tissues during treatment planning, aiming for both functional and aesthetic rehabilitation while creating a prosthetic construction that is in harmony not only with the natural dentition of the patient but also with their face. The patient who came to our notice had a rehabilitative prosthetic implant on the left central incisor area, which did not satisfy any functional or aesthetic parameter. Furthermore, he presented an altered passive eruption in the contralateral hemiarch. *Materials and Methods.* The prosthetic crown was removed, the tissues were studied, and the team decided to proceed with customizing a provisional restoration that would cause the soft tissues to descend. A surgical periodontal procedure was then performed to solve the altered passive eruption condition that was also compromising the aesthetics. In conclusion, a permanent prosthetic crown was fixed into place. *Discussion.* Using a periodontal approach that was both surgical and prosthetic, the patient was rehabilitated correctly regaining both functions and aesthetics. It is of fundamental importance that each step in the procedure is carefully programmed; otherwise, the risk of making mistakes increases and solving the problems becomes less simple or less immediate. In order to do this, one must bear in mind that certain clinical cases can apparently concern just one tooth, yet the mouth must be considered as a whole, both functionally and aesthetically. To perform an optimal implantology, the clinician should be an expert in periodontology so that they can plan and, should it be necessary, perform all the therapeutical options (surgical and nonsurgical) that can lead to the best possible result. *Conclusions.* The resolution of this complex clinical case has been documented in order to share useful advice for the resolution of analogous cases. We strongly advise that each proposed procedure be planned meticulously and that the periodontological aspect of the case never be separated from the prosthetic or the implantological aspects since the integration of the periodontal tissues is of vital importance for both the functional and the aesthetic results.

1. Introduction

Obtaining a functional as well as an aesthetic result is not always immediate, and it can become challenging for dentists. Rehabilitation of a single tooth with a prosthetic crown supported by implants is one of the most frequently performed procedures, thanks also to the high rate of success documented in the literature [1, 2].

To obtain an optimal functional and aesthetic result, the implant should be positioned considering all three dimensions [3, 4, 5]. It is also fundamental not only that there be an adequate bone architecture but also that the hard tissues are correctly handled [6]. Additionally, obtaining optimal aesthetic results involves correct handling of the soft tissue with adequate surgical and nonsurgical procedures. This becomes even more necessary for the anterior teeth [7], where gross errors impede a satisfactory rehabilitation of the patient. It is crucial to emphasize the importance of manufacturing temporary crowns [8] in order to shape the emergent profiles before proceeding with the definitive restoration. A temporary crown with an adequate contour will shape and stabilize the peri-implant soft tissue.

The patient who came to our notice had an implant-supported restoration on element 21, which was not satisfying

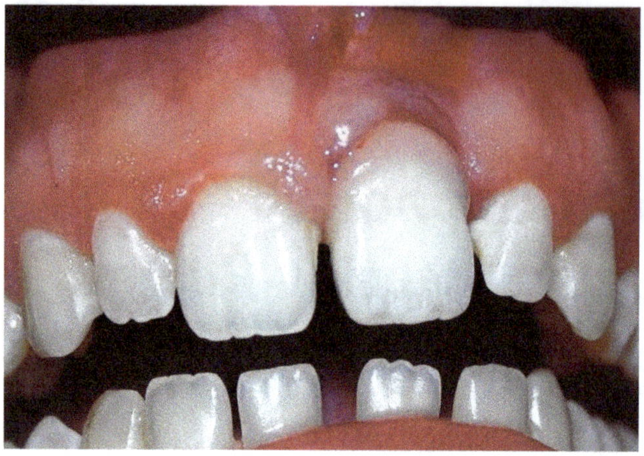

Figure 1: The patient came to us with a prosthetic rehabilitation implant for the 21 that did not satisfy any functional or aesthetic parameter.

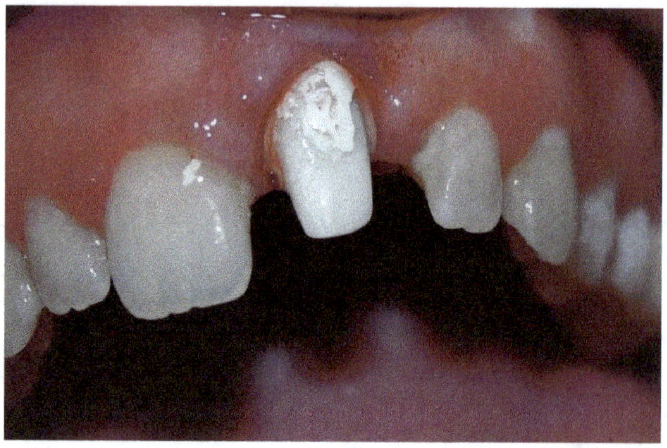

Figure 2: Once the crown was removed, the stump was newly prepared with a diminishing edge in zirconium and a temporary therapeutic element.

any functional or aesthetic parameter. Furthermore, he presented with an altered passive eruption [9] in the contralateral hemiarch (Figure 1).

Specifically, it was clear that the interdental gingiva was not represented [10], and the emergent profile was altered. A poor management of the soft tissues [11] had led to a nonharmonic integration of the prosthetic crown, and it resulted in an excessive retraction of the tissues. The arches were completely unaligned, resulting in an unacceptable rehabilitation.

Furthermore, during the previous treatment, the altered passive eruption [12] on the contralateral arch was not considered; had it been adequately treated together with the implant-prosthetic rehabilitation, it could have contributed to obtaining a satisfactory aesthetical and functional result, obtaining an adequate realignment of the arch.

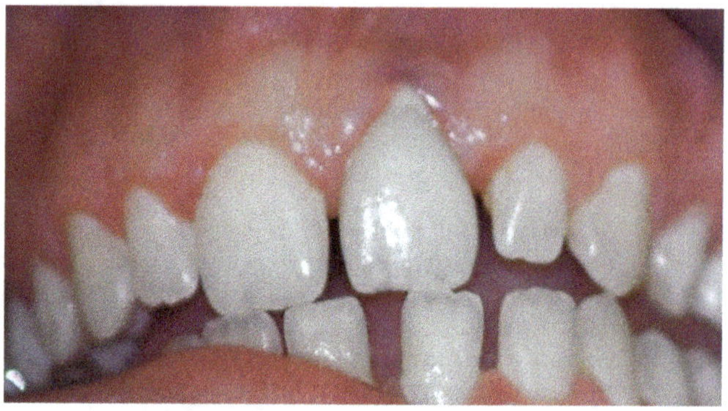

Figure 3: A temporary therapeutic element was inserted.

2. Materials and Methods

The prosthetic crown was removed from the implant, which allowed the study of the peri-implant tissues that were found to be flat and compressed, giving no possibility of reshaping or of adaptation (Figure 2).

Moreover, a horizontal overcontour was emphasized that had contributed to worsening of the aesthetics and the already altered emergent profile, thus not allowing the superficial periodontal tissues to adapt to the prothesis and contributing to the aesthetic deficit [13].

After removing the crown, a zirconia abutment with a decreasing contour was remade and a provisional restoration was placed leaving 2 mm space between it and the free gingival margin, giving the tissues the possibility of descending around the crown and substituting the missing gingival tissue, consequently allowing integration between the periodontal tissues and the provisional prothesis (Figure 3).

After 30 days, the patient was examined, and it was already possible to see that the tissues had descended at least 1.5 mm and that they were defining a new emergent profile, a sign of correct integration between the periodontal area and the prosthetic crown (Figure 4).

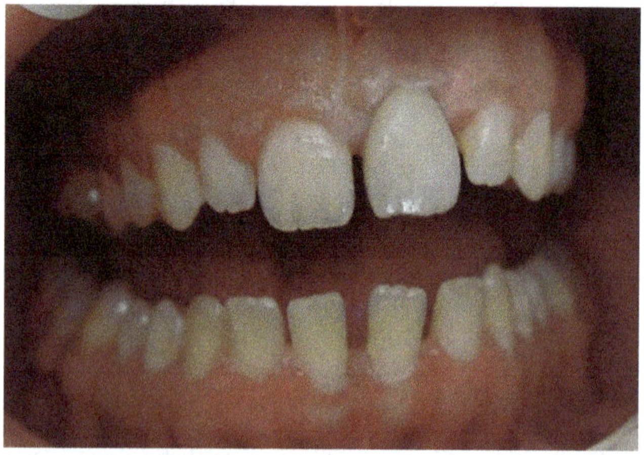

Figure 4: During the day 30 examination it was possible to see that the tissues had descended by at least 1.5 mm and were beginning to define the possibility of a new emergent profile.

The provisional prothesis was then reinserted and the next phase commenced—the redefinition of the arches operating on the altered passive eruption; this allowed functional identical profiles to be obtained, which were also aesthetically pleasant.

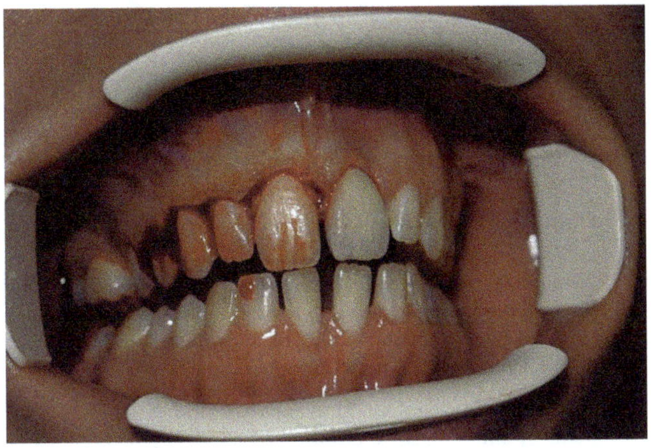

Figure 5: Using a 15c scalpel, a full depth flap was created with a primary nonmarginal incision placed 2 mm from the edge and an intrasulcular fillet incision.

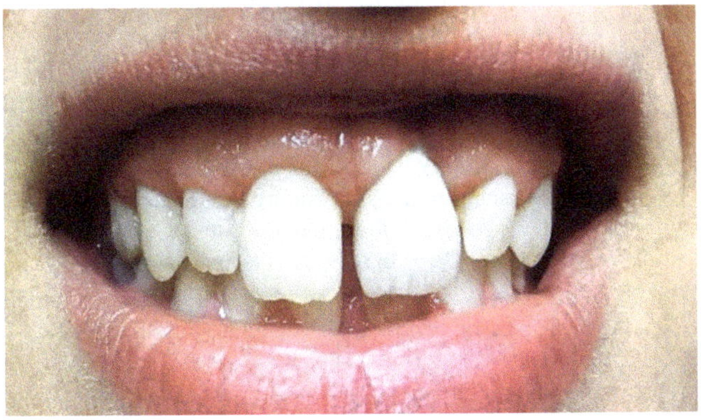

Figure 6: Day 21 examination.

A surgical procedure to restore the periodontium was performed, allowing the realignment of the arches; therefore, to resolve the condition of the altered passive eruption, gingivectomy was carried out according to Goldman [14] but with slight modifications. The patient was anesthetized locally using Optocain 20 mg/ml with adrenalin 1 : 100,000, the bleeding points (BPs) at the apex of the sulcus were located, the operational area was then defined by joining the BPs, and the projection of the future parabolas was determined.

Using a 15c scalpel, a full-thickness flap was performed with a submarginal primary incision at 2 mm from the gingival border, followed by an intrasulcular incision to free the gingival collar, which was then entirely removed with the help of a probe [15, 16] (Figure 5).

At the end of the procedure, the final intrasulcular result could already be envisaged, the new alignment of the emergent profiles, the length of the clinical crown of the dental elements, and the almost perfect adaption of the tissues to the provisional prothesis supported by the implant [17].

Natural, nonabsorbing, monofilament sutures were then applied (Seta 4\0) using separated simple stitches [18].

After 10 days, the suture was removed, and after 21 days, the patient was examined to assess the results of the healing process [19] (Figure 6).

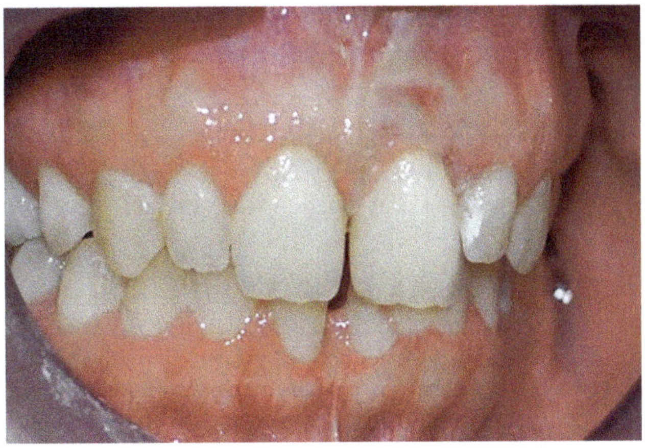

Figure 7: 3 months later, the tissues were properly stabilized and the definitive crown was inserted, completing the rehabilitation.

After 3 months [20], the tissues were adequately stabilized and a permanent prosthetic crown was fitted, finishing the rehabilitation process (Figure 7).

3. Discussion

Through a periodontal approach, both surgical and prosthetic, the patient was correctly rehabilitated, regaining function and aesthetics, balancing the emergent profiles, making the two hemiarches congruent and the prosthetic crown biomimetic and in harmony with the natural dentition.

The lack of planning or inadequate planning, as in this case, exposes treatments to mistakes, and it is not easy to repair the initial error and also obtain an optimal result. To correctly plan a therapeutic program requires certain considerations.

The clinical cases can regard a single tooth, but they should be always seen as a part of the whole mouth. Thus, in the initial evaluation the occlusion, the relationship between the mandible and the maxilla, and both the periodontal and the functional aspects must be taken into account. This allows clinicians to establish if there is any necessary work to be done on both the hemiarches, as in the described case, and to plan and program the therapeutical plan carefully.

To solve such a clinical case, several easily observable periodontal factors must be considered. In this specific case, considering the severe bone deficit of the patient, a space around the crown should have been left without touching the tissue integration. Furthermore, an altered passive eruption on the contralateral arch was present and the elimination of this factor with a simple gingivectomy, operation that is advisable in this sort of situation, allowed us to restore the emergent profiles, renewing the aesthetics and the congruence of the whole of the patient's mouth.

It is important to emphasize that in an aesthetic rehabilitation trough implant, not only the placement of should the implant be guided prosthetically, but it is indisputably necessary that the clinician should be expert in periodontology so that they can plan and perform, when necessary, all the therapeutical options (surgical and nonsurgical) that will lead to the best possible result [21], especially in complex clinical cases like the one just described.

4. Conclusions

This work aimed at showing how to resolve similar cases but also proposing some considerations that are more generally useful:

(1) It is a good idea to always plan every therapeutic intervention with awareness, assessing the whole of the patient's mouth and the patient themselves (state of general health, concomitant conditions, etc.) in order to minimize the risks and to have a choice between possible alternatives.

(2) Consideration of the periodontal factors when one has to resolve similar situations is fundamental; implantology and prosthetics are disciplines that cannot be separated from periodontology; otherwise, the correct or incorrect tissue adaption of the periodontal tissues is left to chance.

References

[1] T. Lindh, J. Gunne, A. Tillberg, and M. Molin, "A meta-analysis of implants in partial edentulism," *Clinical Oral Implants Research*, vol. 9, no. 2, pp. 80–90, 1998.

[2] N. H. Creugers, C. M. Kreulen, P. A. Snoek, and R. J. de Kanter, "A systematic review of single-tooth restorations supported by implants," *Journal of Dentistry*, vol. 28, no. 4, pp. 209–217, 2000.

[3] A. P. Saadoun, M. LeGall, and B. Touati, "Selection and ideal tridimensional implant position for soft tissue aesthetics," *Practical Periodontics and Aesthetic Dentistry*, vol. 11, no. 9, pp. 1063–1072; quiz 1074, 1999.

[4] D. P. Tarnow, S. C. Cho, and S. S. Wallace, "The effect of inter-implant distance on the height of inter-implant bone crest," *Journal of Periodontology*, vol. 71, no. 4, pp. 546–549, 2000.

[5] J. F. Gastaldo, P. R. Cury, and W. R. Sendyk, "Effect of the vertical and horizontal distances between adjacent implants and between a tooth and an implant on the incidence of interproximal Papilla," *Journal of Periodontology*, vol. 75, no. 9, pp. 1242–1246, 2004.

[6] A. P. Saadoun, "The key to peri-implant esthetics: hard- and soft-tissue management," *Dental Implantology Update*, vol. 8, no. 6, pp. 41–46, 1997.

[7] I. Ahmad, "Geometric considerations in anterior dental aesthetics: restorative principles," *Practical Periodontics and Aesthetic Dentistry*, vol. 10, no. 7, pp. 813–822; quiz 824, 1998.

[8] B. Mizrahi, "Temporary restorations: the key to success," *British Dental Journal*, vol. 226, no. 10, pp. 761–768, 2019.

[9] M. Mele, P. Felice, P. Sharma, C. Mazzotti, P. Bellone, and G. Zucchelli, "Esthetic treatment of altered passive eruption," *Periodontology 2000*, vol. 77, no. 1, pp. 65–83, 2018, Epub 2018 Mar 4.

[10] T. Jemt, "Regeneration of gingival papillae after single-implant treatment," *The International Journal of Periodontics & Restorative Dentistry*, vol. 17, no. 4, pp. 326–333, 1997.

[11] F. Cairo, U. Pagliaro, and M. Nieri, "Soft tissue management at implant sites," *Journal of Clinical Periodontology*, vol. 35, pp. 163–167, 2008.

[12] F. Alpiste-Illueca, "Altered passive eruption (APE): a little-known clinical situation," *Medicina Oral, Patología Oral y Cirugía Bucal*, vol. 16, no. 1, pp. e100–e104, 2011.

[13] O. González-Martín, E. Lee, A. Weisgold, M. Veltri, and H. Su, "Contour management of implant restorations for optimal emergence profiles: guidelines for immediate and delayed provisional restorations," *The International Journal of Periodontics & Restorative Dentistry*, vol. 40, no. 1, pp. 61–70, 2020.

[14] H. M. Goldman, "Gingivectomy," *Oral Surgery, Oral Medicine, and Oral Pathology*, vol. 4, no. 9, pp. 1136–1157, 1951.

[15] P. Darakh, Y. Khadtare, P. Waghmare, and A. Mali, "Treatment of altered passive eruption by surgical gingivectomy: a case report," *IP International Journal of Periodontology and Implantology*, vol. 2, pp. 64–68, 2017.

[16] V. A. Patil and J. R. Patel, "Treatment of altered passive eruption related gummy smile—a case report," *Journal of Advanced Medical and Dental Sciences Research*, vol. 5, no. 2, pp. 124–127, 2017.

[17] Y.-D. Cho, K.-H. Kim, Y.-M. Lee, Y. Ku, and Y.-J. Seol, "Periodontal wound healing and tissue regeneration: a narrative review," *Pharmaceuticals*, vol. 14, no. 5, p. 456, 2021.

[18] J. S. Kim, S. I. Shin, Y. Herr, J. B. Park, Y. H. Kwon, and J. H. Chung, "Tissue reactions to suture materials in the oral mucosa of beagle dogs," *Journal of Periodontal & Implant Science*, vol. 41, no. 4, pp. 185–191, 2011, Epub 2011 Aug 31.

[19] G. Polimeni, A. V. Xiropaidis, and U. M. E. Wikesjö, "Biology and principles of periodontal wound healing/regeneration," *Periodontology 2000*, vol. 41, pp. 30–47, 2006.

[20] D. W. Lodding, "Long-term esthetic provisional restorations in dentistry," *Current Opinion in Cosmetic Dentistry*, vol. 4, pp. 16–21, 1997.

[21] G. Zucchelli, P. Sharma, and I. Mounssif, "Esthetics in periodontics and implantology," *Periodontology 2000*, vol. 77, no. 1, pp. 7–18, 2018, Epub 2018 Mar 5.

13

Maxillary Reconstruction with Xenogeneic Bone Graft, Platelet-Rich Fibrin and Titanium Mesh for Rehabilitation with Implants: A 5-year Follow-Up Study

Graziele Parize,[1] Samy Tunchel,[2] Alberto Blay,[2] Eduardo Felippe Duailibi-Neto,[2] Yeon Jung Kim,[1] and Debora Pallos[1]

[1]*University of Santo Amaro, São Paulo, Brazil*
[2]*Private Office, São Paulo, Brazil*

Correspondence should be addressed to Debora Pallos; dpallos@prof.unisa.br

Academic Editor: Giuseppe Alessandro Scardina

Aim. Alveolar deficiency is considered one of the main limitations for placement of osseointegrated implants, as well as for their long-term success, especially in the anterior region of the maxilla. *Objective.* To report a clinical case of reconstruction of atrophic maxilla with deproteinized bovine bone associated with platelet-rich fibrin (PRF) and titanium mesh and to assess the linear and volumetric bone gains and rehabilitation with implants in a 5-year follow-up. *Case.* Patient with bone deficiency in the anterior maxilla region underwent bone reconstruction with deproteinized bovine bone associated with PRF and titanium mesh. After six months, the necessary bone height and volume were obtained for placement of implants, and the bone contour was restored in the anterior region, providing functional and aesthetic improvement. The amount of linear and volumetric bone gains was compared to baseline computed tomography scans. Three implants were placed in the grafted region, and a bone tissue sample was obtained at the time of their placement. Histological analysis showed neo-formed bone tissue in contact with the remaining particles of the biomaterial. After six months, the implants were activated, and the prosthesis was placed on the implants, which were monitored for five years. *Conclusion.* Implants can be placed predictably in regions with vertical and horizontal bone augmentations by using xenogeneic bone grafts associated with titanium mesh and PRF.

1. Introduction

Osseointegrated implants have become a great option to restore lost teeth. The available bone structure will determine the possibility of this rehabilitation [1]. Alveolar ridge resorption can restrict dental implant placement. Normally, bone resorption occurs because of tooth loss resulting from trauma, caries, and periodontal disease. Therefore, bone reconstruction procedures are performed to provide adequate conditions for rehabilitation [2].

In cases of limited amount of bone, the placement of short implants may be a solution in the posterior regions, mainly lower ones. Bone reconstruction may be the best therapeutic choice as it provides an opportunity to restore the lost bone structure, which often leads to better aesthetic results and longer implant survival [2, 3].

Autogenous block graft is considered the gold standard for these cases because it has osteoinductive, osteogenic properties. However, on the other hand, it has limited donor sites, possible morbidities, and reports of unpredictable resorption [4–8]. Therefore, more recent clinical techniques are being developed and advocated by several authors to avoid these problems [9–11].

One of the main complications of bone grafting is bone resorption. To avoid this complication, bone augmentation procedures associated with a non-resorbable membrane can be used to minimize the resorption [10].

Xenogenous bone is used for bone reconstructions with reliable results, reduced morbidity, and low complication

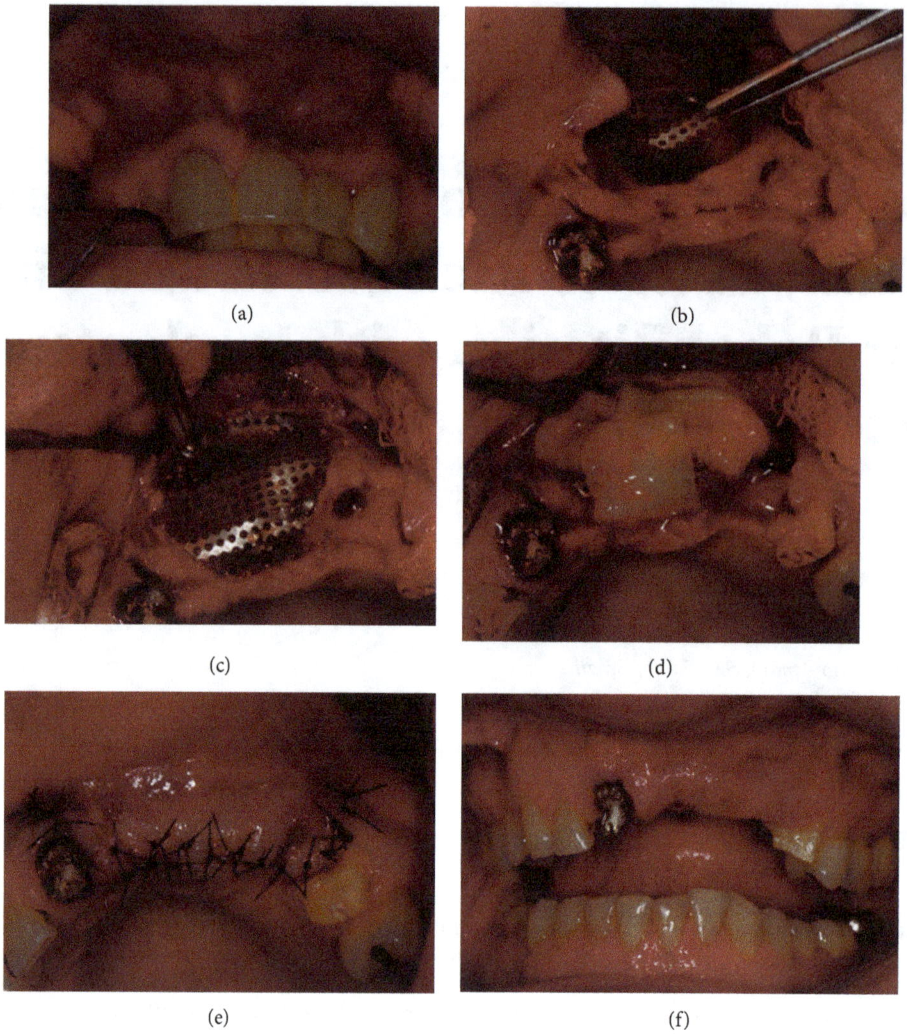

Figure 1: (a) Initial case. (b) Surgical bed preparation. It is possible to observe the bone defect in the region. (c) Xenogeneic bone and mesh in the region correcting the bone defect. (d) Adaptation of PRF membrane to the already-repaired tissue. (e) Surgical bed suture. (f) Removal of stitches without signs of inflammation or infection, good tissue healing.

rate compared to grafts with autogenous bone. Furthermore, they show good long-term stability due to their slow resorption, which is one of their most valuable features [12, 13].

Titanium mesh was chosen, because it has characteristics such as easy handling, allowing the three-dimensional reconstruction of large bone defects both vertically and horizontally [4, 10, 14, 15]. Platelet-rich fibrin (PRF) membrane has a slow release of growth factors, such as transforming growth factors $\beta 1$, platelet-derived growth factor, and vascular endothelial growth factor, all allowing the improvement of wound healing and regeneration of tissues [16].

The objective of this case report was to demonstrate the feasibility of vertical and horizontal bone reconstructions through grafting with deproteinized bovine bone mineral (DBBM) associated with PRF and titanium mesh.

2. Case Presentation

This case report was approved by the Research Ethics Committee of the University of Santo Amaro according to protocol number CAAE 09095619000000081, and the patient read and signed the informed consent form.

A male patient, 56 years old, came to the dental office with the main complaint of absence of teeth #21 and #22. In the initial clinical and radiographic evaluations, it was found that tooth #23 was indicated for extraction. The initial bone and gingival appearance can be seen in Figure 1(a), which shows a depression beneath teeth #21 and #22 indicating a volumetric bone loss in this region.

Computed tomography was used to analyse the bone structure, showing that there was extensive resorption of the alveolar bone in the anterior region of the maxilla, making it impossible to place implants and requiring a reconstruction to increase bone volume and height. For analysis of the linear bone measurement, the patient's upper arch was imaged with TCX Prexion (X Trillion Inc., Tokyo, Japan). To obtain the best image quality, scans were performed at cubic field of view of $8\,\mathrm{cm}^3$, 90 kVp, 4 mA, and 37-second exposure. Next, the images were exported in Diagnostic Imaging and Communication in Medicine

(DICOM) format with a voxel size of 0.160 mm. All files were individually exported to a DICOM directory to allow their visualization by using the OnDemand 3D Dental™ software (Cybermed Co., Tustin, CA, USA) for taking measurements. First, the images were captured and saved in the DICOM system for analysis of the angulation position of the patient's head (axis and reslice), followed by tracing over the region with the Arch/Curve tool to select the area of interest and obtain the measurements. A perpendicular line was also drawn along the slope of the residual bone, and three horizontal lines were recorded in width. This measurement was taken at a distance of 7, 11, and 13 mm from the crest.

The initial thickness was 2.60 mm, and the height was 16.75 mm. The patient did not present any systemic alteration contraindicating the surgical procedures.

A reconstructive surgery was performed by using Bio-Oss® bone graft (Geistlich Pharmaceutical, Wolhusen, Switzerland) as a biomaterial associated with Intralock titanium mesh (i.e., Ti Mesh-Lock® surgical mesh with 0.15 mm thick and spaced 0.8 mm holes designed for allowing cuts without edge) and PRF for obtaining the necessary amount of bone in the region for later placement of the implants and rehabilitation of the patient.

2.1. Site Preparation. Peripheral blood was initially collected in five vacutainer tubes, in which the white one (VACUETTE® Interlock, Intra-Lock, Brasil) was centrifuged in a centrifuge (IntraSpin™, Intra-Lock Iberia, IntraSpin, Intra-Lock, FL, USA) for 3 minutes at a rotation of 2700 rpm. Next, 3 mL of the supernatant was pipetted and stored in a sterile syringe. The other four red tubes (BD Vacutainer®, UKMolt 2/4 Hu-Friedy - Brasil) were centrifuged for 12 minutes at 2700 rpm for preparation of PRF membranes according to the Choukroun technique [17].

The surgical procedure started by infiltrating anesthesia with articaine 4% (Ultracain D®, Sanofi-Aventis, Paris, France) in the region before performing a crestal incision with relaxing incisions for total detachment of the flap and full visualization of the defected region (Figure 1(b)). Next, the recipient area was prepared with small perforations by using #2 spherical drill to allow better vascularization of the bone. Once the PRF membranes were obtained, two ones were perforated and mixed with DBBM before adding 3 mL of the supernatant to this biomaterial mixture. This biomaterial was adjusted to the region by using a molt peeler (Molt 2/4 Hu-Friedy®), and then a 0.15 mm thick Ti mesh-Lock® titanium mesh with 0.8 mm holes was placed onto the region and attached with screws measuring 1.4 and 6 mm. Next, the PRF membranes were placed over the mesh (Figures 1(c) and 1(d)). Suture with 3.0 nylon thread was performed avoiding tension in the operating region (Figure 1(e)). The patient was medicated with amoxicillin 500 mg, anti-inflammatories, dexamethasone 4 mg, and dipyrone 1 g. No changes were observed in the postoperative follow-up, and the suture was removed after 10 days (Figure 1(f)).

After six months, the patient underwent a new computerized tomography scan for evaluation of the bone reconstruction and implant planning (Figures 2(a), 2(b), 2(c), 2(d), 2(e) and 2(f)). The amount of bone was obtained by measuring the bone graft preoperatively and after six months approximately. Tomographic evaluation showed a thickness of 7.54 mm, height of 17.24 mm, and gain of 4.94 mm in thickness (Figures 2(b) and 2(c)).

The titanium mesh was removed for performing the surgery of implant placement, and it was observed that the grafted biomaterial particles were well incorporated into the new bone (Figures 3(a), 3(b), and 3(c)). Three Straumann bone level osseointegrated implants measuring 4.1 mm × 13 mm were inserted (Figure 3(d)), after preparation of the implant placement site with a trephine drill of 2 mm in diameter and 10 in height to remove bone for histological analysis. After six months, a reopening surgery was performed by placing healing caps on each implant. Next, the patient was rehabilitated with metal-ceramic prostheses (Figures 3(e) and 3(f)).

For volumetric analysis, the patient's DICOM files obtained before and after the surgery were exported to the Slicer 5.0.3 software (2022). The images were saved as a DICOM file before being selected for allowing a multiplanar view. Four slices were selected (i.e., axial, coronal, sagittal, and volume), and the volume limit was adjusted according to the area of interest to obtain the volumetric measurement and after creating the surface. These data were obtained from DICOM files before and after the bone grafting surgery, with the difference being the volumetric gain. Therefore, it was possible in which the initial volume was 12.796 mm^3, the volume was 54.090 mm^3 after 6 months, and the volume was 61.913 mm^3 on the final evaluation after 5 years (Figures 2(e) and 2(f)).

At the histological analysis, a newly formed bone was observed in intimate contact with the remaining particles of the biomaterial, where many osteocytes were distributed in fully integrated areas, thus demonstrating biocompatible patterns. No inflammatory cells and multinucleated giant cells were found at the interface with new bone formation (Figures 4(a) and 4(b)). Figure 5 shows the radiographic images of the implants installed after 5 years of follow-up.

3. Discussion

In this case report, it was possible to observe that bone grafting using xenogeneic bone associated with PRF membranes and placement of titanium mesh allowed rehabilitation of the patient with osseointegrated implants as height and volume were obtained. Through the analysis of preoperative and postoperative linear measurements, it was possible to observe linear gain exceeding 8 mm in some regions (Figures 2(b) and 2(c)) and volumetric gain (Figure 2(f)). The clinically obtained gingival contour culminated in a very satisfactory aesthetic result (Figures 3(a) and 3(b)). Histological analysis (Figure 4) showed that the newly formed bone was sound and well-integrated into the region, which is a good alternative compared to the autogenous bone graft.

The choice to use bone of bovine origin without association with other grafting materials was based on its advantages, such as easy availability and lower morbidity. In addition to the good results compared to other related studies, bovine bone has a lower risk of infection compared to

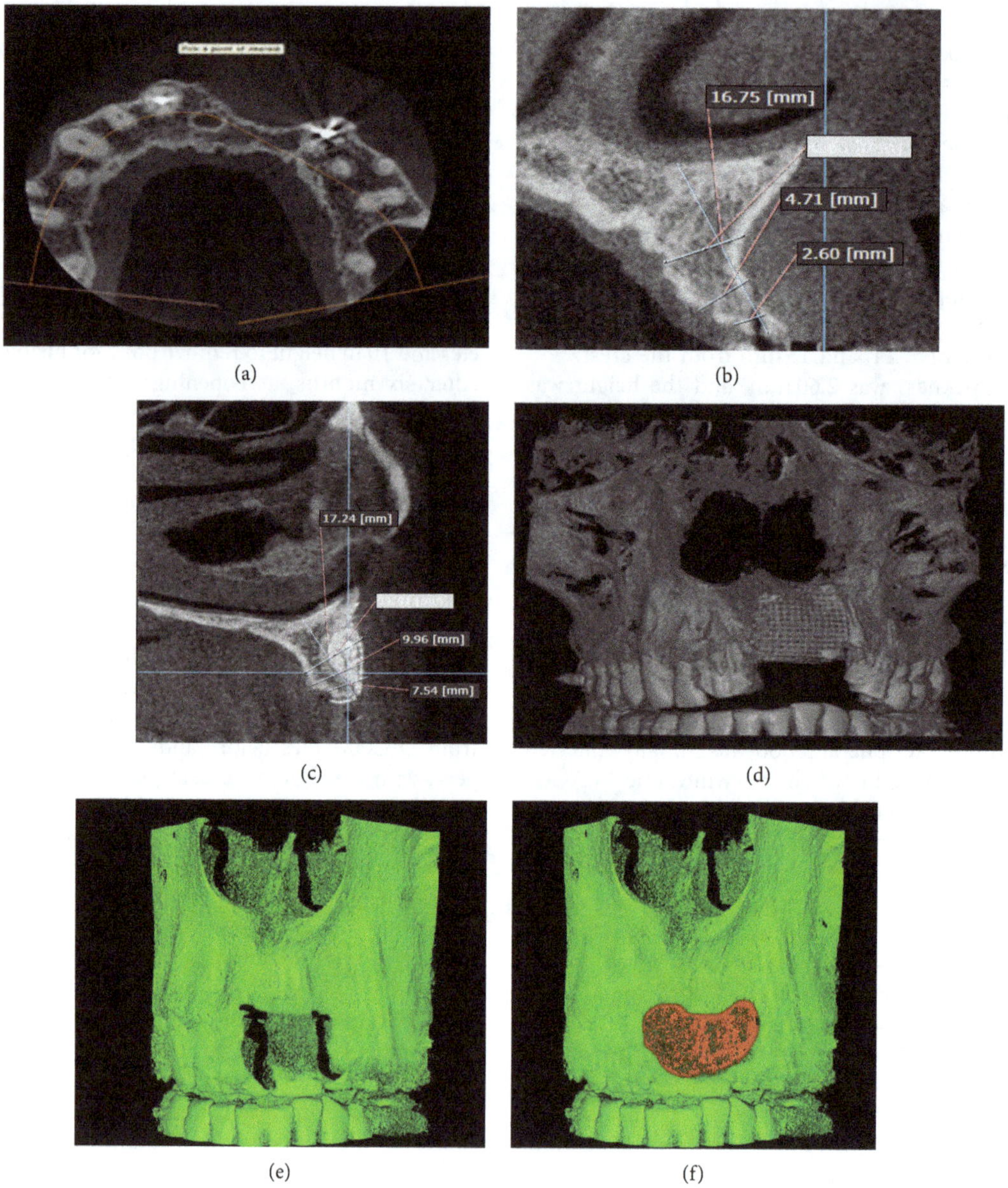

FIGURE 2: (a) Initial image showing sagittal section. (b) Initial image and linear data with measurements. (c) Final image and linear data with measurements. (d) Panoramic view with the adaptive mesh. (e) Initial volumetric image. (f) Volumetric image after grafting.

grafting using autogenous bone [13]. Authors have suggested that the association of autogenous and xenogenous grafts at a ratio of 70 : 30 or 60 : 40 provides good results [11, 15]. In the literature, only one case report of bone reconstruction in a patient with cancer was found, in which bone grafting was performed with xenogenous bone associated with titanium mesh and PRF. The xenogeneic bone was very effective in the case of grafting of large areas, having very promising results [9, 18, 19]. According to Sanz et al. [2], xenogenous bones, also known as DBBM, are the biomaterial most used for bone grafting in the craniomaxillofacial region. The main advantages of this biomaterial lie in its architecture and geometric structure, which are similar to the human bone, and in its slow absorption capacity, which is an important clinical feature to allow the increase in bone volume [3]. As for its limitations, one can cite the lack of biological components, which restricts its activity, and the potential biological risk (e.g., disease transmission) [20, 21]. However, our study has shown that the xenogeneic bone is a good alternative for bone reconstruction with satisfactory and predictable results.

Autogenous bone is the gold standard for grafting procedures due to its characteristics of osteogenesis, osteoinduction, and osteoconduction [11]. However, this biomaterial has some disadvantages, such as high rate of resorption, collection of bone from the donor site, increased surgical morbidity, and limited amount of bone [15]. According to some studies, autogenous grafts seem to have a significantly higher resorption rate compared to xenografts, with averages of 24.4% for autogenous bone and 49% for xenogenous bone [5, 12, 13, 18, 19, 22, 23]. In the study by Proussaefs and Lozada (2006), grafts were performed with a combination

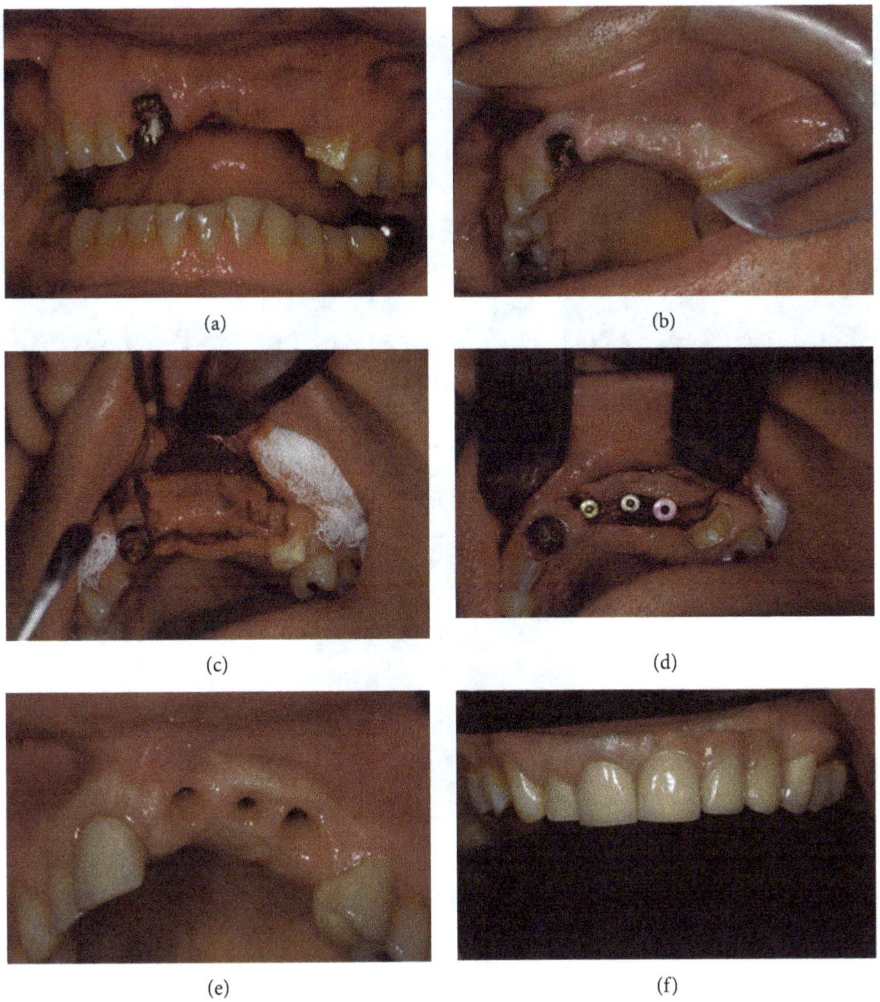

FIGURE 3: (a) Buccal visualization of the bone contour. (b) Bone and gingival contour. (c) Titanium mesh removal surgery. (d) Placement of Straumann implants. (e) Implant follow-up. (f) Permanent denture placement.

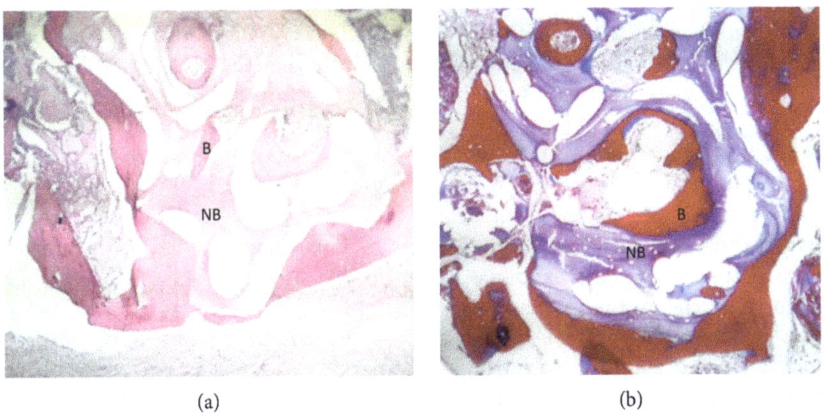

FIGURE 4: Photomicrograph showing newly formed bone in the grafted area at 6 months. (a) Hematoxylin and eosin stain (100×). (b) Masson's trichrome stain (100×). Newly formed bone was observed in intimate contact with remaining particles of biomaterial (b), and many osteocytes were distributed in the newly formed bone and, in some areas, were totally integrated, demonstrating biocompatible patterns.

of autogenous bone and Bio-Oss, and in the histological analysis, it was observed that the mixture of bone with residual particles of Bio-Oss and, in polarized microscopy, the xenograft obtained an active remodeling, and the newly formed bone appeared in firm contact along the structure, and no sign of resorption or active inflammatory process

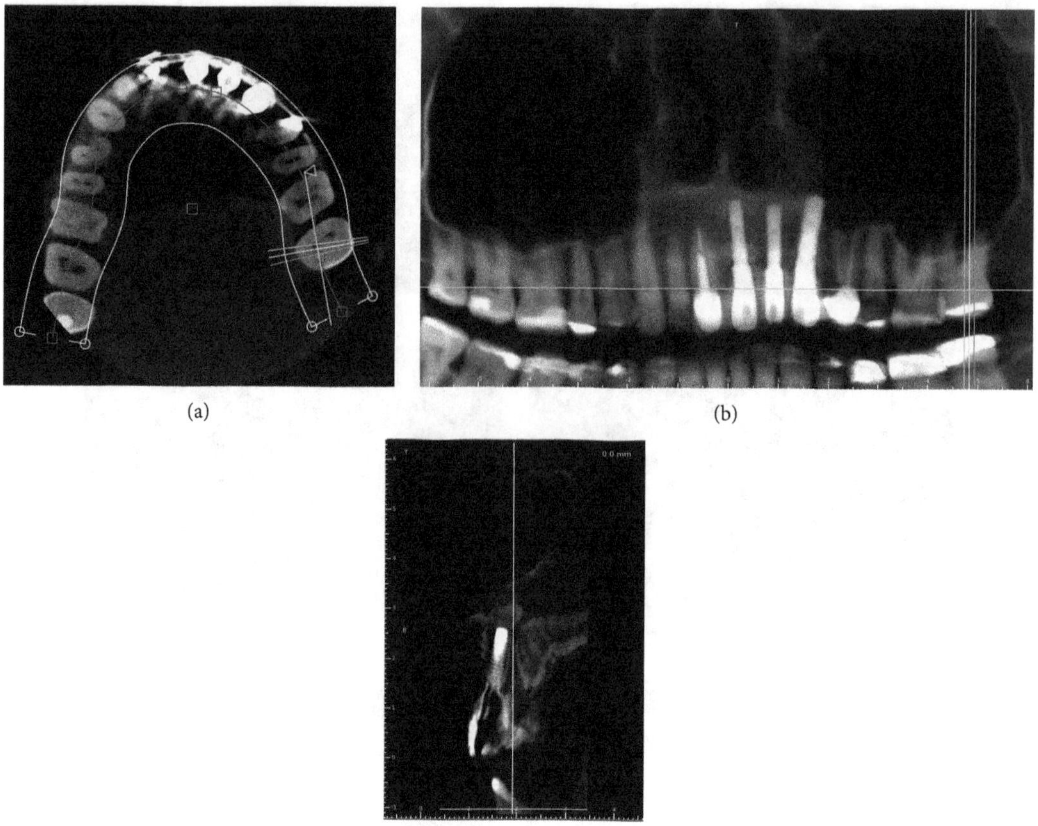

(a) (b) (c)

Figure 5: (a) Image showing sagittal section after 5 years. (b) Panoramic view showing the implant after 5 years. (c) Cone-beam computed tomography after 5-year follow-up.

was seen [24]. The histological analysis of this case report showed that the bone particles appear to be well incorporated.

In the study by Corinaldesi et al. [20], the histological examination showed that the DBBM particles presented as granules well integrated in the regenerated bone. No sign of resorption was observed on the surface of DBBM for 8–9 months after grafting. In the literature, there is no study reporting osteoclastic activity six months after bone reconstruction.

PRF membrane was used to cover the titanium mesh in order to minimize the risk of possible exposure and contamination of the graft material, as the membrane acts on the soft tissue by accelerating the repair process [10]. According to other authors [10, 25, 26], the exposure of the titanium mesh ended up influencing the result of their study.

Boyne [27] suggested the use of titanium mesh for maxillofacial bone reconstruction, reporting positive results in the ridge augmentation obtained before the placement of dental implants.

Other authors pointed to the benefits of titanium mesh, including easy handling, biocompatibility, excellent mechanics, and rigid graft stabilization, thus allowing the treatment of all types and sizes of three-dimensional bone defects [28].

PRF membrane is obtained simply by centrifugation without anticoagulant, but containing platelets and leukocytes as well as a variety of growth factors and cytokines [29]. The key to tissue regeneration lies in its angiogenic potential, which can be explained by its three-dimensional structure, immune system control, cell recruitment potential, and ability to ensure wound closure [30].

The present study corroborates the literature by demonstrating that the bone gain obtained is predictable with less complications, allowing implant stability. This finding was also reported by Briguglio et al. [4], who performed a retrospective study on the association of xenogenous and autogenous grafts with PRF for reconstruction of vertical and horizontal bone defects in the maxilla and mandible.

The gains obtained in the above-mentioned reconstruction made it possible to rehabilitate the patient with implants and ceramic prostheses. It is possible to observe in the clinical images that the prostheses have a gingival margin, which was necessary because the patient's defect was very large and it would not be possible to rehabilitate it without doing so. This allowed the final result to be more aesthetic. In addition, it was possible to minimize the bone defect and prepare the region to receive the osseointegrated implants safely.

As far as we know, this is the first case report on the use of xenogeneic bone in association with titanium mesh and PRF for rehabilitation of patients with insufficient bone volume, presenting low morbidity, low risk of infection, and satisfactory results as well.

4. Conclusion

The present clinical case showed that implants can be placed in bone sites, which were vertically augmented by using only xenogenous grafts associated with titanium mesh and PRF. The result obtained was aesthetically and functionally satisfactory as the patient's oral and emotional health was improved with the use of osseointegrated implants. In addition, further follow-up studies are needed to assess whether osseointegration in this type of augmented bone can be maintained in the long term.

Acknowledgments

This case report was funded by the authors.

References

[1] N. Demetriades, J. I. Park, and C. Laskarides, "Alternative bone expansion technique for implant placement in atrophic edentulous maxilla and mandible," *The Journal of Oral Implantology*, vol. 37, no. 4, pp. 463–471, 2011.

[2] M. Sanz, C. Dahlin, D. Apatzidou et al., "Biomaterials and regenerative technologies used in bone regeneration in the craniomaxillofacial region: consensus report of group 2 of the 15th European Workshop on Periodontology on Bone Regeneration," *Journal of Clinical Periodontology*, vol. 46, Suppl 21, pp. 82–91, 2019.

[3] I. A. Urban, E. Montero, A. Monje, and I. Sanz-Sánchez, "Effectiveness of vertical ridge augmentation interventions: a systematic review and meta-analysis," *Journal of Clinical Periodontology*, vol. 46, Suppl 21, pp. 319–339, 2019.

[4] F. Briguglio, D. Falcomatà, S. Marconcini, L. Fiorillo, R. Briguglio, and D. Farronato, "The use of titanium mesh in guided bone regeneration: a systematic review," *International Journal of Dentistry*, vol. 2019, p. 8, 2019.

[5] S. S. Jensen and H. Terheyden, "Bone augmentation procedures in localized defects in the alveolar ridge: clinical results with different bone grafts and bone-substitute materials," *The International Journal of Oral & Maxillofacial Implants*, vol. 24, suppl, pp. 218–236, 2009.

[6] S. M. Meloni, S. A. Jovanovic, I. Urban, L. Canullo, and T. M. PisanoM, "Horizontal ridge augmentation using GBR with a native collagen membrane and 1:1 ratio of particulated xenograft and autologous bone: a 1-year prospective clinical study," *Clinical Implant Dentistry and Related Research*, vol. 19, no. 1, pp. 38–45, 2017.

[7] A. A. Pelegrine, M. L. Teixeira, M. Sperandio et al., "Can bone marrow aspirate concentrate change the mineralization pattern of the anterior maxilla treated with xenografts? A preliminary study," *Contemporary Clinical Dentistry*, vol. 7, no. 1, pp. 21–26, 2016.

[8] T. Starch-Jensen, H. Aludden, M. Hallman, C. Dahlin, A.-E. Christensen, and A. Mordenfeld, "A systematic review and meta-analysis of long-term studies (five or more years) assessing maxillary sinus floor augmentation," *International Journal of Oral and Maxillofacial Surgery*, vol. 47, no. 1, pp. 103–116, 2018.

[9] M. Hasan Hameed, M. Gul, R. Ghafoor, and F. R. Khan, "Vertical ridge gain with various bone augmentation techniques: a systematic review and meta-analysis," *Journal of Prosthodontics*, vol. 28, no. 4, pp. 421–427, 2019.

[10] I. Miyamoto, K. Funaki, K. Yamauchi, T. Kodama, and T. Takahashi, "Alveolar ridge reconstruction with titanium mesh and autogenous particulate bone graft: computed tomography-based evaluations of augmented bone quality and quantity," *Clinical Implant Dentistry and Related Research*, vol. 14, no. 2, pp. 304–311, 2012.

[11] A. Monje, F. Monje, F. Hernández-Alfaro et al., "Horizontal bone augmentation using autogenous block grafts and particulate xenograft in the severe atrophic maxillary anterior ridges: a cone-beam computerized tomography case series," *The Journal of Oral Implantology*, vol. 41, no. S1, pp. 366–371, 2015.

[12] J. Alayan and S. Ivanovski, "A prospective controlled trial comparing xenograft/autogenous bone and collagen-stabilized xenograft for maxillary sinus augmentation-complications, patient-reported outcomes and volumetric analysis," *Clinical Oral Implants Research*, vol. 29, no. 2, pp. 248–262, 2017.

[13] P. H. De Azambuja Carvalho, G. dos Santos Trento, L. B. Moura, G. Cunha, M. A. C. Gabrielli, and V. A. Pereira-Filho, "Horizontal ridge augmentation using xenogenous bone graft-systematic review," *Oral and Maxillofacial Surgery*, vol. 23, no. 3, pp. 271–279, 2019.

[14] R. Gutta, R. A. Baker, A. A. Bartolucci, and P. J. Louis, "Barrier membranes used for ridge augmentation: is there an optimal pore size?," *Journal of Oral and Maxillofacial Surgery*, vol. 67, no. 6, pp. 1218–1225, 2009.

[15] F. Pieri, G. Corinaldesi, M. Fini, N. N. Aldini, R. Giardino, and C. Marchetti, "Alveolar ridge augmentation with titanium mesh and a combination of autogenous bone and anorganic bovine bone: a 2-year prospective study," *Journal of Periodontology*, vol. 79, no. 11, pp. 2093–2103, 2008.

[16] S. Najeeb, Z. Khurshid, M. A. S. Agwan, S. A. Ansari, M. S. Zafar, and J. P. Matinlinna, "Regenerative potential of platelet rich fibrin (PRF) for curing intrabony periodontal defects: a systematic review of clinical studies," *Tissue Engineering and Regenerative Medicine*, vol. 14, no. 6, pp. 735–742, 2017.

[17] J. Choukroun and S. Ghanaati, "Reduction of relative centrifugation force within injectable platelet-rich-fibrin (PRF) concentrates advances patients' own inflammatory cells, platelets and growth factors: the first introduction to the low speed centrifugation concept," *European Journal of Trauma and Emergency Surgery*, vol. 44, no. 1, pp. 87–95, 2017.

[18] M. Esposito, M. G. Grusovin, P. Felice, G. Karatzopoulos, H. V. Worthington, and P. Coulthard, "The efficacy of horizontal and vertical bone augmentation procedures for dental implants—a Cochrane systematic review," *European Journal of Oral Implantology*, vol. 2, no. 3, pp. 167–184, 2009.

[19] H. B. Nielsen and T. Starch-Jensen, "Lateral ridge augmentation in the posterior part of the mandible with an autogenous bone block graft harvested from the ascending mandibular ramus. A 10-year retrospective study," *Journal of Stomatology, Oral and Maxillofacial Surgery*, vol. 122, no. 2, pp. 141–146, 2021.

[20] G. Corinaldesi, F. Pieri, C. Marchetti, M. Fini, N. N. Aldini, and R. Giardino, "Histologic and histomorphometric evaluation of alveolar ridge augmentation using bone grafts and titanium micromesh in humans," *Journal of Periodontology*, vol. 78, no. 8, pp. 1477–1484, 2007.

[21] N. Esfahanizadeh, P. Daneshparvar, N. Takzaree, M. Rezvan, and N. Daneshparvar, "Histologic evaluation of the bone regeneration capacities of Bio-Oss and MinerOss X in rabbit calvarial defects," *The International Journal of Periodontics & Restorative Dentistry*, vol. 39, no. 6, pp. e219–e227, 2019.

[22] G. Mendoza-Azpur, A. de la Fuente, E. Chavez, E. Valdivia, and I. Khouly, "Horizontal ridge augmentation with guided bone regeneration using particulate xenogenic bone substitutes with or without autogenous block grafts: a randomized controlled trial," *Clinical Implant Dentistry and Related Research*, vol. 21, no. 4, pp. 521–530, 2019.

[23] C. C. Osorio, L. M. Escobar, M. C. González, L. F. Gamboa, and L. Chambrone, "Evaluation of density, volume, height and rate of bone resorption of substitutes of autologous bone grafts for the repair of alveolar clefts in humans: a systematic review," *Heliyon*, vol. 6, no. 9, article e04646, 2020.

[24] P. Proussaefs and J. Lozada, "Use of titanium mesh for staged localized alveolar ridge augmentation: clinical and histologic-histomorphometric evaluation," *The Journal of Oral Implantology*, vol. 32, no. 5, pp. 237–247, 2006.

[25] M. Chiapasco, P. Casentini, and M. Zaniboni, "Bone augmentation procedures in implant dentistry," *The International Journal of Oral & Maxillofacial Implants*, vol. 24, Suppl, pp. 237–259, 2009.

[26] K. Sagheb, E. Schiegnitz, M. Moergel, C. Walter, B. Al-Nawas, and W. Wagner, "Clinical outcome of alveolar ridge augmentation with individualized CAD-CAM-produced titanium mesh," *International Journal of Implant Dentistry*, vol. 3, no. 1, p. 36, 2017.

[27] P. J. Boyne, "Restoration of osseous defects in maxillofacial casualties," *Journal of the American Dental Association*, vol. 78, no. 4, pp. 767–776, 1969.

[28] G. E. Salvi, A. Monje, and C. Tomasi, "Long-term biological complications of dental implants placed either in pristine or in augmented sites: a systematic review and meta-analysis," *Clinical Oral Implants Research*, vol. 29, Suppl 16, pp. 294–310, 2018.

[29] E. Anitua, "Plasma rich in growth factors: preliminary results of use in the preparation of future sites for implants," *The International Journal of Oral & Maxillofacial Implants*, vol. 14, no. 4, pp. 529–535, 1999.

[30] R. J. Miron, G. Zucchelli, M. A. Pikos et al., "Use of platelet-rich fibrin in regenerative dentistry: a systematic review," *Clinical Oral Investigations*, vol. 21, no. 6, pp. 1913–1927, 2017.

14

Canalis Sinuosus Damage after Immediate Dental Implant Placement in the Esthetic Zone

Roman Volberg[1] **and Oleg Mordanov**[2]

[1]*Private Practice, Moscow, Russia*
[2]*Department of Prosthodontics, Central Research Institute of Dental and Maxillofacial Surgery, Moscow, Russia*

Correspondence should be addressed to Oleg Mordanov; mordanov19@gmail.com

Academic Editor: Hüsamettin Oktay

Dental implant failure in the anterior maxilla can be caused by the range of the features. One of them is neighboring neurovascular structure damage, such as the canalis sinuosus (CS), that carries the superior anterior alveolar nerve. The aim of the report is to demonstrate clinical symptomatology and radiographic signs of CS damage in a 45-year-old female patient who underwent upper left lateral incisor extraction and immediate implant placement and implant removal in 16 days secondary to pain and paresthesia in the maxillary left region.

1. Introduction

Immediate implant placement has been considered as an effective treatment for partially edentulous patients with a high implant survival rate [1]. However, not all implants that survive are necessarily successful [2]. Implant failure may be primary or secondary nature [3]. One of the examples of the secondary implant failure and, as a result, untoward consequence of performing implant dentistry could be the implant removal due to the damage to the infraorbital nerve and its branches [4].

The anterior superior alveolar nerve (ASAN) is a branch of infraorbital nerve that enters in the infraorbital canal, which has a side intrabony branch called the *canalis sinuosus* (CS) [5, 6]. The canalis sinuosus goes through the anterior wall of the maxilla and then along the lateral wall of the nasal cavity [7], residing in the alveolar process of the maxilla [8–12]. CS nerves and vessels supply anterior teeth and adjacent soft tissues [13].

The proximity to the neurovascular bundle of the CS can compromise dental implant treatment [8, 14, 15] with potential bleeding and temporary or permanent sensory disturbances [9, 16]. For example, Machado et al. [9] presented two case reports where patients suffered from pain and it was immediately relieved after implant extractions that had been placed with CS damage. Also, McCrea [14] and Arruda et al. [17] reported different cases in which dental implant placement in the anterior maxilla in the CS led to persistent pain, and the patient's symptoms were resolved with the following removal of the implant. However, Shaeffer [18] reported a case of intractable pain following implant placement in the upper left first premolar region and the pain did not subside following the extraction of the implant.

When planning dental implants, carrying out radiographic examinations, alongside clinical examinations, has become necessary to reduce the risk of implant procedure failure and complications. The cone-beam computed tomography (CBCT) imaging is a valuable tool to determine the anatomic structures before any surgery, including implant surgery [19]. The recent literature review stated that CBCT exams were the best way to evaluate the CS [16].

Also, it was shown that the terminal portion of CS is more prevalent in the anterior region of the maxilla, more specifically in the incisor and canine regions near the palate [16]. On the other hand, the widely recommended direction for immediate implant placement in the anterior maxilla is

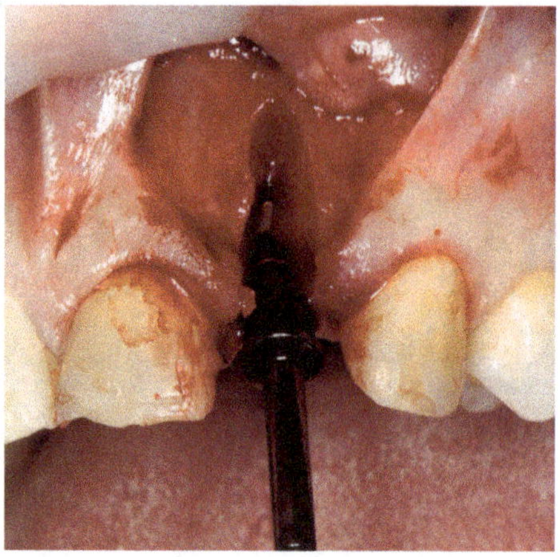

FIGURE 1: Intraoperative view. Implant site preparation after upper left lateral incisor extraction. No excessive bleeding was presented during the surgery.

palatal to the extracted root axis to engage more native bone in order to achieve maximum bony support and favorable esthetic outcome [20].

The aim of this article is to report a case with clinical and radiographic signs of CS damage after immediate dental implant placement in the maxillary left lateral incisor region.

2. Case Report

A 45-year-old female patient underwent maxillary left lateral incisor extraction secondary to severe horizontal tooth fracture below the cementoenamel junction (CEJ). Preoperative CBCT examination was provided and evaluated before the procedure.

The CBCT scan was obtained with a 3D eXam (KaVo, Biberach, Germany) with standard exposure settings (23 cm × 17 cm field of view, 0.3 mm voxel size, 110 kV, and 1.6–20 s) and was analyzed with the I-CAT viewer software (Version 10, Hatfield, England).

The patient gave written consent before all procedures. Extraction was provided atraumatically with the luxators. The flap was reflected. Immediate implant placement was performed with the simultaneous guided bone regeneration (GBR) without corticotomy and soft tissue grafting (so-called "Burger technique" by Urban et al. [21, 22]). The implant placement and GBR procedures went without any complications (Figure 1); primary stability of the implant was 35 N cm (Dentium Implantium 3.5 mm * 10 mm). The GBR was provided using a mixture of the autogenous bone and a Bio-Oss® particulate graft (Geistlich) and Bio-Gide membrane (Geistlich). The site was sutured with Prolene 6/0. No excessive bleeding, as in the case of vessel damage, was noted during the surgery (Figure 2).

In a few hours after the procedure, the patient started complaining about the pain and paresthesia in the left maxilla. First week pain was insignificant, and 400 mg of ibuprofen was prescribed twice a day and it relieved the pain. In one week, the pain started increasing and became so strong and continuous that none of the painkillers could relieve it.

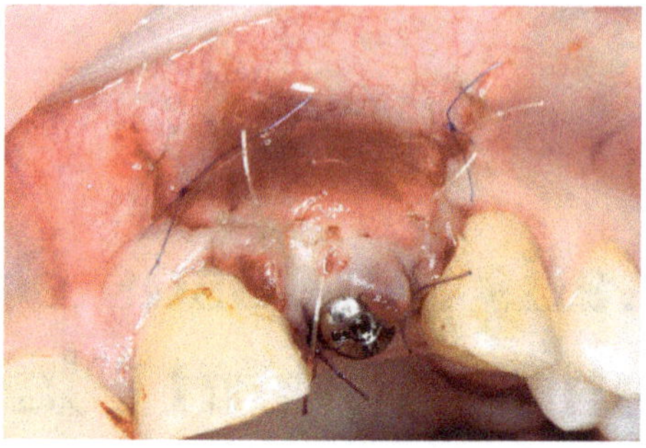

FIGURE 2: Intraoperative view. Immediate implant placement in the upper left lateral incisor region after GBR and soft tissue grafting. The healing abutment was placed and flaps were sutured.

The pain generally was located in the area of the maxillary left canine. All sensitive disorders were not located in the area of implant site—they spread out around the maxillary left canine, the palate, and the nasal region. Also, the patient complained about burning in the back of the head in the occipital region. Painkillers, tranquilizers, and neurotropic agents were ineffective at this moment. However, no significant findings were noted during extraoral and intraoral clinical examinations.

After the clinical examinations, it was suspected to be a neurological disorder, so differential diagnostic procedures were held. During these procedures, different types of the nerve blocks were performed on the patient. Palatal, incisive, and infraorbital nerve blocks were used one by one; however, only the infraorbital block relieved the pain.

No other symptoms of inflammation were found such as pain, fever, exudation, or excessive bleeding in the area of implant placement and GBR. Neither the patient nor her relatives presented neurological disease in the medical history.

New CBCT evaluation was performed after the surgery with the same equipment. During precise examination of the CBCT scans before and after the implant placement, CS was found with the diameter 2.3 mm in size with two small branches. One of them was found close to the palatal side with the diameter 1.9 mm in size; the other was found close to the buccal side in the maxillary left lateral incisor/implant region (Figures 3 and 4) with the diameter 0.7 mm in size in the most coronal point (both were referred to the lateral incisor region according to the de Oliveira-Santos et al. classification [5]).

The implant was extracted in two weeks and two days. Then, the pain and paresthesia started slowing down. However, an area of necrosis was found by the end of the third week on the palatal mucosa (Figure 5) even though the palatal flap was not reflected and no palatal and nasopalatine anesthesia was provided, so palatal blood supply was not compromised. Also, bony contours of the left greater palatal artery and nerve were visualized on the CBCT scans in the anterior maxilla 10.1 mm from the implant (Figure 5); thus, the damage of the greater palatal artery was excluded. The implant was 5.62 mm from the incisive foramen and 5.66 mm from the nasopalatine canal according to CBCT data, so the intervention to these structures is excluded as well.

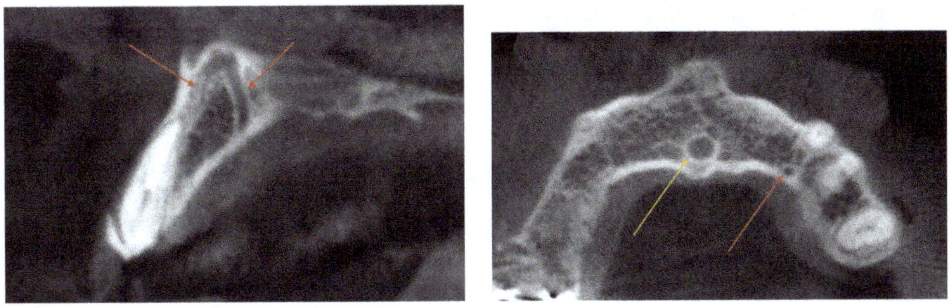

(a) (b)

FIGURE 3: Preoperative CBCT scan. (a) Sagittal view. Accessory branches of CS (red arrows) have palatal and buccal directions close to the maxillary left lateral incisor. (b) Axial view. CS (red arrow) near the maxillary left canine and nasopalatine canal (yellow arrow).

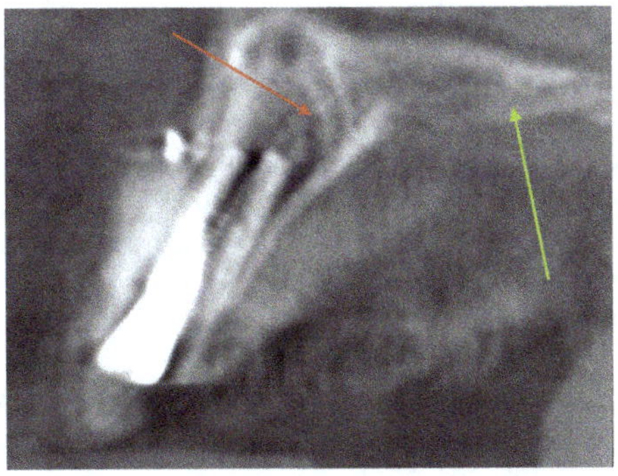

FIGURE 4: Postoperative CBCT scan, sagittal view in the left maxillary incisor region. The dental implant in situ. The diagnosis is difficult due to artefacts caused by the titanium implant; however, the major palatal branch of the CS could be seen (red arrow). Also, the bony contours of the left greater palatal artery and nerve are visualized (green arrow).

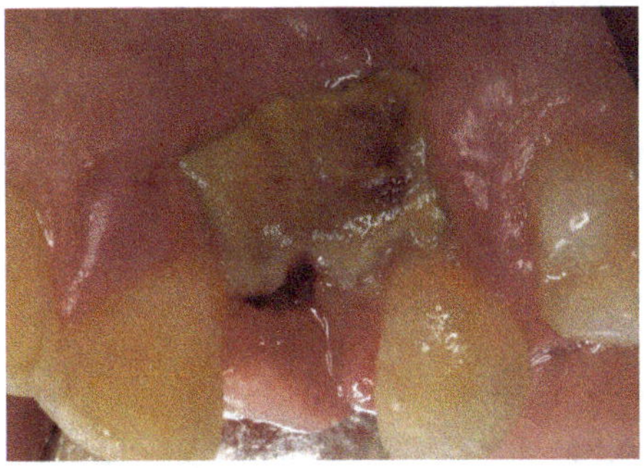

FIGURE 5: Palatal mucosa necrosis after dental implant extraction.

The bony defect after implant removal healed under a blood clot as an alveolar socket after tooth extraction. The patient was prescribed antiseptics for local application. Further treatment and follow-ups of the patient were impossible, because the patient decided to change the clinical practice.

3. Discussion

The CS, first described by Jones [23], carries an anterior superior neurovascular bundle through the anterior maxilla that innervates the central and lateral incisors and the canines. This small, poorly recognized bony canal is not known by surgeons unless complications such as paresthesia happen [11].

Several studies and clinical cases showed that CBCT is the best radiographic technique for CS visualization [16]. The CBCT examinations in the case showed that the accessory damaged canal of canalis sinuosus was buccal to the lateral incisor; according to von Arx et al. [12] and Machado et al. [9], the end of the CS was most frequently found palatal to the anterior maxillary teeth especially to the central incisors.

Though CBCT provides accurate three-dimensional images of dentomaxillofacial hard tissues [24], its limitation is the presence of image artefacts—deviations between the reconstructed image and the real content of the studied object [25]. A dental implant is a high-density structure that is the source of beam hardening resulting in the artefacts [26]. That is why after suspecting CS damage in the postoperative CBCT scans, it was decided to evaluate the preoperative CBCT scan for better diagnosis without the implant artefact.

During the preoperative CBCT evaluation and dental implant planning, none of the nerve structures around left lateral incisor were noticed. This demonstrates the necessity of knowing the existence of CS and its characteristics, which may influence treatment outcomes.

There are several case reports with dental implants placed in the anterior maxilla and CS damage, presenting the same neurological symptomatology [9, 17]; however, this case additionally contributes the symptoms of trigeminal neuralgia [27] as pain irradiation in the back of the head and no intraoperative excessive bleeding rather than the usual one during the implant site preparation. The tests with the different types of local nerve blocks showed a good diagnostic efficacy indicating the damaged infraorbital nerve branch.

As the damage of the greater palatal and nasopalatine nerve and blood supply was excluded, the palatal mucosa necrosis that appeared after implant extraction could be explained by the contraction of smooth muscle within the arterial wall during the neurovascular bundle constriction that leads to transient ischemia of structures and tissue necrosis [28]. However, the definite terms of the necrosis manifestation are still unclear.

To avoid sensory disturbance in the anterior maxilla in the case of CS detection, Shelley et al. [29] in their case offered a realistic fixed alternative: an adhesive cantilever bridge that had the advantage of very low risk, rapidity of production, and low cost, to potentially damaging implant therapy.

4. Conclusion

This clinical report of immediate implant placement showed the importance of anatomical structure knowledge and accurate and precise preoperative CBCT scan estimation, especially in the esthetic zone. The damage of CS can lead to neurological symptomatology and implant extraction.

We suggest that single-tooth defects with the risk of CS damage in the region should be restored without implant treatment or with the use of surgical guides designed for fully guided implant placement.

Consent

Written consent was signed by the patient for every procedure.

References

[1] N. P. Lang, L. Pun, K. Y. Lau, K. Y. Li, and M. C. M. Wong, "A systematic review on survival and success rates of implants placed immediately into fresh extraction sockets after at least 1 year," *Clinical Oral Implants Research*, vol. 23, Suppl. 5, pp. 39–66, 2012.

[2] D. Clark and L. Levin, "Dental implant management and maintenance: how to improve long-term implant success?," *Quintessence International*, vol. 47, no. 5, pp. 417–423, 2016.

[3] B. R. Chrcanovic, T. Albrektsson, and A. Wennerberg, "Reasons for failures of oral implants," *Journal of Oral Rehabilitation*, vol. 41, no. 6, pp. 443–476, 2014.

[4] G. Greenstein, J. R. Carpentieri, and J. Cavallaro, "Nerve damage related to implant dentistry: incidence, diagnosis, and management," *The Compendium of Continuing Education in Dentistry*, vol. 36, no. 9, pp. 652–659, 2015.

[5] C. Oliveira-Santos, I. R. F. Rubira-Bullen, S. A. C. Monteiro, J. E. León, and R. Jacobs, "Neurovascular anatomical variations in the anterior palate observed on CBCT images," *Clinical Oral Implants Research*, vol. 24, no. 9, pp. 1044–1048, 2012.

[6] A. M. V. Wanzeler, C. G. Marinho, S. M. A. Junior, F. R. Manzi, and F. M. Tuji, "Anatomical study of the canalis sinuosus in 100 cone beam computed tomography examinations," *Oral and Maxillofacial Surgery*, vol. 19, no. 1, pp. 49–53, 2015.

[7] T. von Arx and S. Lozanoff, "Anterior superior alveolar nerve (ASAN)," *Swiss Dental Journal*, vol. 125, no. 11, pp. 1202–1209, 2015.

[8] F. S. Neves, M. Crusoé-Souza, L. C. S. Franco, P. H. F. Caria, P. Bonfim-Almeida, and I. Crusoé-Rebello, "Canalis sinuosus: a rare anatomical variation," *Surgical and Radiologic Anatomy*, vol. 34, no. 6, pp. 563–566, 2012.

[9] V. D. C. Machado, B. R. Chrcanovic, M. B. Felippe, L. R. C. Manhães Júnior, and P. S. P. de Carvalho, "Assessment of accessory canals of the canalis sinuosus: a study of 1000 cone beam computed tomography examinations," *International Journal of Oral and Maxillofacial Surgery*, vol. 45, no. 12, pp. 1586–1591, 2016.

[10] L. R. C. Manhães Júnior, M. F. L. Villaça-Carvalho, M. E. L. Moraes, S. L. P. de Castro Lopes, M. B. F. Silva, and J. L. C. Junqueira, "Location and classification of canalis sinuosus for cone beam computed tomography: avoiding misdiagnosis," *Brazilian Oral Research*, vol. 30, no. 1, pp. 1–8, 2016.

[11] G. Gurler, C. Delilbasi, E. E. Ogut, K. Aydin, and U. Sakul, "Evaluation of the morphology of the canalis sinuosus using cone-beam computed tomography in patients with maxillary impacted canines," *Imaging Science in Dentistry*, vol. 47, no. 2, pp. 69–74, 2017.

[12] T. Von Arx, S. Lozanoff, P. Sendi, and M. M. Bornstein, "Assessment of bone channels other than the nasopalatine canal in the anterior maxilla using limited cone beam computed tomography," *Surgical and Radiologic Anatomy*, vol. 35, no. 9, pp. 783–790, 2013.

[13] M. G. G. Torres, L. de Faro Valverde, M. T. A. Vidal, and I. M. Crusoé-Rebello, "Branch of the canalis sinuosus: a rare anatomical variation – a case report," *Surgical and Radiologic Anatomy*, vol. 37, no. 7, pp. 879–881, 2015.

[14] S. J. J. McCrea, "Aberrations causing neurovascular damage in the anterior maxilla during dental implant placement," *Case Reports in Dentistry*, vol. 2017, Article ID 5969643, 10 pages, 2017.

[15] R. Jacobs, M. Quirynen, and M. M. Bornstein, "Neurovascular disturbances after implant surgery," *Periodontol 2000*, vol. 66, no. 1, pp. 188–202, 2014.

[16] R. Ferlin, B. S. C. Pagin, and R. Y. F. Yaedú, "Canalis Sinuosus: A Systematic Review of the Literature," *Oral Surgery, Oral Medicine, Oral Pathology and Oral Radiology*, vol. 127, no. 6, pp. 545–551, 2019.

[17] J. A. Arruda, P. Silva, L. Silva et al., "Dental implant in the canalis sinuosus: a case report and review of the literature," *Case Reports in Dentistry*, vol. 2017, Article ID 4810123, 5 pages, 2017.

[18] W. Shaeffer, "A case of intractable pain in the anterior maxilla following dental implant placement," in *Association of Dental Implantology Members' National Forum*, London, UK, 2015.

[19] T. Genç, O. Duruel, H. Kutlu, E. Dursun, E. Karabulut, and T. Tözüm, "Evaluation of anatomical structures and variations in the maxilla and the mandible before dental implant treatment," *Dental and Medical Problems*, vol. 55, no. 3, pp. 233–240, 2018 Jul-Sep.

[20] S. H. Chung, Y. S. Park, S. H. Chung, and W. J. Shon, "Determination of Implant Position for Immediate Implant Placement in Maxillary Central Incisors Using Palatal Soft Tissue Landmarks," *The International Journal of Oral & Maxillofacial Implants*, vol. 29, no. 3, pp. 627–633, 2014 May-Jun.

[21] I. Urban, *Vertical and horizontal ridge augmentation: new perspectives*, Quintessence Publishing, Germany, 1st Edition edition, 2017.

[22] I. A. Urban, H. Nagursky, J. L. Lozada, and K. Nagy, "Horizontal ridge augmentation with a collagen membrane and a combination of particulated autogenous bone and anorganic bovine bone-derived mineral: a prospective case series in 25 patients," *The International Journal of Periodontics and Restorative Dentistry*, vol. 33, no. 3, pp. 299–307, 2013.

[23] F. W. Jones, "The anterior superior alveolar nerve and vessels," *Journal of Anatomy*, vol. 73, Part 4, pp. 583–591, 1939.

[24] K. Abramovitch and D. D. Rice, "Basic principles of cone beam computed tomography," *Dental Clinics of North America*, vol. 58, no. 3, pp. 463–484, 2014.

[25] S. R. Makins, "Artifacts Interfering with Interpretation of Cone Beam Computed Tomography Images," *Dental Clinics of North America*, vol. 58, no. 3, pp. 485–495, 2014.

[26] A. Parsa, N. Ibrahim, B. Hassan, P. van der Stelt, and D. Wismeijer, "Influence of object location in cone beam computed tomography (NewTom 5G and 3D Accuitomo 170) on gray value measurements at an implant site," *Oral Radiology*, vol. 30, pp. 153–159, 2014.

[27] J. M. Zakrzewska and M. E. Linskey, "Trigeminal neuralgia," *BMJ*, vol. 348, no. feb17 9, p. g474, 2014.

[28] N. Gogna, S. Hussain, and S. Al-Rawi, "Case reports: palatal mucosal necrosis after administration of a palatal infiltration," *British Dental Journal*, vol. 219, no. 12, pp. 560-561, 2015.

[29] A. Shelley, J. Tinning, J. Yates, and K. Horner, "Potential neurovascular damage as a result of dental implant placement in the anterior maxilla," *British Dental Journal*, vol. 226, no. 9, pp. 657–661, 2019.

15

Novel use of Silicone Sheets for Immediate Implant Placement in Fresh Molar Extraction Sockets

Won-Pyo Lee,[1] Jae-Heung Choi,[2] Sang-Joun Yu,[1] and Byung-Ock Kim[1]

[1]*Department of Periodontology, School of Dentistry, Chosun University, 309 Pilmun-daero, Dong-gu, Gwangju 61452, Republic of Korea*
[2]*Department of Preventive and Public Health Dentistry, School of Dentistry, Chosun University, 309 Pilmun-daero, Dong-gu, Gwangju 61452, Republic of Korea*

Correspondence should be addressed to Byung-Ock Kim; bobkim@chosun.ac.kr

Academic Editor: Asja Celebic

In the recent years, the immediate placement of dental implants into fresh extraction sites has become an acceptable treatment approach. However, immediate molar implant placement presents specific challenges because of the anatomical and physiologic limitations. Such implant surgeries commonly require procedures that use a barrier membrane to generate bone and soft tissue or one that seals the molar extraction socket through a coronally advanced flap. Here, as an alternative, we report a method for treating molar extraction socket wounds in the hard and soft tissues after immediate placement of an implant using a silicone sheet.

1. Introduction

In the recent years, the immediate placement of an implant into the fresh extraction socket has become a popular surgical procedure, as it improves patient comport and shortens treatment period. This not only reduces the time until the implant can be restored but also results in fewer surgical procedures and has a high success rate [1–3].

However, because of anatomical and physiological limitations, the immediate placement of dental implants into fresh molar extraction sockets may be adversely affected by the osseous socket anatomy, lack of soft tissue closure, and flap dehiscence over the extraction site [4]. Such an implant surgery commonly requires procedures that use bone graft material and a barrier membrane to generate bone and soft tissue between the fixture and extraction socket [5] or one that seals the extraction socket through a coronally advanced flap [6]. However, these procedures require vast clinical experience, and the use of a barrier membrane is accompanied by an increase in the cost and risk of infection [7, 8]. Furthermore, additional flap manipulation involves a time-consuming series of procedures that causes unnecessary stress to patients [9, 10].

Medical grade silicone sheets have been widely used in the medical field. Because silicone sheets are available in a wide range of sizes and thicknesses, these sheets can be customized by the surgeon into different configurations and sizes to meet individual procedure requirements to provide flexibility for each patient [11–13].

Therefore, we hereby report a method for treating molar extraction socket wounds in hard and soft tissues after immediate placement of an implant using medical grade U-shaped silicone sheets.

2. Case Reports

2.1. Silicone Cap. The silicone cap was a custom-made silicone fragment. We used a commercially available, elastic, sterile, and U-shaped medical grade 1 mm thick silicone sheet (Kuwotech, Gwangju, Korea) (Figure 1(a)). Using an Irish scissor, we cut the silicone sheet at least 2–3 mm longer than the extraction socket in both the buccal and lingual directions, covering the extraction socket completely. We then made a hole with a diameter smaller than that of the healing abutment using a custom-made punching tool (Kuwotech, Gwangju, Korea) (Figure 1(b)). The diameter of

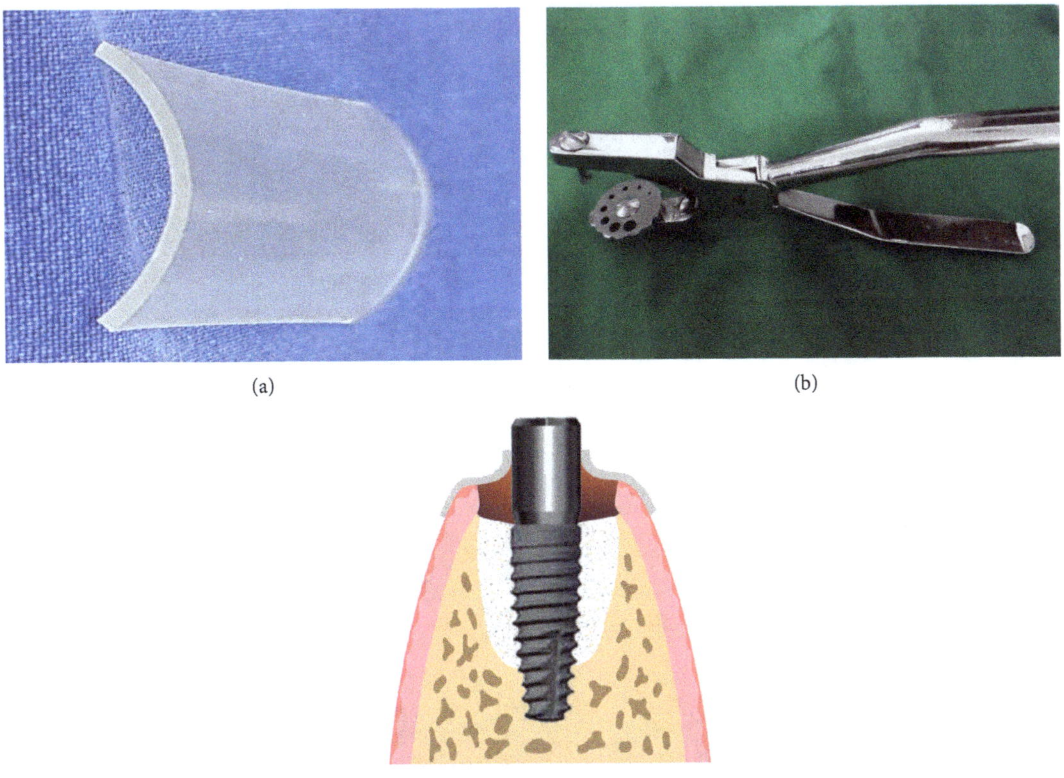

FIGURE 1: (a) Medical grade U-shaped silicone sheet. (b) Punching tool to produce silicone caps. (c) A schematic diagram of a silicone cap placed over a cylinder-type healing abutment.

the cylinder-type healing abutment (Kuwotech, Gwangju, Korea) was 4.5 mm and that of the hole in the silicone cap was 2.5 mm. When the silicone cap, stretched using pincettes, is placed over the healing abutment fastened to an implant fixture, the hole portion of the silicone cap that touches the healing abutment is pulled upward by frictional force. In response, a compressive force is generated in the soft tissue around the extraction socket at the margin of the U-shaped silicone cap (Figure 1(c)) [14].

2.2. Case 1. A 56-year-old female patient with an overall healthy oral state visited the clinic for implant placement after the removal of a retained right mandibular 1st molar (tooth 46) root (Figures 2(a) and 2(b)). After local anesthesia, the dental root was separated using a high-speed handpiece and #558 bur, followed by careful atraumatic extraction using an elevator. After drilling into the interradicular septum using only a 4 mm diameter trephine bur to obtain autologous bone, a 10 mm long and 5 mm diameter implant (Any-One, Megagen Implant Co., Seoul, Korea) was inserted 1 mm deeper than the height of the buccolingual alveolar ridge. The gap between the inserted fixture and extraction socket was about 4 mm in both the buccolingual and mesiodistal directions (Figure 2(c)). The gap between the extraction socket and implant was filled with autologous particulate bone obtained by grinding the bone core made by the trephine bur (Figure 2(d)). After equipping it with a cylinder-type healing abutment (Figure 2(e)), a silicone cap was fabricated as described earlier and then placed over the healing abutment because it was easily stretched using the pincettes (Figure 2(f)). Except for the force that exerted light pressure on the soft tissues around the extraction socket, the installed silicone cap showed no movement (Figure 2(g)). Thus, without making an incision or using sutures and a barrier membrane, the extraction socket was sealed using only autologous bone and a silicone cap. The silicone cap is seen as a radiopacity on a radiograph (Figure 2(h)).

The patient was instructed to be careful not to dislodge the cap with their tongue, masticatory movements, or by brushing. The patient was advised to rinse with a 0.1% chlorhexidine digluconate solution (Hexomedine solution, Bukwang Pharm. Co., Seoul, Korea) twice daily for 2 weeks. Additionally, the patient was prescribed with antibiotics (Augmentin 625 mg, Ilsung Pharm. Co., Seoul, Korea) three times a day for 7 days. On clinical images taken at 2 weeks postinsertion, plaque bacteria were observed adhering to the healing abutment, but not the silicon cap, with only slight discoloration (Figure 3(a)). The cap also did not create a foreign body reaction or cause pain to the patient. Although the surrounding gingival margin was temporally suppressed by compression due to the silicon cap, healthy soft tissue regenerated, completely sealing the extraction socket (Figure 3(b)). At 2 months after the removal of the cap, the suppressed soft tissue had healed completely (Figure 3(c)). A final prosthesis was provided at 6 months after implant insertion, and healthy attached gingiva formed around the final prosthesis (Figure 3(d)), showing integration with the surrounding gingival margin, including the mucogingival junction (MGJ)

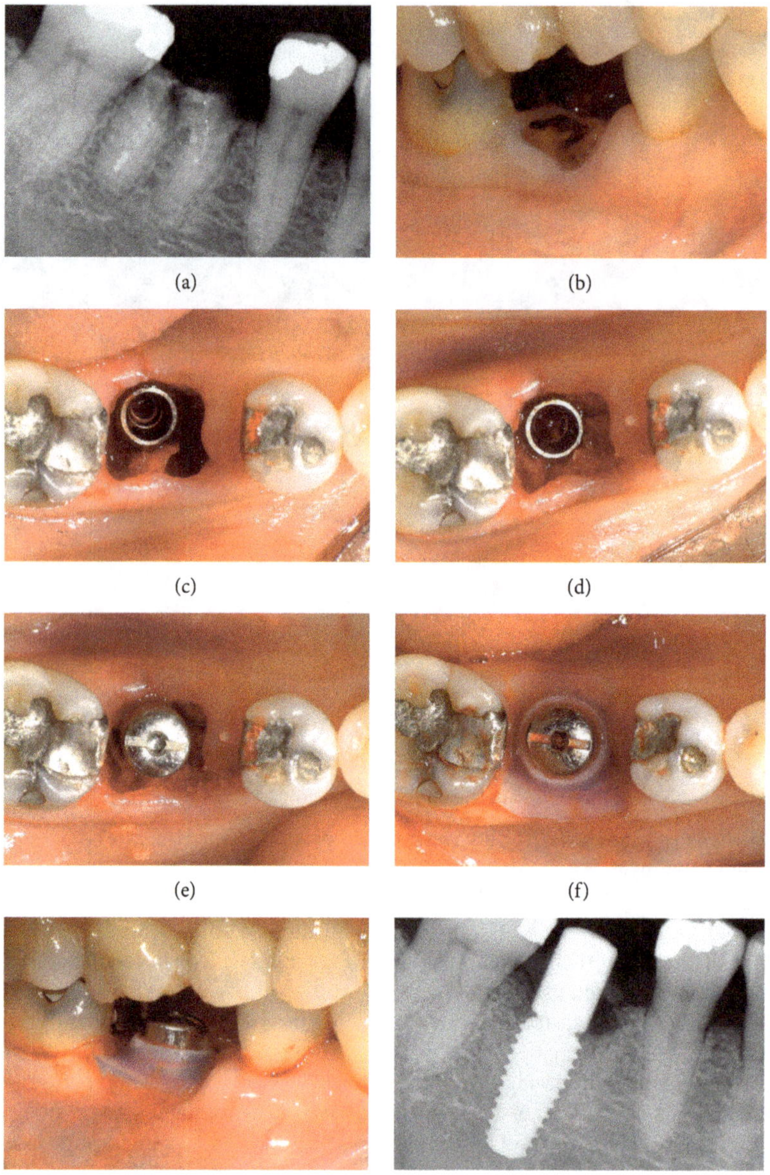

(a) (b) (c) (d) (e) (f) (g) (h)

FIGURE 2: (a) Periapical radiograph of tooth 46 from the initial examination. (b) Buccal view of tooth 46 at the initial examination. (c) Implant inserted into interradicular septum. (d) Clinical condition after gap filling with autologous particulate bone. (e) Clinical condition after the installation of a cylinder-type healing abutment. (f) Occlusal view after the application of silicone cap on healing abutment. (g) Buccal view after the application of silicone cap on healing abutment. (h) Periapical radiograph immediately after surgery.

line (Figure 3(e)). Furthermore, regenerated bone tissue was observed on the radiograph (Figure 3(f)). A radiograph taken at 22 months postoperatively also showed a well-maintained alveolar bone height (Figure 3(g)).

2.3. Case 2. A 42-year-old male patient was admitted for a retained dental root and root apex lesion at tooth 16 and required an implant prosthesis for an extracted tooth 17 (Figure 4(a)). Computed tomography (Figure 4(b)) revealed that the retained bone height was insufficient due to the large root apex lesion of tooth 16. After atraumatic extraction of tooth 16, bone-added osteotome sinus floor elevation (BAOSFE) was performed using allogenic bone (SureOss, Osstem Implant Co., Seoul, Korea) to enhance the primary fixation of the implant. This BAOSFE procedure was performed using a drill and osteotome according to Summers' original technique [15]. A 13 mm long and 6 mm diameter implant (AnyOne, Megagen Implant Co., Seoul, Korea) was then immediately inserted with insertion torque exceeding 40 N cm (Figure 4(c)); the implant was inserted 1 mm deeper than the height of the alveolar ridge of the extraction socket. After collecting 10 cm^3 of peripheral blood, platelet-rich fibrin (PRF) was prepared using a centrifuge (MF550, Hanil Science Industrial Co., Incheon, Korea). After application of the cylinder-type healing abutment, the gap in the extraction socket was filled with allograft material (SureOss, Osstem Implant Co., Seoul, Korea) up to the height of the alveolar ridge of the extraction socket, followed by filling with the

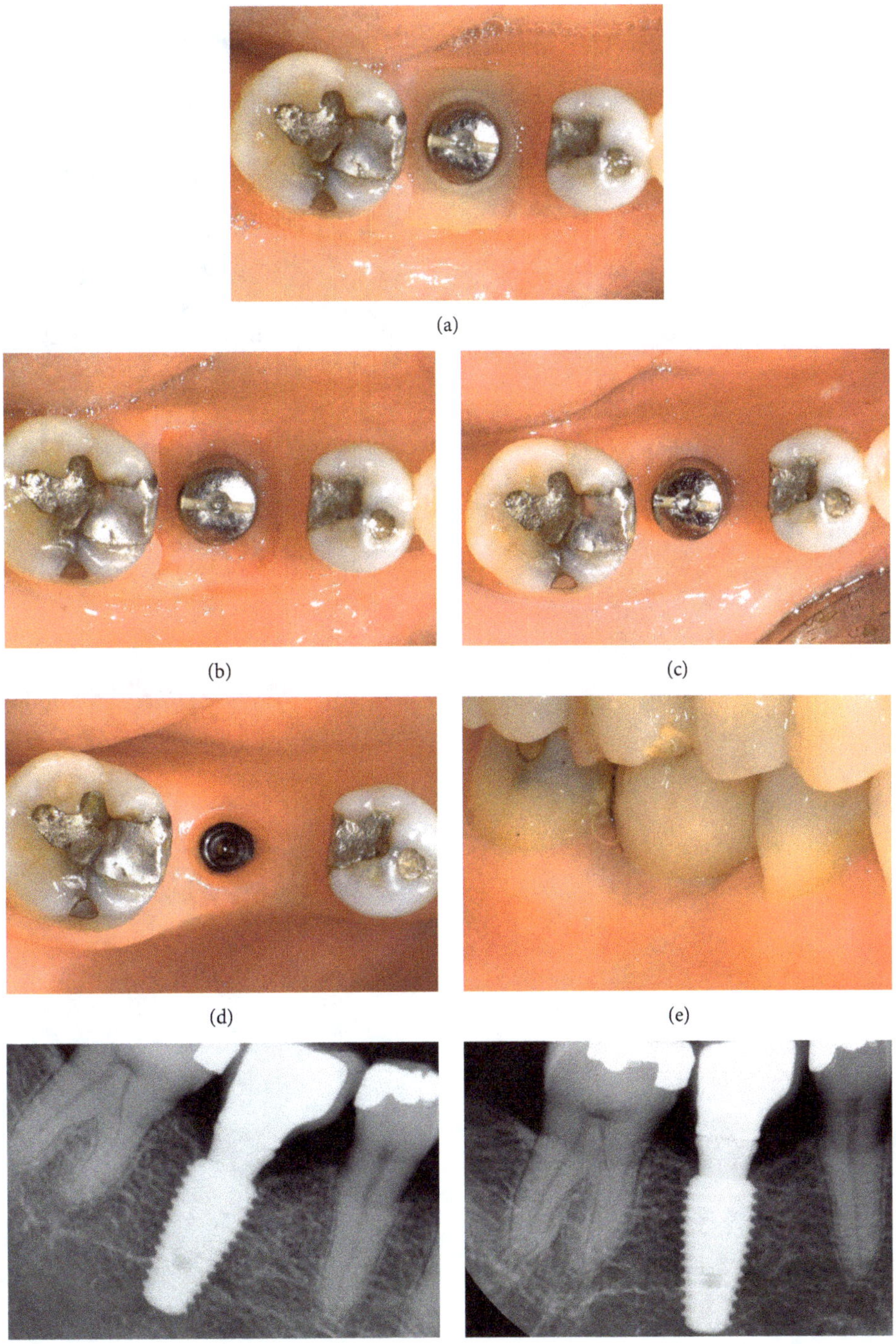

(a) (b) (c) (d) (e) (f) (g)

Figure 3: (a) Clinical condition before the removal of the silicone cap at 2 weeks postoperatively. (b) Soft tissue condition after the removal of the silicone cap at 2 weeks postoperatively. (c) Clinical condition at 2.5 months postoperatively. (d) Clinical condition at 6 months postoperatively before the application of the final prosthesis. (e) Buccal view at 6 months postoperatively with the final prosthesis. (f) Radiograph at 6 months postoperatively. (g) Radiograph at 22 months postoperatively.

PRF membrane up to the height of the soft tissue in the extraction socket (Figure 4(d)). Due to gingival tearing during extraction, two interrupted nonabsorbable sutures (Dafilon 5-0, B. Braun, Melsungen, Germany) were inserted. After fabricating a silicone cap as described earlier, it was placed over the healing abutment (Figures 4(e) and 4(f)). Using a flapless technique, a nonsubmerged 13 mm long and 5 mm diameter implant (AnyOne, Megagen Implant Co., Seoul, Korea) was inserted into the region of tooth 17, where the ridge had healed, accompanied by BAOSFE to enhance the primary fixation of the implant.

At 2 weeks postinsertion, the cleanly maintained silicone cap and sutures were removed (Figure 5(a)); the extraction socket showed satisfactory healing, with soft tissue formation

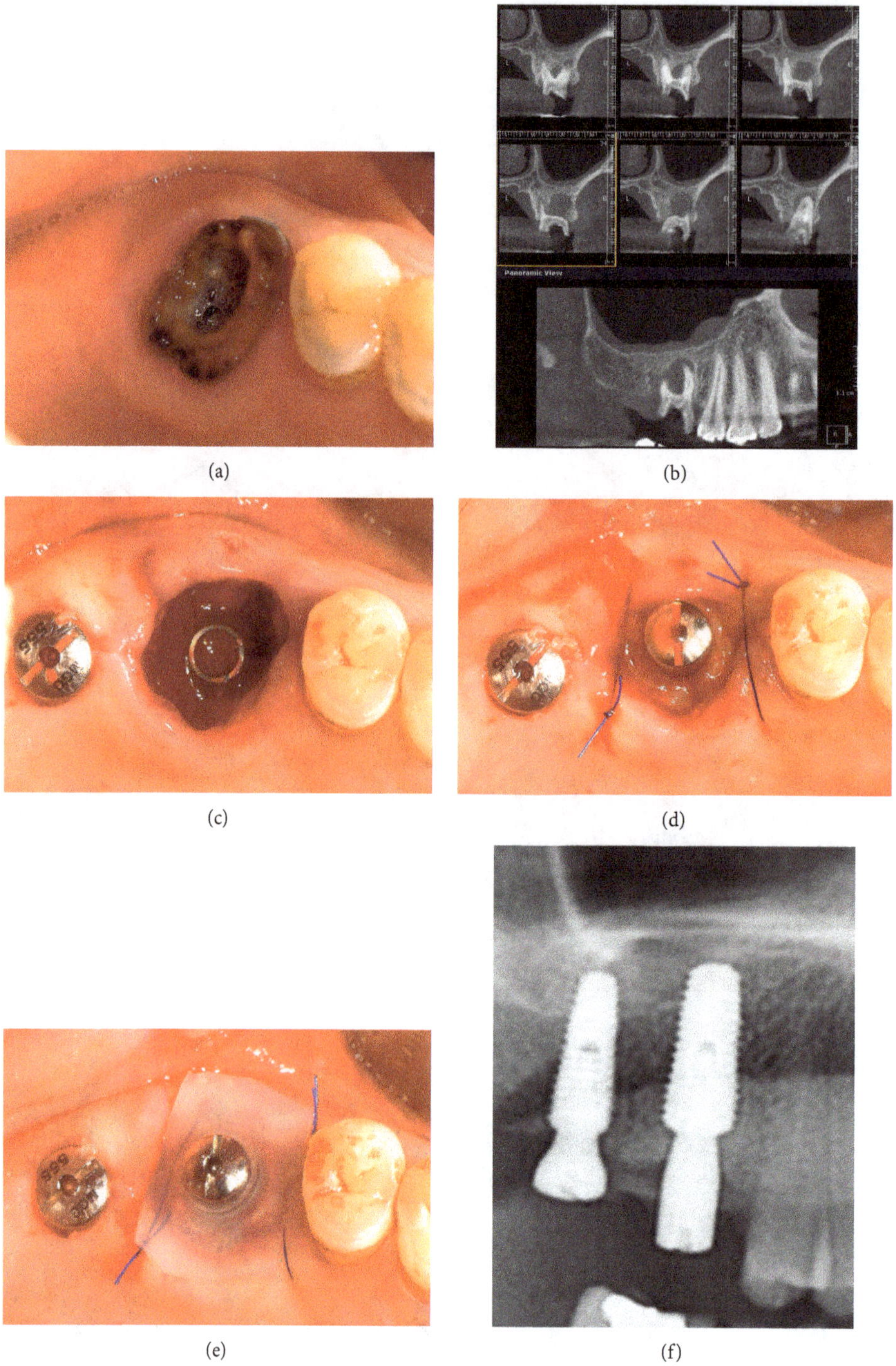

FIGURE 4: (a) Occlusal view at the initial examination. (b) Cone beam computerized tomography image at the initial examination. (c) Occlusal view immediately after the insertion of the implant. (d) Clinical condition of the interrupted sutures after gap filling of the extraction socket with allogenic bone and PRF. (e) Application of the silicone cap. (f) Radiograph taken immediately after implant insertion.

(Figure 5(b)). The final prosthesis was applied 8 months postoperatively. The soft tissue initially suppressed by the silicone cap was restored, and a well-formed attached gingiva was observed (Figure 5(c)). In addition, stable bone tissue was observed around the inserted implant neck, and increased vertical alveolar bone was observed under the implant (Figure 5(d)). Clinical and radiographic evaluation at 2 years postoperatively revealed a healthy gingival margin and satisfactory stability (Figures 5(e) and 5(f)).

3. Discussion

These cases demonstrate the potential for the application of a silicone cap in the immediate placement of molar implants. A silicone sheet is durable, flexible, thin, and easily manipulated and can completely cover the extraction socket or surgical area. Thus, it can prevent infection and protect the blood clot that is required for soft tissue healing at the extraction socket [13]. This can simplify the surgery required for

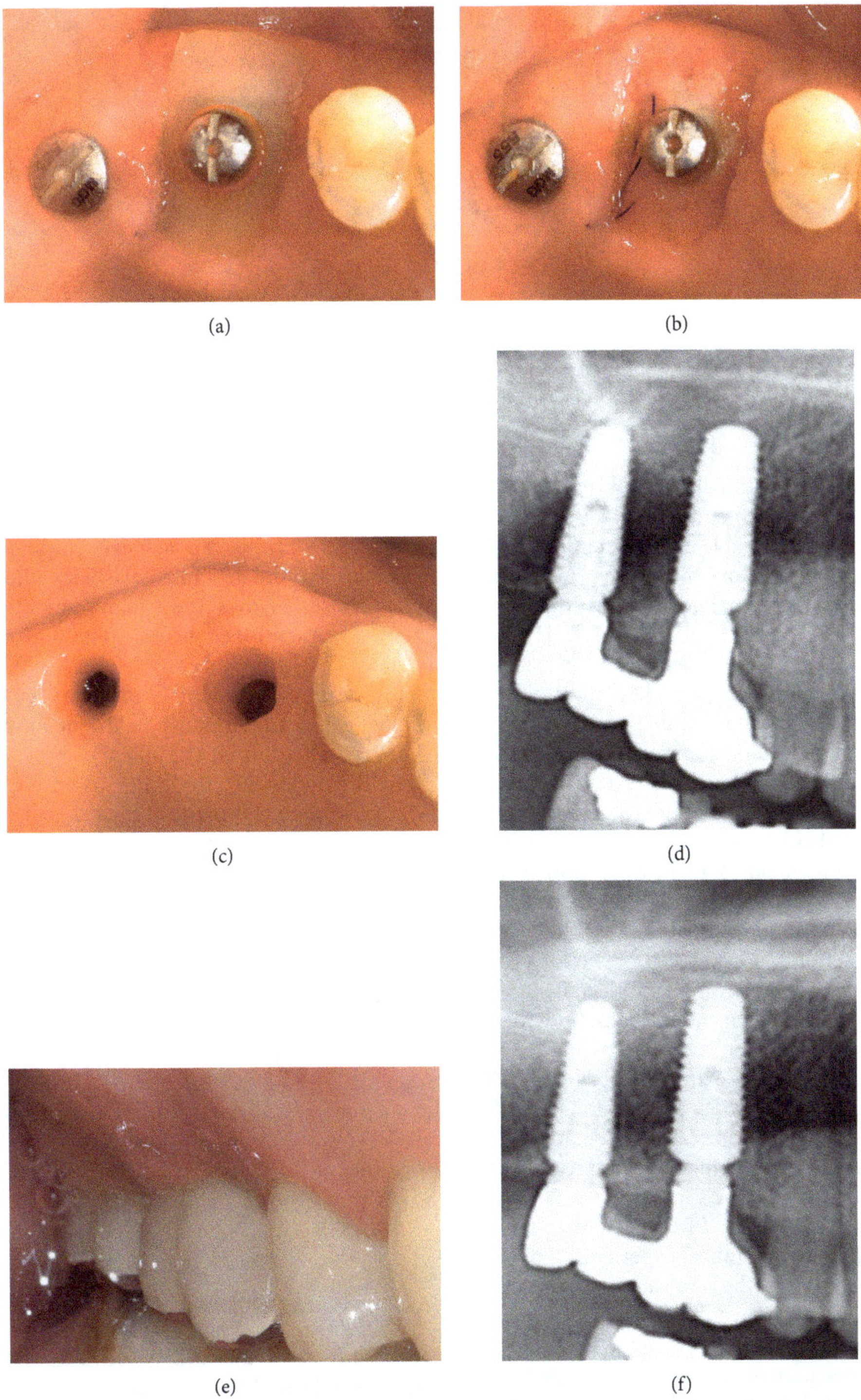

FIGURE 5: (a) Clean silicone cap at 2 weeks postoperatively. (b) Healing condition of the extraction socket at 2 weeks postoperatively. (c) Clinical condition before the application of the final prosthesis at 8 months after surgery. (d) Radiograph taken after the application of the final prosthesis at 8 months after surgery. (e) Buccal view at 2 years after surgery. (f) Radiographic view at 2 years after surgery.

the immediate placement of a dental implant, because the need for incision, dissection, periosteal-releasing incision, and suturing of the flap is eliminated or minimized. Additionally, since a coronally advanced flap is not required for extraction socket closure, the physiological MGJ line is preserved prior to extraction, enhancing the attachment of the gingiva.

Many previous attempts at sealing extraction sockets after immediate molar implant placement have been reported. Zafiropoulos et al. reported the use of a nonresorbable high-density polytetrafluoroethylene covering membrane in an open membrane technique [16]. Cafiero et al. reported that immediate transmucosal implant placement using a resorbable collagen membrane was a predictable treatment option

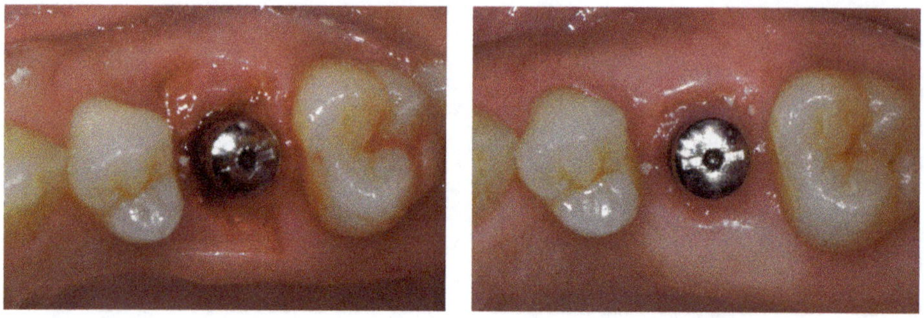

(a) (b)

FIGURE 6: Other case that PRF membrane was not used for immediate implant placement in fresh maxillary molar extraction socket (tooth 26). (a) Poor healing condition of the extraction socket at 2 weeks postoperatively. (b) Healing condition of the extraction socket at 8 weeks postoperatively.

[17]. However, both methods require flap elevation and complex sutures to place each barrier membrane precisely. Additionally, in the case of a nonresorbable membrane, additional invasive surgery is required to remove the barrier membrane. Jiansheng et al. attempted to seal the molar extraction socket by using a healing abutment with a wide diameter [18]. In this study, one of the 162 implants failed before prosthetic restoration, resulting in a success rate of 99.4%. However, this also required additional flap manipulation and sutures to attach the flap closely to the healing abutment, which caused some loss of gingival attachment. For full-mouth implant-supported rehabilitation of the upper jaw, Malchiodi et al. inserted immediately loaded implants after tooth extraction [19]. In this case, they attempted to attain extraction socket sealing using a temporary prosthesis. However, the indication for an immediately loaded implant is limited in the molar region, unlike in the anterior region. Thus, silicone caps may be an alternative to immediate molar implant placement.

There are several points requiring attention in immediate implant placement using a silicone cap. The use of a PRF membrane is recommended for the extraction socket of both maxillary and mandibular molars when performing immediate implant placement using a silicone cap. For a mandibular molar, desirable healing of the soft tissue is observed only when a clot is present in the extraction socket at 2 weeks postoperatively, even without using PRF membrane under the silicone cap according to our clinical experience. For this reason, we generally recommend the removal of silicone caps at 2 weeks postoperatively. However, when the PRF membrane was not used for maxillary molars, poor healing was observed when the upper part of the extraction socket was filled with a mixture of new soft tissue and graft material used for gap filling (Figure 6(a)). Furthermore, it took 4-8 weeks longer for appropriate soft tissue healing in the extraction socket (Figure 6(b)). It has been postulated that this poor healing was caused by inhibition of soft tissue healing, because graft material from the maxilla was moved to the upper region of the extraction socket by gravity. In contrast, when a PRF membrane was used to cover the graft material, these issues were resolved (Figure 5(b)). In particular, the PRF membrane produced more favorable results due to the healing-promoting effect of growth factors on soft tissue in the extraction socket [20].

Moreover, it has been recommended that a cylinder-type healing abutment, rather than the tapered type, should be used. The silicone cap achieves sealing of the extraction socket due to the generated elasticity when a small punched hole is inserted over the healing abutment, requiring it to stretch as mentioned before (Figure 1(c)). However, it is impossible to obtain a complete seal of the extraction socket if the healing abutment is of the tapered type, where the diameter becomes smaller in the downward direction, and there is a chance that the silicone cap will be pushed inside the extraction socket, inhibiting its healing. In contrast, when using a healing abutment of the cylinder type, with the same diameter in its upper and lower parts, a stable extraction socket sealing effect is maintained over a period of time according to our clinical experience.

4. Conclusion

In these case reports, we have presented a new method for immediate implant placement after molar extraction using a silicone cap. Although it has been suggested that a good clinical outcome can be obtained with this technique, further investigation with long-term data and a larger sample size is needed to verify this approach.

Acknowledgments

This study was supported by the research fund from Chosun University Dental Hospital, 2018.

References

[1] S. Valenzuela, J. M. Olivares, N. Weiss, and D. Benadof, "Immediate implant placement by interradicular bone drilling before molar extraction: clinical case report with one-year follow-up," *Case Reports in Dentistry*, vol. 2018, Article ID 6412826, 5 pages, 2018.

[2] T. Urban, L. Kostopoulos, and A. Wenzel, "Immediate implant placement in molar regions: risk factors for early failure," *Clinical Oral Implants Research*, vol. 23, no. 2, pp. 220–227, 2012.

[3] D. Botticelli, T. Berglundh, and J. Lindhe, "Hard-tissue alterations following immediate implant placement in extraction sites," *Journal of Clinical Periodontology*, vol. 31, no. 10, pp. 820–828, 2004.

[4] T. J. Griffin and W. S. Cheung, "The use of short, wide implants in posterior areas with reduced bone height: a retrospective investigation," *The Journal of Prosthetic Dentistry*, vol. 92, no. 2, pp. 139–144, 2004.

[5] O. Hoffmann, B. K. Bartee, C. Beaumont, A. Kasaj, G. Deli, and G. G. Zafiropoulos, "Alveolar bone preservation in extraction sockets using non-resorbable dPTFE membranes: a retrospective non-randomized study," *Journal of Periodontology*, vol. 79, no. 8, pp. 1355–1369, 2008.

[6] B. Rosenquist, "A comparison of various methods of soft tissue management following the immediate placement of implants into extraction sockets," *The International Journal of Oral & Maxillofacial Implants*, vol. 12, no. 1, pp. 43–51, 1997.

[7] W. Becker, P. Hujoel, and B. E. Becker, "Effect of barrier membranes and autologous bone grafts on ridge width preservation around implants," *Clinical Implant Dentistry and Related Research*, vol. 4, no. 3, pp. 143–149, 2002.

[8] H. D. Barber, J. Lignelli, B. M. Smith, and B. K. Bartee, "Using a dense PTFE membrane without primary closure to achieve bone and tissue regeneration," *Journal of Oral and Maxillofacial Surgery*, vol. 65, no. 4, pp. 748–752, 2007.

[9] C. E. Nemcovsky, Z. Artzi, and O. Moses, "Rotated palatal flap in immediate implant procedures. Clinical evaluation of 26 consecutive cases," *Clinical Oral Implants Research*, vol. 11, no. 1, pp. 83–90, 2000.

[10] B. Rosenquist and M. Ahmed, "The immediate replacement of teeth by dental implants using homologous bone membranes to seal the sockets: clinical and radiographic findings," *Clinical Oral Implants Research*, vol. 11, no. 6, pp. 572–582, 2000.

[11] J. S. Baek, S. Lee, J. H. Lee, H. S. Choi, J. W. Jang, and S. J. Kim, "Predictors of silicone tube intubation success in patients with lacrimal drainage system stenosis," *Korean Journal of Ophthalmology*, vol. 30, no. 3, pp. 157–162, 2016.

[12] M. Kabuto, T. Kubota, H. Kobayashi et al., "Long-term evaluation of reconstruction of the sellar floor with a silicone plate in transsphenoidal surgery," *Journal of Neurosurgery*, vol. 88, no. 6, pp. 949–953, 1998.

[13] J. R. Parry, H. D. Stupak, and C. M. Johnson, "The immediate use of a silicone sheet wound closure device in scar reduction and prevention," *Ear, Nose, & Throat Journal*, vol. 95, no. 2, pp. E27–E33, 2016.

[14] W. P. Lee, "How to make a silicone cap [video file]," December 2018, https://www.youtube.com/watch?v=eI5zsWExDDk&feature=youtu.be.

[15] R. B. Summers, "The osteotome technique: part 3: less invasive methods of elevating the sinus floor," *Compendium*, vol. 15, no. 6, pp. 698–708, 1994.

[16] G. G. Zafiropoulos, A. Kasaj, and O. Hoffmann, "Immediate implant placement in fresh mandibular molar extraction socket: 8-year results. A case report," *The Journal of Oral Implantology*, vol. 36, no. 2, pp. 145–151, 2010.

[17] C. Cafiero, S. Annibali, E. Gherlone et al., "Immediate transmucosal implant placement in molar extraction sites: a 12-month prospective multicenter cohort study," *Clinical Oral Implants Research*, vol. 19, no. 5, pp. 476–482, 2008.

[18] H. Jiansheng, X. Dongying, W. Xianfeng, X. Baoyi, L. Qiong, and Z. Jincai, "Clinical evaluation of short and wide-diameter implants immediately placed into extraction sockets of posterior areas: a 2-year retrospective study," *The Journal of Oral Implantology*, vol. 38, no. 6, pp. 729–737, 2012.

[19] L. Malchiodi, G. Corrocher, A. Cucchi, P. Ghensi, G. Bissolotti, and P. F. Nocini, "Long-term results of immediately loaded fast bone regeneration-coated implants placed in fresh extraction sites in the upper jaw," *The Journal of Oral Implantology*, vol. 36, no. 4, pp. 251–261, 2010.

[20] M. Arunachalam, S. J. Pulikkotil, and N. Sonia, "Platelet rich fibrin in periodontal regeneration," *The Open Dentistry Journal*, vol. 10, no. M4, Supplement 1, pp. 174–181, 2016.

16

Full-Mouth Screw-Retained Implant-Supported Rehabilitation with Multiunit Abutments Using Virtual Guided Surgery and Digital Prosthetics Protocol

Igor Ashurko,[1] Artem Trofimov,[2] Svetlana Tarasenko,[1] and Sabina Mekhtieva[1]

[1]*Department of Surgery Dentistry Institute of Dentistry, Federal State Autonomous Educational Institution of Higher Training I.M. Sechenov First Moscow State Medical University of the Ministry of Health of the Russian Federation (Sechenov University), 8-2 Trubetskaya St., 119991 Moscow, Russia*
[2]*Dental Clinic(Rio-Stom), 9 Veliyaminovskaya St., 105318 Moscow, Russia*

Correspondence should be addressed to Igor Ashurko; ashurko@yandex.ru

Academic Editor: Mariano A. Polack

Total rehabilitation is one of the most sophisticated kinds of dental implant-supported prosthetics. The usage of multiunit abutment system allows the clinician an accurate and passive fitting of screw-retained full-arch construction. In addition, it retains a condition of soft and bone tissues around prosthetic construction. The aim of this case is to demonstrate a modern approach in planning and realisation of full-mouth screw-retained dental implant prosthetics. A 59-year-old patient had an extraction of all failed teeth on upper and lower jaws with immediate 16 implant placement (8 implants on maxilla and 8 implants on mandible) using surgical template. Multiunit abutments were installed intraoperatively. Temporary constructions were fixed immediately after surgery. After 3 months of dental impressions, plaster models and their scan were prepared to make final screw-retained zirconium dioxide constructions. Reevaluation of functional and aesthetic result of the treatment was made after 12 months.

1. Background

Dental implantation is a well-documented treatment of partial or full adentia [1, 2]. Success indications of total rehabilitation with dental implants are high and directly depend on preoperative planning [3, 4]. Modern CAD/CAM technologies give maximally accurate choice of size and position of dental implants and furthermore allow precise placement according to preoperative planning. However, the choice of cement or screw fixation of prosthetic construction is still a subject of discussion [5–8]. One of the significant problems of full-arch implant-supported prosthesis is to reach the passive fitting. Perfect passive fit is achieved when the opposing surfaces of the implants and the framework intaglio are in maximal spatial congruency, without strains in the components after tightening of all screws, provided the implant and framework surfaces are fabricated perfectly plain [9]. Screw retaining from bone level platform may not secure the passive fitting of construction. Moreover, at this type of fixation, complications may vary from a fracture of various components in implant suprastructure system to an implant fracture or failure of its osseointegration [6, 10]. On the other side, cement retaining can provide passive fitting due to cement space between the abutment and prosthesis, but this type of fixation may provide other complications like the absence of maintenance service possibility and risk of peri-implantitis development because of excess cement in the peri-implant area, more specifically in soft tissues [11–13]. In this regard, the use of multiunit abutment system is an option for making screw-retained implant-supported prosthetic constructions. The multiunit abutments provide absolutely passive fitting of prosthesis even with significant divergence of placed implant axes. Furthermore, intraoperative multiunit abutment placement protects peri-implant soft tissues from damaging by multiple screwing/unscrewing implant suprastructures, because all manipulations will

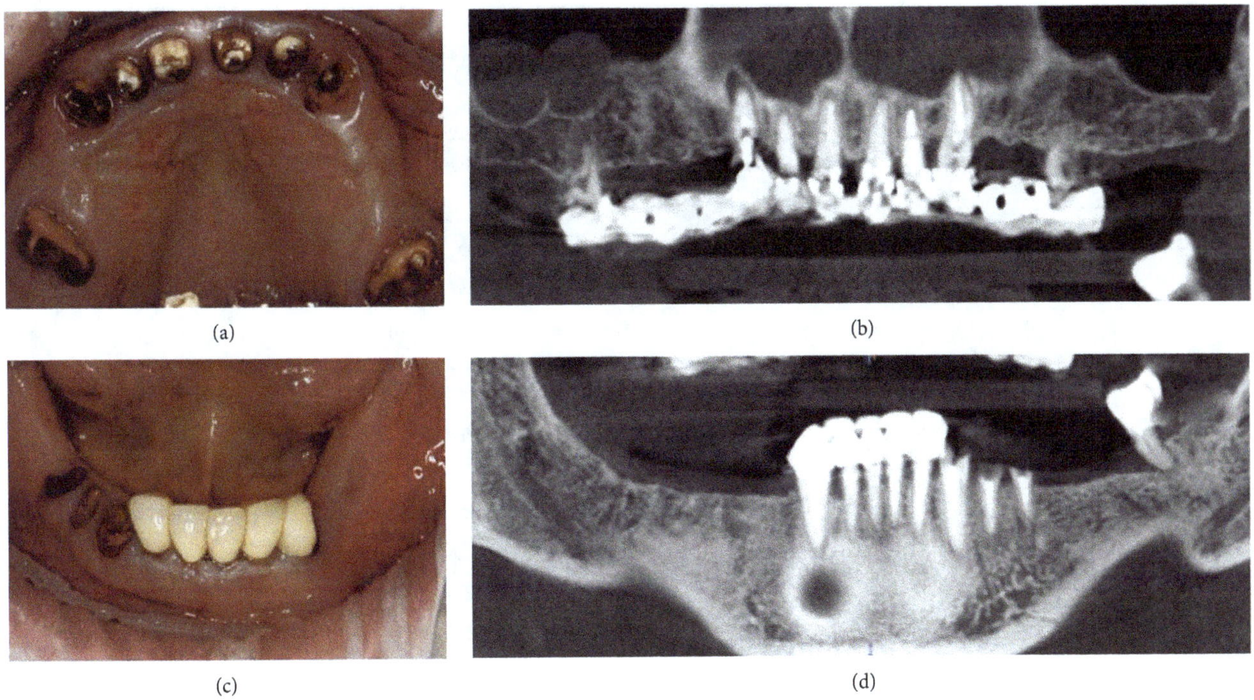

FIGURE 1: Maxillary (a, b) and mandibular (c, d) teeth condition: multiple carious lesions, absence of ferrule-effect, and periodontal and other changes, which demands for extraction of all decayed teeth.

happen above the bone level and implant platform. This clinical case shows predictable treatment protocol of full-arch implant-supported rehabilitation using guided surgery, intraoperative multiunit abutment choosing, immediate loading, and final prosthetics.

2. Case Presentation

A 59-year-old male patient came to department of surgery dentistry at the Institute of Dentistry (Sechenov University) complaining about partial teeth absence, difficulty in chewing, and dissatisfaction in teeth aesthetics. According to the patient, he loses his teeth gradually over 20 years due to caries and its complications (Figure 1). Prosthetic constructions were made about 10 years ago.

3. Planning

Supporting teeth failure was revealed after cone-beam computed tomography and removal of old prosthetic constructions. The treatment plan was composed under functional and aesthetic analysis, which included the extraction of all teeth with immediate 16 dental implant placement (8 implants for each jaw) and intraoperative multiunit abutments installed with immediate loading. The making of zirconium dioxide fixed screw-retained prosthesis by multiunit abutment level was planned after a period of osseointegration. Received CBCT images and scanned plaster models were exported into programme application Implant Studio (3Shape, Denmark). Placement and sizes of dental implants were chosen after evaluation of bone situation and position of virtual prosthetic construction (Figure 2).

Two surgical templates were made for each jaw. The first template was positioning the teeth-supported surgical template containing sleeves for drilling intraosseous holes for the placement of fixation pins. The localisation of these holes fully matches similarly in the second, full-guided surgical template attached on the edentulous jaw by fixation pins in the same intraosseous holes after extraction of all teeth. Thus, maximum accuracy of the full-guided template was achieved on working on edentulous jaws (Figure 3). The patient reviewed the treatment plan and signed the informed procedure agreement.

4. Surgical Procedure

The patient received a prophylactic dose of antibiotic (875 mg/125 mg augmentin+clavulanic, GSK GlaxoSmithKline, London, UK) 1 hour before surgery. All procedures were performed with local anaesthetics. Intravenous sedation was patient's request. After local anaesthesia by Ubistesin (articaine 4% with 1 : 200000 adrenaline solution for local anaesthesia, 3 M ESPE, St. Paul, MN, USA), positioning the surgical template was attached on each jaw, and intraosseous holes for fixing pins were drilled to a specified depth, and then, the templates were removed. Afterwards, all of patient's teeth were extracted by using Periotome (Hu-Friedy, USA/-Germany) and gentle elevation with forceps to prevent a fracture of the facial alveolar bone. All extraction sockets were thoroughly treated with aggressive curettage. Before immediate implant placement, a decontamination protocol was performed by packing extraction sockets soaked in 0.2% chlorhexidine gluconate gauze and keeping there for 5 min in situ. Then, on each edentulous jaw, the full-guided surgical

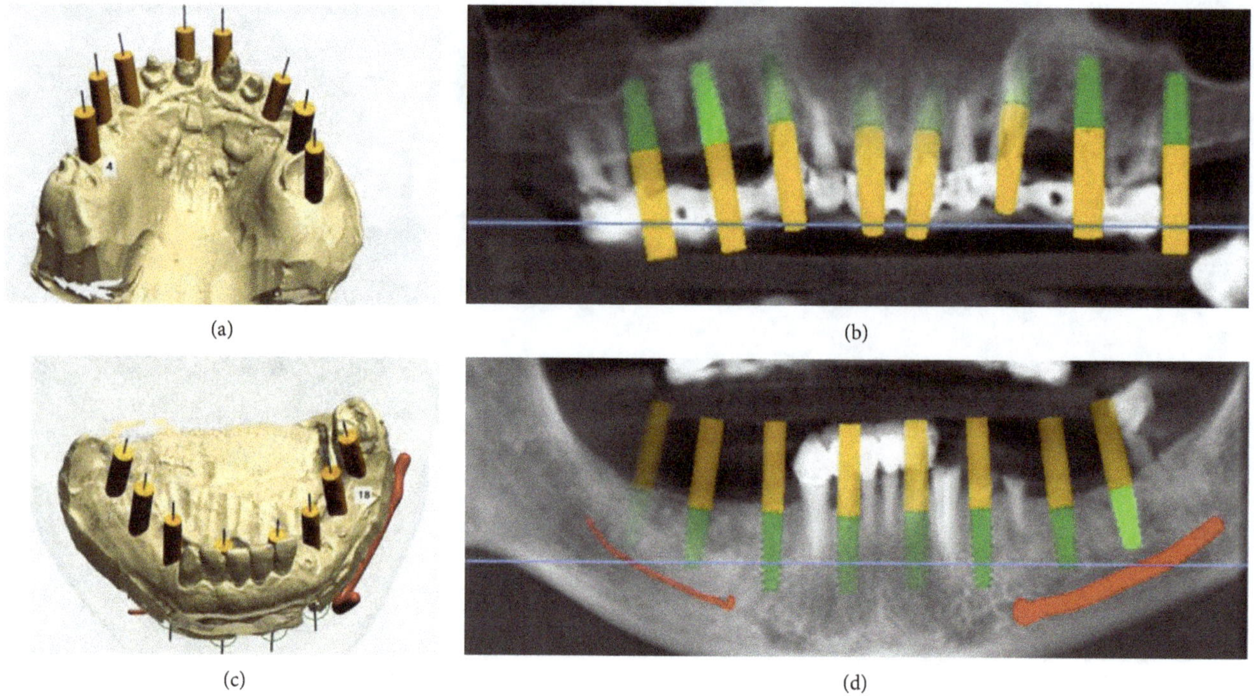

FIGURE 2: Dental implants positions on maxilla (a, b) and mandible (c, d).

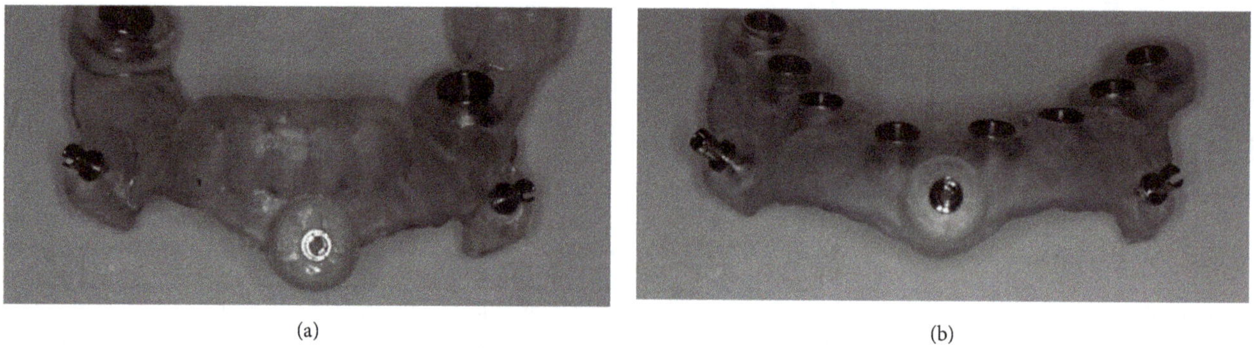

FIGURE 3: Positioning surgical template (a) and full-guided surgical template (b).

template was attached tightly by fixing pins to previously prepared intraosseous holes. Placement of 16 SGS dental implants (SGS Dental Implant System Holding, Switzerland) (8 implants on each jaw) was performed under standard protocol. Eight SGS implants were used on the maxilla with aggressive thread (P7), and they were placed transmucosally (flapless). The criteria for the flapless surgery were an adequate amount on the bone for implant placement, the presence of 2 mm thickness each bone on buccal and palatal sides around implant as planned in a favourable prosthetic position (which defined by using CBCT analysis), and the presence of sufficient keratinised attached gingiva (it must be at least 3 mm around the each implant) (Figure 4).

SGS implants P1 were used on the mandible with parallel surfaces and placed by forming mucoperiosteal flap and standard protocol drilling, excluding places where extraction sockets were located, as immediate implantation was made there using the flapless method (Figure 5).

All the implants were placed with minimal torque above 50 Ncm. Afterwards, the selection of multiunit abutments (SGS Dental Implant System Holding, Switzerland) was made intraoperatively. For the four implants in the front of maxilla, two-component 30-degree multiunit abutments were chosen, and left over on the distal side are four direct one-component multiunit abutments. All of these multiunit abutments have the height of the transgingival part equal to 2 mm. For the mandibular implants, direct one-component multiunit abutments were chosen with the height of the transgingival part equal to 1 mm. Thus, all of the multiunit abutments were installed intraoperatively with a torque equal to 25 Ncm, and their removal was not performed in the future (Figure 6).

Then on multiunit abutments were installed healing abutments and made 6-0 Prolene (Ethicon W8005, Johnson & Johnson) monofilament interrupted sutures to close the flaps. Augmentation of extraction sockets by xenograft was not performed. Full-arch maxillary and mandibular

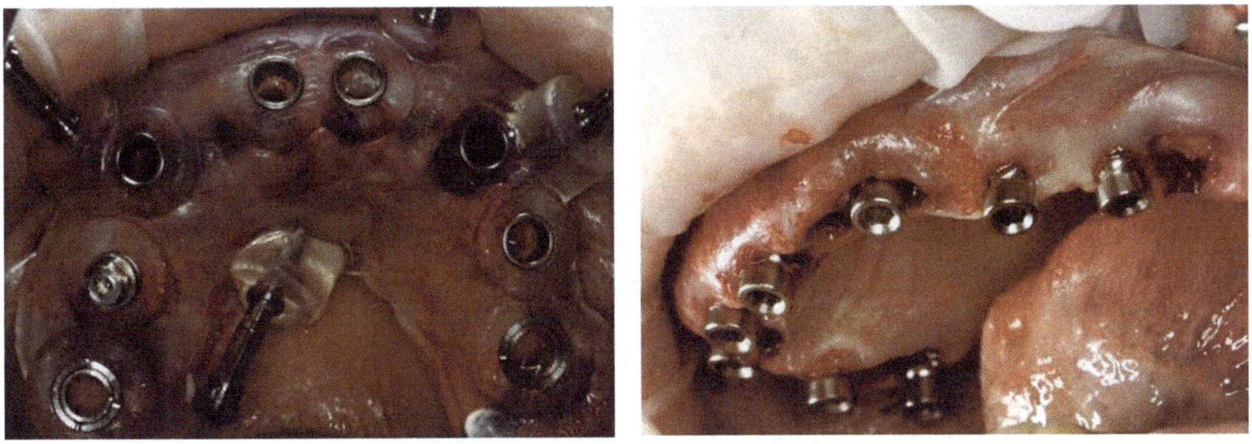

(a) (b)

FIGURE 4: Full-guided surgical template attaching to the upper jaw (a). The condition of the jaw after placement of 8 dental implants by using flapless method with installed implant drivers (b).

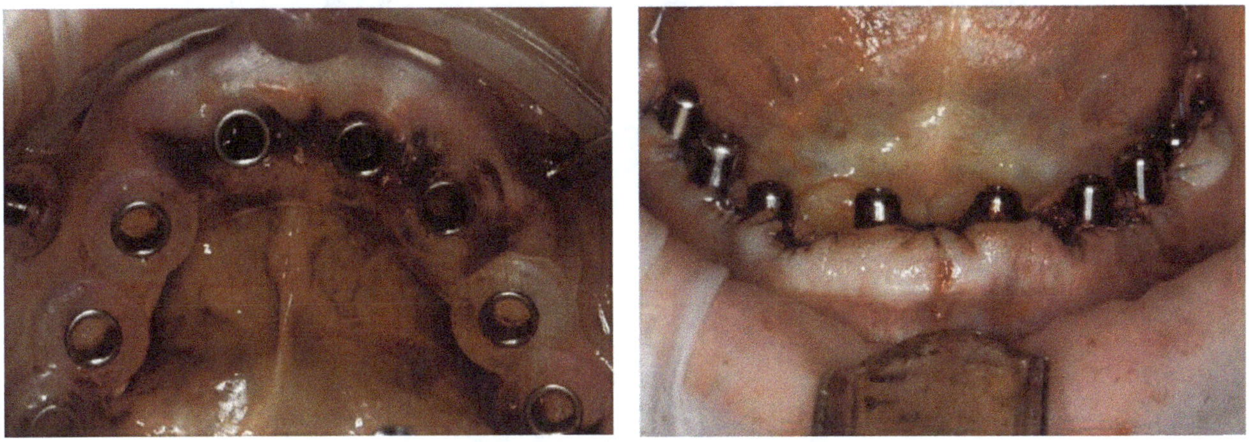

(a) (b)

FIGURE 5: Full-guided surgical template attaching to the mandible (a). The condition of the jaw after placement of 8 dental implants by using standard protocol (b).

impressions were made from multiunit abutment platform with appropriate transfers for open tray with polyether impression material (Impregum, 3 M ESPE, St. Paul, MN, USA) and sent to the laboratory for making first temporary constructions in centric occlusion relationship. The prepared temporary restorations were attached after 4 h with recommended torque equal to 10 Ncm, and target X-rays of the implant suprastructure systems were performed.The patient was instructed for postoperative oral care like rinsing oral cavity with 0.2% (by volume) chlorhexidine gluconate mouthwash (Corsodyl, GlaxoSmithKline) solution twice a day for a week and cleaning the temporary restorations with an extra fine toothbrush. The patient received an antibiotic (1 g amoxiclav, LEK, d.d., Slovenia) twice a day for 5 days. For pain control, the patient was prescribed a 100 mg of nimesulide (Nise; Dr. Reddy's Laboratories Ltd., India). The patient was also advised to minimise trauma at the surgery site; no special diet was recommended. The sutures were removed 10 days after the surgery.

5. Prosthetic Procedure

Further prosthetic procedures were initiated after 2 months of soft and bone tissue healing. For centric relation (CR) definition, Kois Deprogrammer was prepared and recommended to wear for 8 h each day for a week. After that, second temporary constructions in CR relationship were prepared. Another month later (3-month postoperative), the impression was taken on a multiunit abutment level with transfers for open tray with polyether impression material (Impregum, 3M ESPE, St. Paul, MN, USA). Temporary prosthetic constructions were installed to prepared plaster models, which were mounted on the articulator SAM 3 (SAM PRÄZISIONSTECHNIK GmbH, Gauting, Germany) (Figure 7).

The prostheses were designed on the ExoCAD software (ExoCAD GmbH, Darmstadt, Germany). An epoxy resin prototype was printed and sent to verify the lip support, midline position, incisal edge position and teeth display, occlusal

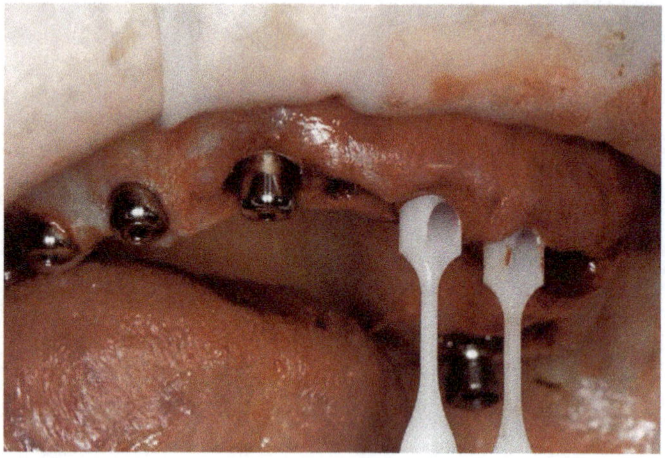

Figure 6: Intraoperative selection of 30 degrees multiunit abutments at the front side of maxilla and installation healing caps at the distal side.

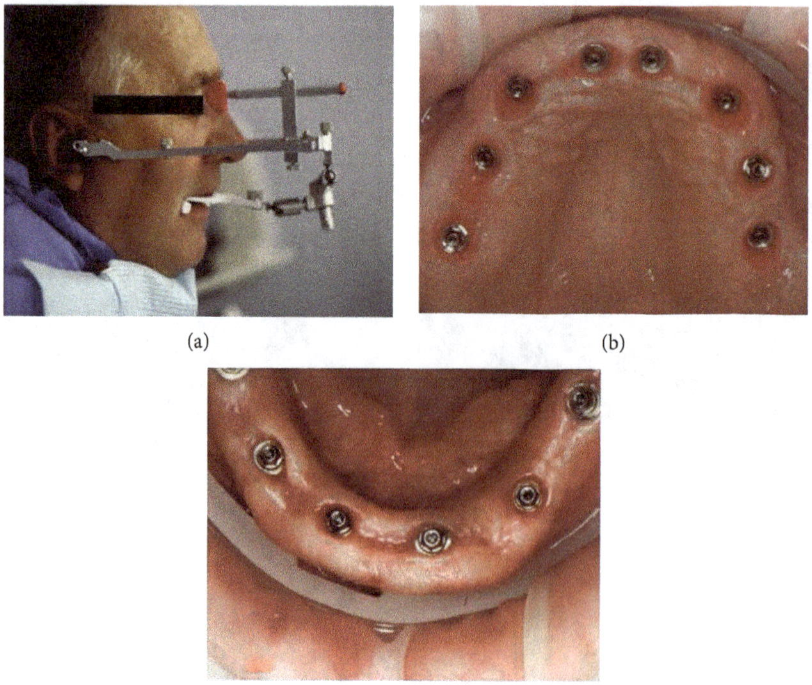

(a) (b) (c)

Figure 7: Final prosthetics after 3 month healing (a). Good condition of soft tissues on maxilla (b) and mandible (c) after wearing temporary screw-retained multiunit abutment-supported restorations.

plane orientation, centric relation, phonetics, and aesthetics for the sake of patient's satisfaction. After some adjustments, the restorations in full anatomy were milled in monolithic zirconia block (KATANA Zirconia STML, Kuraray Noritake Dental Inc., Aichi, Japan) (Figure 8) and were sintered, colourised, and then glazed. Each part of restoration was bonded with titanium base in the following ways: both surfaces were treated with 50 microns of aluminium oxide particles at 2 bar pressure (0.25 MPa) for 20 s at a distance of 10 mm (RONDOflex Plus 360, KaVo, Germany). After that, a universal single-component priming agent (Monobond Plus, Ivoclar Vivadent, Liechtenstein) was applied to the zirconia and titanium bases accordingly. Dual-curing luting composite for the aesthetic and permanent cementation of ceramic (Variolink Esthetic DC, Ivoclar Vivadent, Liechtenstein) was used to lute the two components extraorally according to the manufacturer's recommendations.

The final full-arch prostheses were clinically verified with a one-screw test for passive fitting. The prosthesis screws were tightened following the instructions to 15 Ncm. The screw access holes were filled with temporary material. Functional specificities, including group function, interocclusional contacts, no contacts on protrusive and lateral excursions, were achieved by minor selective modifications, central fossa expansions on premolars and molars and teeth appearance reduction (Figures 9 and 10).

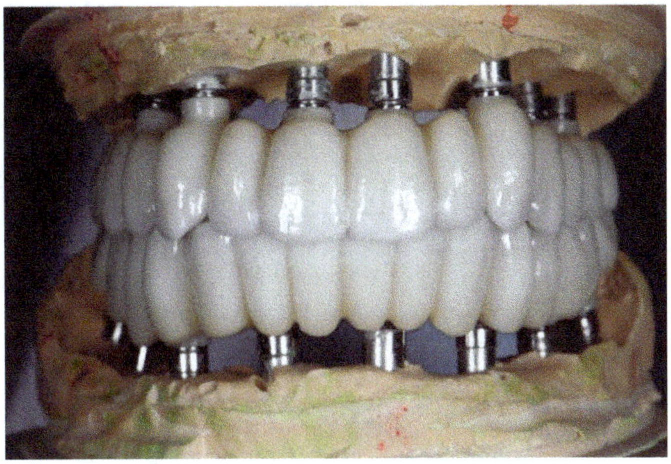

Figure 8: Final look of the zirconia full-arch prostheses. Afterwards, the titanium bases were inserted.

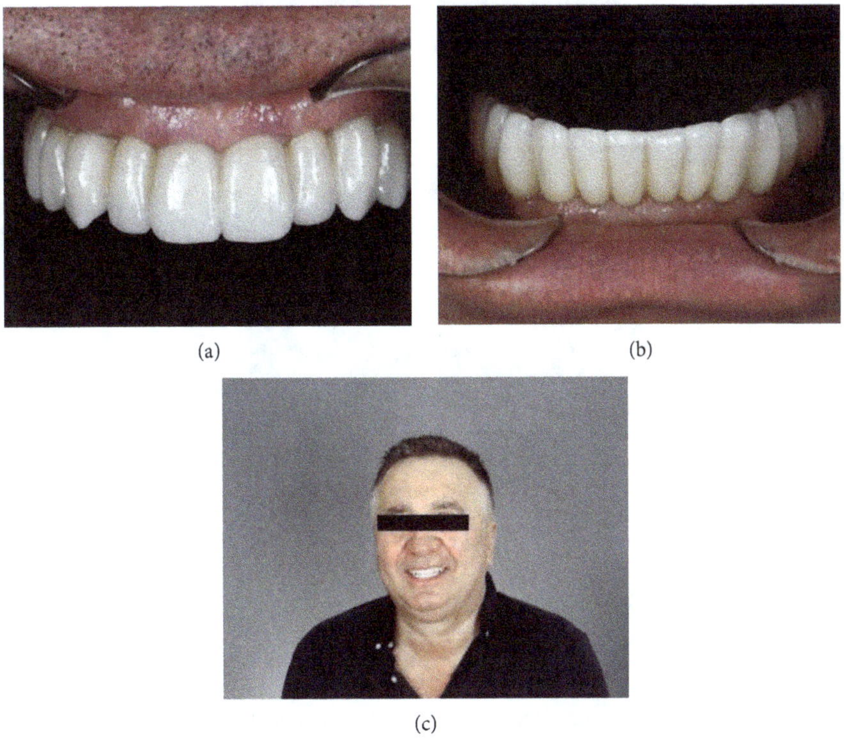

Figure 9: Final look of the prostheses on maxilla (a) and mandible (b). Patient's joyful smile (c).

Finally, the aesthetics and phonetics were verified. Occlusion check was made by articulation paper 100-micron thickness (BAUCSH, Germany). Three days later, the occlusion recheck was made by articulation paper 48-micron thickness (BAUCSH, Germany). Front teeth in full contact 8-micron disocclusion were achieved. Screw access holes were filled with the flowable resin Filtek Ultimate Flow (3 M ESPE, USA). Postoperative instructions including hygiene care were advised to the patient. For outcome and follow-up, the patient was surveyed after 6 weeks and 12 weeks postoperatively for monitoring the stability of the implants and assessing the health of the peri-implant tissues. Postoperative instructions including hygiene care were advised to the patient. Multidisciplinary regular check-up was emphasised. The patient was followed at 1, 3, 6, and 12 months post loading. CBCT scanning was taken after 12 months, and no any bone resorption around implant platform was found (Figure 11). Soft tissues were completely healthy at the follow-up time.

6. Discussion

Zirconium as a material for permanent restorations has many beneficial characteristics such as low temperature conductivity and corrosion potential, low bacterial contamination, and high biocompatibility [14]. The main complication in the prosthetics was the risk of porcelain fracture or chipping. The short-term clinical results show that

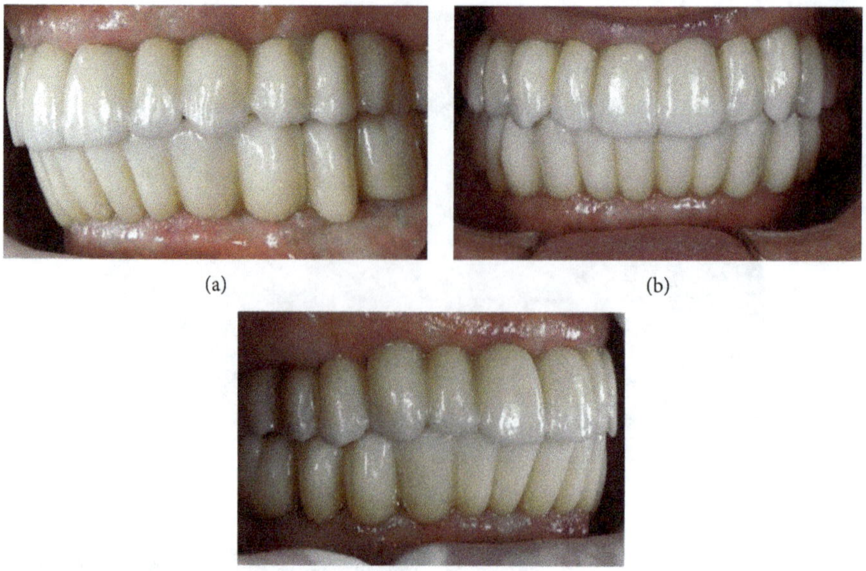

(a) (b) (c)

FIGURE 10: Occluding prostheses: left side (a), front side (b), and right side (c).

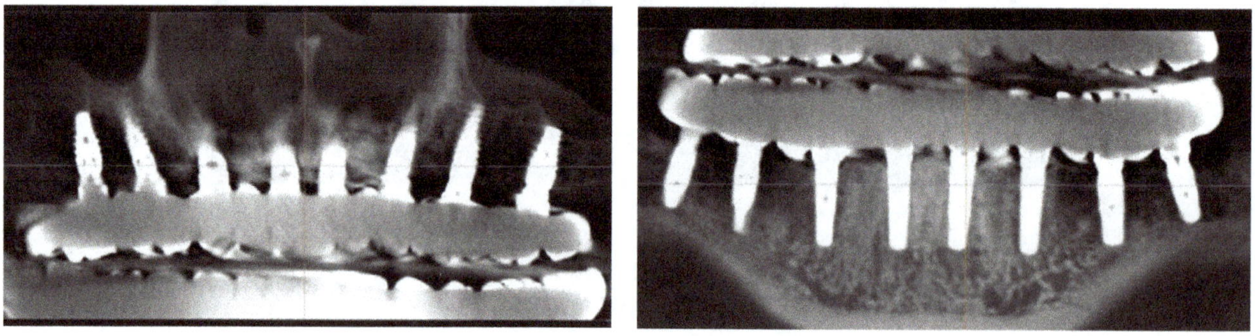

(a) (b)

FIGURE 11: Condition and level stability of the bone tissue around dental implants after 12 month of prosthetics. (a) Is maxilla and (b) is mandible.

this type of constructions may be a viable prosthetic option for the edentulous patient [15–17]. In this clinical case, priority was given to monolithic zirconia implant-supported fixed dental prosthesis with titanium bases. Despite the fact that the full-zirconium construction without bonded titanium bases has the potential of a more favourable soft tissue response, zirconia chipping, as seen in this prosthesis, can occur at a higher rate [18]. Patient's requirement was full-arch fixed restoration up to the second molars. It is well known that excessive cantilever can negatively influence proper biomechanics in implant-supported prosthesis and can result in overloading which may lead to the fracture of the prosthesis and/or abutment screws [14]. In addition, higher length and more quantity of implant supporting a full-arch prosthesis promoted less stress concentration during the simulated load, which is especially important with the use of zirconium. Decreasing the number of implants in rehabilitation is more harmful than decreasing their length for the stress and strain distribution [19, 20]. That is why our team decided for using eight-implant-supported full-arch fixed prosthesis. Advantages of virtual guided technologies for treatment planning are beneficial for the surgeon, orthopaedist-prosthetist, and patient, because it allows performing the operation quickly with maximum accuracy of implant placement into the right position and reducing the trauma of the surgery. Nowadays, CAD/CAM technologies are so far to provide maximum accuracy specifically in edentulous patients. However, the new improvements and trends reduce this gap each time [21, 22]. Implant placement on edentulous jaws is difficult in case of the attaching a surgical template on soft tissues cannot give us accuracy of positioning, even when using intraosseous fixing pins. In this regard, the approach of using strategic teeth in combination with two surgical templates (positioning and full-guided) allows surgery according to preoperative planning. In this case, clinical and CBCT results confirm the fact that the usage of virtual guided technologies can reduce the incidence of complications associated with dental implantation, help the doctor with choosing the most appropriate option of surgery (e.g., flapless method), and reduce the time of operation and healing time after due to minimal trauma of the soft tissues. Dental implant positioning accuracy is an important factor in full-arch implant-supported rehabilitation. However, the choice of retaining type of prosthetic construction is highly important. Cement-retained prosthesis has some advantages like a simpler construction technology, a compensation of placed implants absence of parallel axes, and a passive fitting of prosthesis due to cement space between construction and abutment [5, 12]. However, this type of fixation may provide other complications like the absence of maintenance service possibility and the risk of peri-implantitis development because of excess cement in the peri-implant area, more specifically in soft tissues [23]. Therefore, most clinicians agree that in full-arch implant-supported prosthetics, preference should be given to screw retaining. This type of retaining ensures the maintainability of prosthesis and the possibility of its removal for monitoring and hygienic procedures, and more importantly, screw retaining completely eliminates cement in the peri-implant tissues. The last is most important, because excess cement control is difficult due to fake gingiva on prosthetic construction [24, 25]. On the other side, screw-retained prosthesis may not give passive fitting of construction in case of differences of screwing axes, exactly of them significant divergence. Moreover, at this type of fixation, complications may vary from a fracture of various components in system implant suprastructure to an implant fracture or failure of its osteointegration [6, 10]. In this clinical case, implant placements were made by using surgical template, but this construction may not guarantee implants' parallel axes in need for preparing a screw-retained prosthesis from bone level platform, because of 1–2-degree divergence may result in tension in implant suprastructure system. In this case, four implants were placed in the front side of the maxilla with significant vestibular axes tilt due to bone anatomy specificity. Furthermore, this. situation complicates performing a screw-retained full-arch prosthetic construction from the bone level. The usage of 30-degree multiunit abutments in combination with direct multiunit abutments guaranteed absolutely passive fitting of full-arch prosthesis. The use of multiunit abutments has other advantages. It is well-known that any factor disrupting soft tissue integrity of the biological width may affect the bone level around the implant. Standard protocol of implant-supported rehabilitation includes frequent unscrewing the healing abutment or temporary abutment until the final construction will be retained. Multiple suprastructure unscrewing leads to permanent failure of poor hemidesmosomal soft tissue connection around an implant with following reduction of connective tissue circle. This contributes to a formation of a newer connection and less strong and narrower hemidesmosomal attachment. All of this could be a reason for bone resorption, especially at patients with thin mucosa biotype. Some studies show that multiple abutment screwing-unscrewing series could affect the oral mucosa barrier and could lead to bone loss [26–28]. The meta-analysis by Koutouzis T et al. [29] showed that multiple screwing-unscrewing truly leads to marginal bone loss despite the controversy of results from other studies. In this clinical case, CBCT scanning 1 year after prosthetics shows the consistent bone level around dental implants without remodelling of the peri-implant bone. Moreover, implants were used with six-sided connection and without platform switching system. Intraoperative installation of multiunit abutments allows to seal an implant neck and create a new, stronger, and wider hemidesmosomal connection on the multiunit abutment neck level. Further prosthetic manipulations were made by multiunit abutment level, which is higher than peri-implant bone. This made it possible to avoid multiple screwing/unscrewing by implant neck level and to preserve hemidesmosomal connection. All of this enabled the stability of periimplant bone tissues.

7. Conclusion

Dental implant positioning accuracy is an important factor in full-arch implant-supported rehabilitation, especially when the final restoration should be prepared without any ceramic gingiva ("nature-like" teeth). Virtual-guided technologies provide optimal implant placement according to the correct prosthetic position and minimise intraoperative trauma and procedure time.

Screw retaining prostheses have some advantages against cement-retained constructions like an absence of cement in peri-implant tissues and a maintenance service possibility (construction monitoring and its unscrewing, professional hygiene procedures, etc.). The multiunit abutments provide absolutely passive fitting of prosthesis even with significant divergence of placed implants axes.

Intraoperative installation of multiunit abutments allows to seal an implant neck and to create a new, stronger, and wider hemidesmosomal connection on the multiunit abutment neck level and makes it possible to avoid multiple screwing/unscrewing, preserving the stability of peri-implant tissues.

References

[1] R. Adell, B. Eriksson, U. Lekholm, P. I. Brånemark, and T. Jemt, "Long-term follow-up study of osseointegrated implants in the treatment of totally edentulous jaws," *The International Journal of Oral & Maxillofacial Implants*, vol. 5, no. 4, pp. 347–359, 1990.

[2] P. I. Branemark, B. Svensson, and D. van Steenberghe, "Ten-year survival rates of fixed prostheses on four or six implants ad modum Branemark in full edentulism," *Clinical Oral Implants Research*, vol. 6, no. 4, pp. 227–231, 1995.

[3] S. U. Rajgiri and M. Dayalan, "Full-mouth. Rehabilitation with implant-supported fixed prosthesis," *International Journal of Oral Implantology & Clinical Research*, vol. 7, no. 3, pp. 73–80, 2016.

[4] G. A. Zarb, J. Hobkirk, S. Eckert, and R. Jacob, *Prosthodontic Treatment for Edentulous Patients: Complete Dentures and*

Implant-Supported Prostheses, Elsevier Health Sciences, Missouri, 13th ed. edition, 2013.

[5] K. X. Michalakis, H. Hirayama, and P. D. Garefis, "Cement-retained versus screw-retained implant restorations: a critical review," *The International Journal of Oral & Maxillofacial Implants*, vol. 18, no. 5, pp. 719–728, 2003.

[6] I. Sailer, S. Mühlemann, M. Zwahlen, C. H. F. Hämmerle, and D. Schneider, "Cemented and screw-retained implant reconstructions: a systematic review of the survival and complication rates," *Clinical Oral Implants Research*, vol. 23, suppl 6, pp. 163–201, 2012.

[7] S. Sherif, S. M. Susarla, J. W. Hwang, H. P. Weber, and R. F. Wright, "Clinician- and patient-reported long-term evaluation of screw- and cement-retained implant restorations: a 5-year prospective study," *Clinical Oral Investigations*, vol. 15, no. 6, pp. 993–999, 2011.

[8] J. G. Wittneben, T. Joda, H. P. Weber, and U. Brägger, "Screw retained vs. cement retained implant-supported fixed dental prosthesis," *Periodontology 2000*, vol. 73, no. 1, pp. 141–151, 2017.

[9] J. Katsoulis, T. Takeichi, G. A. Sol, L. Peter, and K. Katsoulis, "Misfit of implant prostheses and its impact on clinical outcomes. Definition, assessment and a systematic review of the literature," *European Journal of Oral Implantology*, vol. 10, Supplement 1, pp. 121–138, 2017.

[10] C. Millen, U. Bragger, and J. G. Wittneben, "Influence of prosthesis type and retention mechanism on complications with fixed implant-supported prostheses: a systematic review applying multivariate analyses," *The International Journal of Oral & Maxillofacial Implants*, vol. 30, no. 1, pp. 110–124, 2015.

[11] T. Linkevicius, A. Puisys, E. Vindasiute, L. Linkeviciene, and P. Apse, "Does residual cement around implant-supported restorations cause peri-implant disease? A retrospective case analysis," *Clinical Oral Implants Research*, vol. 24, no. 11, pp. 1179–1184, 2013.

[12] T. G. Wilson Jr., "The positive relationship between excess cement and peri-implant disease: a prospective clinical endoscopic study," *Journal of Periodontology*, vol. 80, no. 9, pp. 1388–1392, 2009.

[13] J.-G. Wittneben, C. Millen, and U. Brägger, "Clinical Performance of Screw- Versus Cement-Retained Fixed Implant-Supported Reconstructions—A Systematic Review," *The International Journal of Oral & Maxillofacial Implant*, vol. 29, Supplement, pp. 84–98, 2014.

[14] V. F. Rojas, "Retrospective 2- to 7-year follow-up study of 20 double full-arch implant-supported monolithic zirconia fixed prostheses: measurements and recommendations for optimal design," *Journal of Prosthodontics*, vol. 27, no. 6, pp. 501–508, 2018.

[15] A. Pozzi, S. Holst, G. Fabbri, and M. Tallarico, "Clinical reliability of CAD/CAM cross-arch zirconia bridges on immediately loaded implants placed with Computer-Assisted/Template-Guided surgery: a retrospective study with a follow-up between 3 and 5 years," *Clinical Implant Dentistry and Related Research*, vol. 17, Suppl 1, pp. e86–e96, 2015 Jan;17.

[16] A. A. Abdulmajeed, K. G. Lim, T. O. Närhi, and L. F. Cooper, "Complete-arch implant-supported monolithic zirconia fixed dental prostheses: a systematic review," *The Journal of Prosthetic Dentistry*, vol. 115, no. 6, pp. 672–677.e1, 2016.

[17] A. S. Bidra, P. Rungruanganunt, and M. Gauthier, "Clinical outcomes of full arch fixed implantsupported zirconia prostheses: a systematic review," *European Journal of Oral Implantology*, vol. 10, Suppl 1, pp. 35–45, 2017.

[18] P. Papaspyridakos and K. Lal, "Computer-assisted design/-computer-assisted manufacturing zirconia implant fixed complete prostheses: clinical results and technical complications up to 4 years of function," *Clinical Oral Implants Research*, vol. 24, no. 6, pp. 659–665, 2013.

[19] J. P. M. Tribst, A. M. de Oliveira Dal Piva, A. L. S. Borges, and M. A. Bottino, "Effect of implant number and height on the biomechanics of full arch prosthesis," *Brazilian Journal of Oral Sciences*, vol. 17, no. June 2019, article e18222, 2018.

[20] G. Dimililer, S. Kücükkurt, and S. Cetiner, "Biomechanical effects of implant number and diameter on stress distributions in maxillary implant-supported overdentures," *The Journal of Prosthetic Dentistry*, vol. 119, no. 2, pp. 244–249.e6, 2018.

[21] K. El Kholy, R. Lazarin, S. F. M. Janner, K. Faerber, R. Buser, and D. Buser, "Influence of surgical guide support and implant site location on accuracy of static computer-assisted implant surgery," *Clinical Oral Implants Research*, vol. 30, no. 11, pp. 1067–1075, 2019.

[22] A. Gintaute, N. Papatriantafyllou, M. Aljehani, and W. Att, "Accuracy of computerized and conventional impression-making procedures for multiple straight and tilted dental implants," *The International Journal of Esthetic Dentistry*, vol. 13, no. 4, pp. 550–565, 2018.

[23] C. Wadhwani, D. Rapoport, S. La Rosa, T. Hess, and S. Kretschmar, "Radiographic detection and characteristic patterns of residual excess cement associated with cement-retained implant restorations: a clinical report," *The Journal of Prosthetic Dentistry*, vol. 107, no. 3, pp. 151–157, 2012.

[24] J. Cosyn, L. Van Aelst, B. Collaert, G. R. Persson, and H. De Bruyn, "The peri-implant sulcus compared with internal implant and suprastructure components: a microbiological analysis," *Clinical Implant Dentistry and Related Research*, vol. 13, no. 4, pp. 286–295, 2011.

[25] W. Keller, U. Bragger, and A. Mombelli, "Peri-implant microflora of implants with cemented and screw retained suprastructures," *Clinical Oral Implants Research*, vol. 9, no. 4, pp. 209–217, 1998.

[26] I. Abrahamsson, T. Berglundh, and J. Lindhe, "The mucosal barrier following abutment dis/reconnection. An experimental study in dogs," *Journal of Clinical Periodontology*, vol. 24, no. 8, pp. 568–572, 1997.

[27] I. Abrahamsson, T. Berglundh, S. Sekino, and J. Lindhe, "Tissue reactions to abutment shift: an experimental study in dogs," *Clinical Implant Dentistry and Related Research*, vol. 5, no. 2, pp. 82–88, 2003.

[28] K. Becker, I. Mihatovic, V. Golubovic, and F. Schwarz, "Impact of abutment material and dis-/re-connection on soft and hard tissue changes at implants with platform-switching," *Journal of Clinical Periodontology*, vol. 39, no. 8, pp. 774–780, 2012.

[29] T. Koutouzis, F. Gholami, J. Reynolds, T. Lundgren, and G. Kotsakis, "Abutment disconnection/reconnection affects peri-implant marginal bone levels: a metaanalysis," *The International Journal of Oral & Maxillofacial Implants*, vol. 32, no. 3, pp. 575–581, 2017 May/June.

17

Implant Treatment with 12-Year Follow-Up in a Patient with Severe Chronic Periodontitis: A Case Report and Literature Review

Keisuke Seki[1,2] **and Yoshiyuki Hagiwara**[1]

[1]*Implant Dentistry, Nihon University School of Dentistry Dental Hospital, Tokyo, Japan*
[2]*Department of Comprehensive Dentistry and Clinical Education, Nihon University School of Dentistry, Tokyo, Japan*

Correspondence should be addressed to Keisuke Seki; seki.keisuke@nihon-u.ac.jp

Academic Editor: Jose López-López

Tooth loss among adults is associated with progressive periodontitis. Implant prosthetic treatment has long been utilized in periodontal patients. Even when the implants are applied, ongoing management of periodontal disease and control of inflammation is necessary to maintain a healthy oral cavity. Lack of appropriate periodontal treatment can result in recurrence of periodontal disease during a maintenance period; loss of the supportive capacity of the periodontal tissues will increase the susceptibility of residual teeth to traumatic force. For this reason, it is worthwhile to improve oral function by applying implants as a fixed device. Here, we report that implant treatment in a patient with generalized severe chronic periodontitis helped maintain the periodontal and peri-implant tissue for a long term. We propose that initial periodontal treatment and ongoing supportive therapy can help maintain implants in patients with severe periodontitis. In addition, we reviewed case reports in the English literature so far.

1. Introduction

Periodontitis is an endogenous multibacterial infectious disease in which the periodontal tissues break down as a result of the interactions between specific anaerobic bacteria and host immune mechanisms [1–3]. Additionally, it is a multifactorial disease, involving bacterial, environmental, and biological factors [4]. For the periodontal treatment, it is effective for improving a local environment by removal of plaque retention factors while improving systemic factors like diabetes treatment and smoking cessation. Severe periodontitis is characterized by progressive destruction of the periodontal tissues resulting in over 5 mm of clinical attachment loss. A correlation between periodontitis and a weakened immune response has been reported, and the accumulated destruction of periodontal tissues with age can result in progressive attachment loss and bone resorption [5]. A recent study reported that severe periodontitis is the sixth most prevalent disease worldwide [6]. Due to the loss of teeth caused by this disease, the burden imposed on the physical, mental, and financial state of the patient increases. This also causes the patient's QOL to decrease markedly.

While a history of periodontitis is considered a localized risk indicator for implant failure at the start of maintenance, it has also been recognized as an important risk indicator for peri-implantitis [7]. It has been reported that a history of periodontitis decreases the success rate of implants. Therefore, appropriate periodontal treatment must be implemented for long-term implant stability [8]. In this regard, it is necessary to investigate previous reports related to long-term outcomes in severe chronic periodontitis patients with applied implant treatment. The purpose of this case report is to show the necessity of implant treatment for severe periodontitis and to include a review showing that the implant is useful for long-term conservation of residual teeth. The patient was maintained successfully for 12 years, suggesting that implants following initial periodontal treatment may contribute to maintaining good oral function.

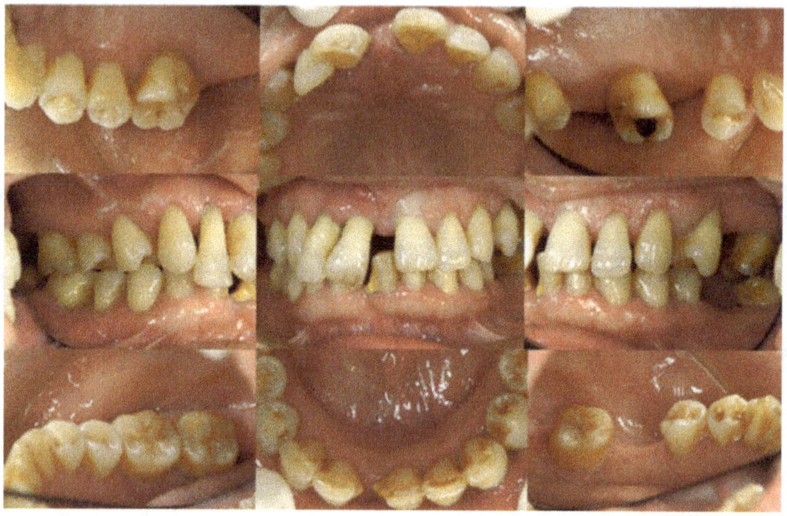

(a)

	7	6	5	4	3	2	1	1	2	3	4	5	6	7
Prognosis		H	Q	Q	Q	H	H	H	H	F	Q		Q	
Mobility		I		I	I	III	III	III	II	I	I		I	
Furcation		II II II											I I	
PPD B		3 8 6	6 4 3	4 3 8	4 3 6				8 3 4	4 3 4	4 3 4		6 6 7	8 8 6
PPD P		6 7 7	7 6 6	8 6 8	5 4 4				6 4 4	3 3 3	6 6 4		5 4 4	6 4 4
Tooth no. (upper)	7	6	5	4	3	2	1	1	2	3	4	5	6	7
Tooth no. (lower)	7	6	5	4	3	2	1	1	2	3	4	5	6	7
PPD L	6 6 6	5 5 8	3 3 4	3 3 3	3 3 4	3 4 4		4 3 4	3 3 5	4 3 6	6 6 6	5 3 5		4 4 6
PPD B	9 9 4	4 8 8	5 3 4	4 4 3	3 3 4	4 3 4		6 2 3	2 3 6	6 3 4	6 2 3	3 3 5		6 5 5
Furcation		III III												
Mobility		I												I
Prognosis	P	Q	F	F	F	F		Q	Q	Q	Q	F		Q

(b)

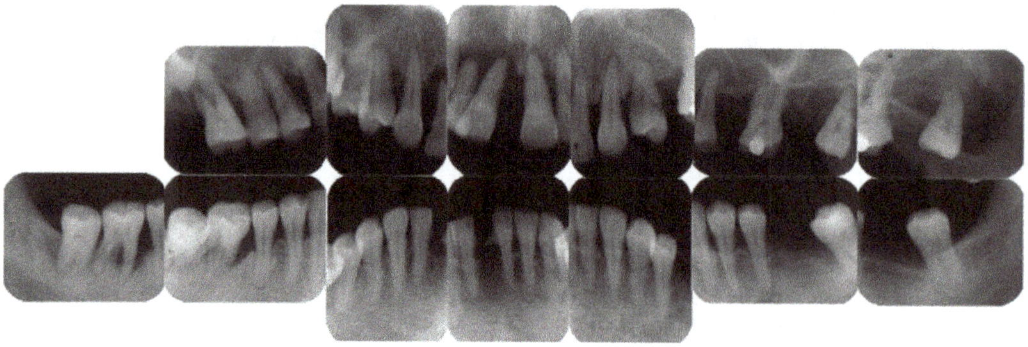

(c)

Figure 1: (a) Pretreatment intraoral photographs (April 2004). Generalized inflammation is observed, particularly between tooth #11 and tooth #12, where a fistula is present. (b) Pretreatment periodontal chart. Teeth #11, #12, #16, #21, and #22 were evaluated as "hopeless"; #46 and #47 were "poor" (PPD: periodontal probing depth; G: good; F: fair; Q: questionable; P: poor; H: hopeless, red: bleeding). (c) Pretreatment radiographs. Thirteen dental X-ray films show severe bone loss in the maxillary anterior and mandibular right molar regions.

2. Case Presentation

A nonsmoking 51-year-old woman visited Nihon University School of Dentistry Dental Hospital in April 2004 with a chief complaint of mobility in the maxillary teeth. The patient was in good general health. Her past medical and dental history was unremarkable, as was her family history. A few months before presentation, she developed difficulty eating as a result of tooth mobility and increased sensitivity to cold water.

2.1. Examination Findings. On intraoral examination, diffuse redness and swelling were observed in the marginal gingiva and interdental papillae. Bleeding and purulent discharge from the pockets were found mainly in the right molar region. The patient had halitosis. The deposition of supragingival calculus was observed in the mandibular anterior segment. Pathologic tooth migration was observed in teeth #11 and #12 (overjet 5 mm, overbite 7 mm) (Figure 1(a)). Teeth #11, #12, and #21 exhibited class III mobility. Tooth #46 had a class III furcation lesion. Sixty-one percent of the teeth had a deep periodontal probing depth (PPD) over 4 mm (PPD ≥ 4), 61% had bleeding on probing (BOP) (Figure 1(b)), and all teeth scored 100% on O'Leary's plaque control record. Radiographic examination revealed periodontal tissue destruction, generally with 3 to 5 mm of horizontal bone resorption and 4 to 6 mm of vertical bone resorption in teeth #16, #14, #26, and #46 (Figure 1(c)). Occlusal examination showed Eichner's index B1. Based on these results, we diagnosed generalized moderate-to-severe chronic periodontitis.

2.2. Treatment Plan. The treatment plan consisted of the following items:

(1) Initial periodontal treatment

- (i) Oral hygiene instruction
- (ii) Scaling and root planing
- (iii) Tooth extraction (teeth #16, #12, #11, #21, #22, and #27)
- (iv) Therapeutic partial denture (teeth #12–#22)
- (v) Root canal treatment and hemisection (tooth #46)
- (vi) Occlusal adjustment (teeth #13 and #23)

(2) Reevaluation

(3) Treatment of oral functional rehabilitation

- (i) Implant prostheses (site of #16, #12, #22, #36, and #41)

(4) Reevaluation

(5) Supportive periodontal and implant therapy

2.3. From the First Visit to Initial Periodontal Treatment (2004–2005). Prior to initial periodontal treatment, we informed the patient of her current periodontal status and the necessity of treatment. The patient gave her consent to the treatment plan. We instructed the patient to use the Bass brushing method and recommended using dental floss or a tufted toothbrush. Following gross scaling, confirming that redness and swelling had improved, the teeth of chief complaint (teeth #11, #12, and #21) were extracted. A therapeutic partial denture was prepared and applied immediately. Scaling and root planing were performed under local anesthesia for all teeth with PPD over 4 mm. At the first reevaluation, the patient's oral hygiene had improved (BOP: 12%; PPD ≥ 4: 12%; PCR: around 20%). However, tooth #47 was determined to be unsalvageable and was extracted. Root canal treatment was performed for the distal root of tooth #46; while the medial root was prognosed to be impossible to preserve due to furcation involvement, trisection was adopted (Figure 2).

2.4. Implant Treatment (2005–2007). Implants were chosen respecting the patient's desire to avoid using a removable device and further cutting of natural teeth. We created a diagnostic template based on setup models and used it at X-ray and CT examination. Following administration of local anesthetic (Xylocaine®; 2% lidocaine with 1 : 100,000 epinephrine, DENTSPLY SANKIN, Tokyo, Japan), an incision was made on the alveolar crest and a full-thickness flap was raised. Root form-type implants (Replace® Select Tapered; Nobel Biocare AB, Göteborg, Sweden) were placed with the aid of surgical guides (at #41: NP 3.5 × 13 mm; at #36: WP 5.0 × 10 mm; at #12 and #22: RP 4.3 × 13 mm). Considering the lack of maxillary bone at the site of #16, a 4.0 × 8 mm implant (4.0ST; ASTRA TECH AB, Mölndal, Sweden) was installed using osteotome sinus floor elevation. Primary stability was achieved for all implants. The sites were closed with interrupted 5-0 sutures (MONOCRYL® 5.0; Ethicon, Inc., Somerville, NJ, USA). After these procedures, medications (cephalexin, 1000 mg twice daily for 3 days and diclofenac, 50 mg, three times daily as needed for pain) and postoperative care were prescribed. No adverse postoperative sequelae were observed.

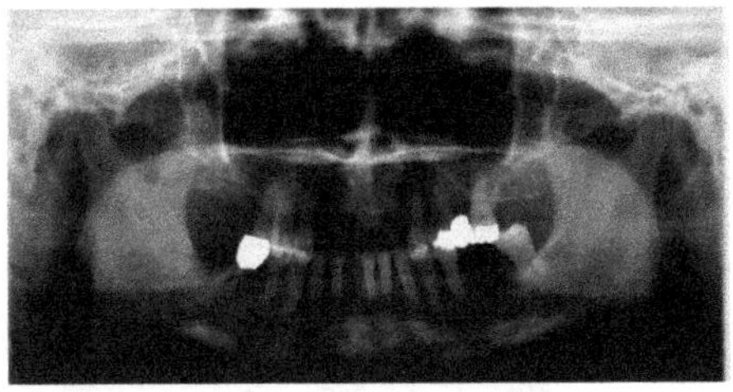

FIGURE 2: Reevaluation radiographs. Panoramic radiography revealed partially edentulous maxilla and mandible.

All surgical procedures were conducted with a two-stage surgical approach. During the 5-month relief period, a partial denture was used in the maxillary anterior region. With regard to the reevaluation for 3 months later in the mandibular, abnormal findings such as drainage or bleeding were not observed.

Secondary surgery was performed after an adequate healing period, with confirmed osseointegration during surgery. After 1 month of soft tissue healing, the superstructure was made. All custom abutments and porcelain-fused-to-metal crowns were retained with side screws (Figures 3(a)–3(e)). In addition, the palatal surface at sites #13 and #23 was adjusted, molding both in composite resin, to obtain disclusion during lateral movement, according to the pretreatment setup model (Figure 4).

2.5. Supportive Periodontal and Implant Treatment (2007–2018). After superstructure setting, the patient was given supportive periodontal and implant therapy and scheduled for follow-up appointments at 3-month intervals which is the most appropriate time to destroy the microflora in the periodontal pocket. Throughout the follow-up period, probing depths of both natural teeth and implants were monitored carefully. For the areas of plaque accumulation, we instructed the patient on the use of interdental brushes (Interprox® Plus; DENTAID, Barcelona, Spain) and enhanced her oral hygiene with regular professional cleanings. To remove dental plaque, we used hand instruments for the implants and an ultrasonic scaler for natural teeth. For professional tooth cleaning, a polishing paste not containing fluoride (Hawe

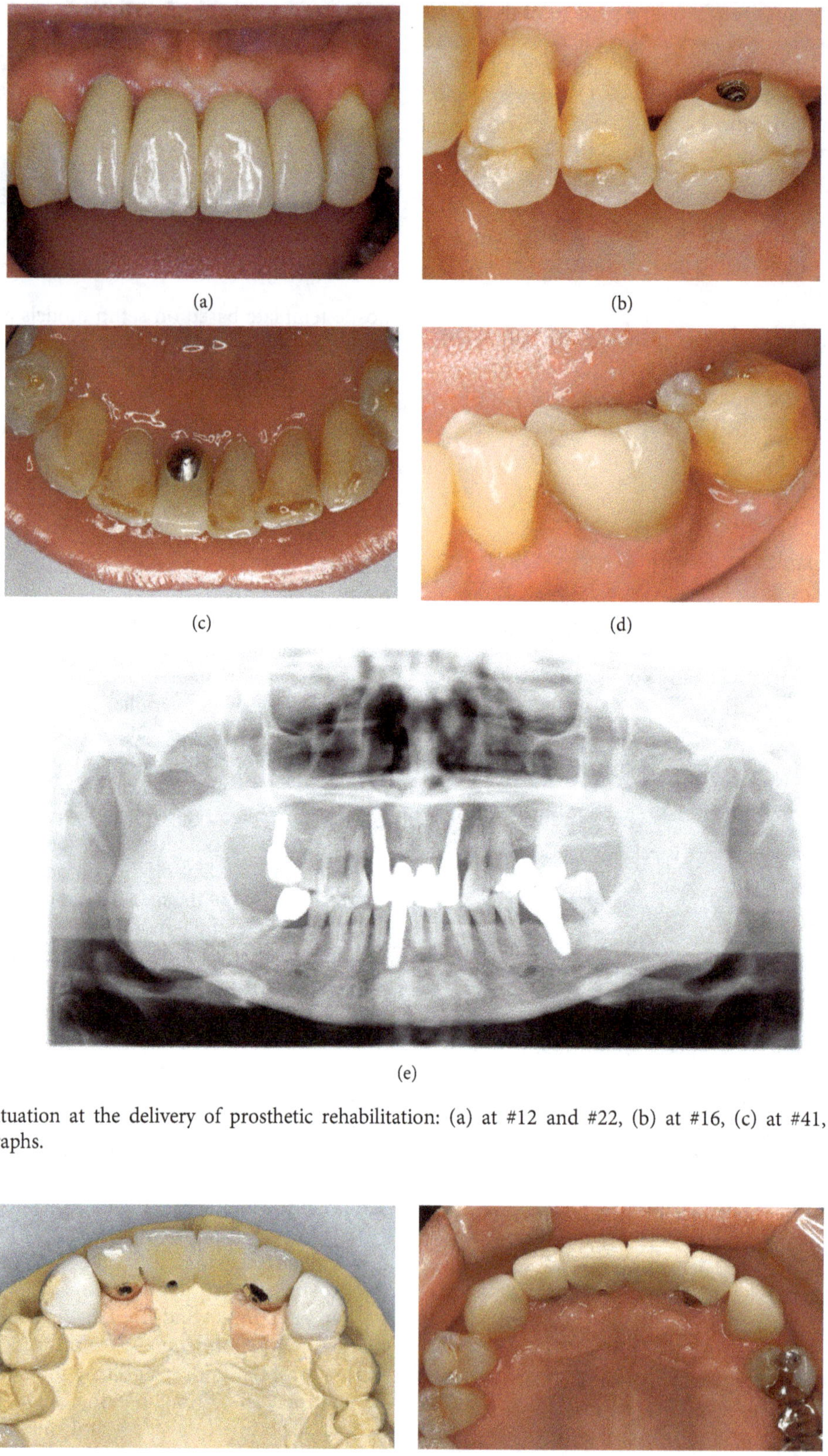

FIGURE 3: Clinical situation at the delivery of prosthetic rehabilitation: (a) at #12 and #22, (b) at #16, (c) at #41, (d) at #36, and (e) postoperative radiographs.

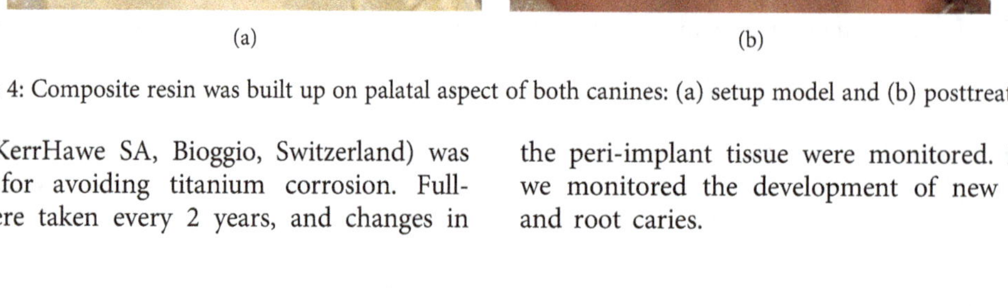

FIGURE 4: Composite resin was built up on palatal aspect of both canines: (a) setup model and (b) posttreatment.

Implant paste®; KerrHawe SA, Bioggio, Switzerland) was used in regard for avoiding titanium corrosion. Full-mouth X-rays were taken every 2 years, and changes in the peri-implant tissue were monitored. In natural teeth, we monitored the development of new bone resorption and root caries.

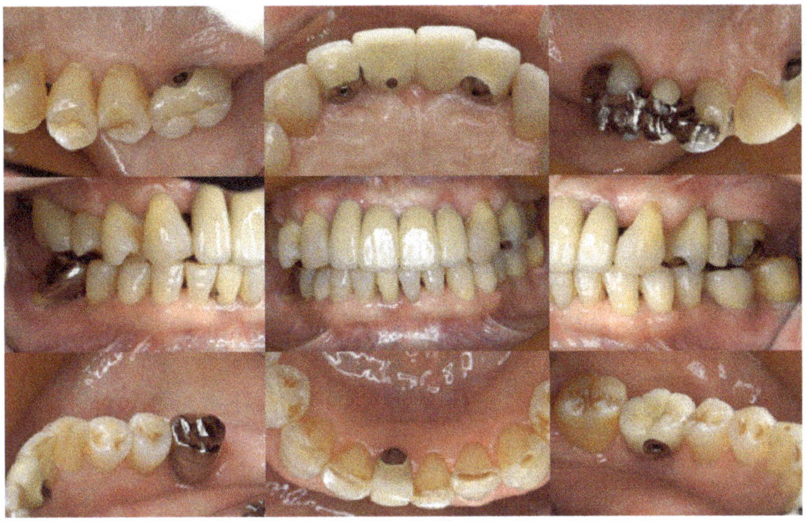

(a)

Prognosis		F	G	F	F	G			G	G	F		G	
Mobility		none	0	I	I	none			none	0	I		0	
Furcation														
PPD B		3 3 3	2 2 3	3 3 3	3 3 2	2 2 3			4 3 3	2 2 2	3 2 2		2 2 2	
PPD P		3 3 3	2 2 2	3 3 3	3 3 3	4 3 3			3 3 3	2 2 2	2 2 2		2 2 2	
Tooth no. (implant)	7	6	5	4	3	2	1	1	2	3	4	5	6	7
	7	6	5	4	3	2	1	1	2	3	4	5	6	7
PPD L		3 3 3	2 2 2	2 2 2	2 2 2	2 2 3	3 3 3	2 2 2	3 3 2	2 2 3	2 2 2	3 3 3	3 3 4	2 2
PPD B		2 2 2	2 2 2	2 2 2	2 2 2	2 2 2	3 3 3	2 2 2	2 2 2	2 2 2	2 2 2	3 3 3	3 3 4	3 2 2
Furcation														
Mobility		0	0	0	0	0	none	0	0	0	0	0	none	I
Prognosis		F	G	G	G	G	G	G	G	G	G	G	G	F

(b)

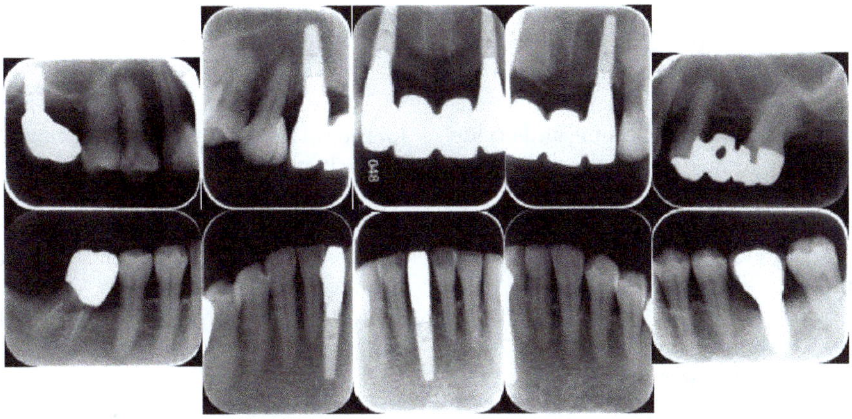

(c)

Figure 5: (a) 12-year postoperative intraoral photographs (April 2016). Intraoral view after completion of care. The gingival texture and peri-implant mucosa appear healthy. (b) 12-year postoperative periodontal chart. Prognoses ranged from "fair" to "good" (PPD: periodontal probing depth; yellow: implant). (c) 12-year postoperative radiographs. Posttreatment radiographs suggest improvement of the severe bone resorption lesions. No bone resorption is seen around the five implants.

We did not observe inflammatory signs such as redness, swelling, pus, or other dysfunctions in the peri-implant mucosa during the maintenance period (Figure 5(a)). Periodontal pockets have been maintained with less than 3 mm PPD and below 10% BOP in natural teeth (Figure 5(b)). All implant sites have maintained PPD of 3 to 4 mm, with slight BOP observed. The modified Silness–Löe plaque index was below a score of 1 for all implants. No pathological finding of remodeling surrounding implants was recognized on radiographic examination (Figure 5(c)). In oral microbiological examination using quantitative real-time PCR, *Porphyromonas gingivalis* was below the detection limit. With regard to prosthetic complications, the patient experienced tipping of the porcelain at site #31 shortly after starting

Table 1: Case reports of implant treatment in a patient with periodontitis.

Authors (y)	Patient	Diagnosis	Therapy	Implants (n)	Maintenance interval	Follow-up (y)
Brezavšček et al. (2014)	71 M	Chronic generalized periodontitis (severe form)	(i) Extraction of 16 hopeless teeth (ii) Scaling and root planing (iii) Temporary RPDs (iv) Tooth- and implant-supported telescope-retained PRDs	Astra® (2)	3 months	1
Zafiropoulos et al. (2011)	39 F	Severe periodontitis	(i) Initial treatment, periodontal surgery (previous dentist) (ii) Extraction of hopeless tooth	Straumann® (12)	3-6 months	7
Zafiropoulos and Rebbe (2010)	47 M	Advanced chronic periodontitis	(i) Scaling and root planing (ii) Antibiotic treatment (iii) GTR (iv) Extraction of 7 teeth after 2 years (v) Overdenture, PFM crown (vi) 1 tooth fracture during 9-year maintenance	Straumann® (6)	6 months	15
Naert and Quirynen (2007)	47 F	Diagnosed "full extraction"	(i) Comprehensive treatment (Department of Periodontology, 30 years before) (ii) Recurrence of tooth fracture	NR (5)	NR	28
Kreissl (2007)	51 F	Severe periodontitis	(i) Extraction of hopeless tooth (ii) CTG	XIVE (5)	NR	NR
Hofer et al. (2002)	22 M	Rapid generalized early-onset periodontitis (1993 AAP definition)	(i) Scaling, gingivectomy (previous dentist) (ii) Hygiene phase, FOP (referred specialist)	Straumann® (4)	3 months	2

RPD: removable partial denture; GTR: guided tissue regeneration; PFM: porcelain-fused-to-metal; CTG: connective tissue graft; FOP: flap operation; NR: not reported.

function; because this tipping did not cause problems, we followed the course. Similarly, the abutment screw at site #16 loosened twice during the 12-year maintenance period. In each case, the screw was restored after cleaning and occlusal adjustment. The patient's oral hygiene has been well maintained, with no recurrence or worsening of periodontal disease among natural teeth.

3. Literature Review

The present study searched for articles published until 2018. The database Medline via PubMed was searched using the following terms: ("Dental Implants" [Mesh] OR "Dental Implantation" [Mesh]) OR ("Dental Prosthesis, Implant-Supported" [Mesh] OR implant [Title/Abstract]) AND (periodontitis [MeSH Terms] OR periodontitis [Title/Abstract]) AND (case reports [Publication Type] OR "case reports" [Title/Abstract] OR "case report" [Title/Abstract]) AND long-term [Title/Abstract]. Case reports on rare diseases or specific syndrome and edentulous patients and literature except for English were omitted with manual search. Six case reports were hit in the past 12 years (Table 1). Many reports showed that the majority of the interval maintenance period was 3 months [9–16]. In these reports, obtaining favorable healing process following periodontal initial treatment and surgical procedure was mentioned.

4. Discussion

This report describes the successful implant treatment and long-term management of a patient with severe periodontitis. To achieve successful periodontal treatment, both the removal of inflammatory factors and the improvement of occlusal factors are needed. In this case, these goals were obtained through oral hygiene instruction, scaling and root planing, occlusal adjustment, and application of a partial denture. A supportive therapy after active periodontal therapy is effective in maintaining the health of periodontal tissues [17].

Comprehensive treatment including maintenance or supportive therapy contributes to a decreased incidence of tooth loss [18]. A previous study found that the incidence of tooth loss among periodontal patients ranged from 0.09 to 0.16 per year [19–21]. That finding suggests that tooth loss can be minimized to only one tooth every 10 years with maintenance treatment. In this case, six hopeless teeth were extracted out of 24 present at the initial visit. Five implants were placed as prosthesis for seven missing teeth, and the patient did not lose any teeth during the maintenance period. In this regard, our results were better than those of similar reports.

To improve Eichner's index from B1 to A1, the occlusal supporting area was increased while stability of the periodontal tissue was achieved. Due to improved Eichner's index from B1 to A1, the occlusal supporting area was increased while stability of the periodontal tissue was achieved. It was prospected that periodontal tissue was protected by applying implants to provide a vertical stop and proper anterior guidance. In contrast, the reason for the loosening of the abutment screw was considered to be the wearing of the composite resin, which altered the occlusal condition and lateral forces on the superstructure at site #16.

It has been reported that long-term maintenance therapy for implants can prevent other complications and improve success rates [22]. Among the frequent problems with implants, prosthetic and biological complications are common [23]. In particular, peri-implantitis has gained attention as one major biological complication in recent years. *Aggregatibacter actinomycetemcomitans, Porphyromonas gingivalis, Prevotella intermedia*, and *Fusobacterium* spp. are implied to be pathological bacteria related to peri-implantitis. Likewise, their role in periodontitis has been studied [24, 25]. Moreover, natural teeth can act as reservoirs of microorganisms for colonization of oral implants [26].

A reliable treatment of peri-implantitis has not yet been established, and managing peri-implant tissue remains difficult. Nevertheless, it is clear that the risk factors for peri-implantitis include poor oral hygiene, a history of periodontitis, and smoking [7]. While the mechanisms and pathology of peri-implantitis are similar to those of periodontitis [27], much remains unknown about the condition [28]. Although periodontitis has been reported to decrease implant success rate [29], peri-implantitis can be prevented among patients with severe periodontitis. This success mainly relies on appropriate initial periodontal treatment, which allows us to maintain the patient's oral health during long-term maintenance therapy [30].

In this case, inflammatory remarkable symptoms were not detected during the maintenance period. Although it was previously established that BOP is evidence of inflammation [31], implant BOP is an uncertain clinical parameter for diagnosing the health of these tissues because of greater sensitivity than natural teeth [32] and depends on the shape of the superstructure and measuring technique. However, although it is not a completely established method, implant probing and accompanying bleeding are considered useful for diagnosing peri-implantitis [33]. Moreover, the absence of periodontal bacteria during supportive therapy confirmed that removal of inflammatory factors was successful and continuous.

In the present case, we eliminated inflammatory factors and improved the oral environment with comprehensive periodontal treatment. In the future, careful monitoring of alteration of occlusion and trauma force for teeth with altered crown-root ratios will be necessary. By applying implants to stabilize occlusion, the mobility of natural teeth was decreased. The course of this patient is good, with no deep PPD. Ongoing supportive therapy is necessary.

5. Conclusion

The patient diagnosed with generalized severe chronic periodontitis underwent comprehensive treatment involving implants. A long-term maintenance has been achieved, with no recurrence of periodontitis and with stability of the peri-implant tissues. With appropriate initial periodontal treatment and ongoing supportive therapy, oral health can be maintained soundly and longitudinally in patients with implants.

Consent

Written informed consent was obtained from the patient and her relative for publication. The written consent is available for review.

Authors' Contributions

KS wrote this manuscript and treated the patient. YH advised the possible treatment and gave valuable comments to this manuscript.

References

[1] P. J. Pérez-Chaparro, C. Gonçalves, L. C. Figueiredo et al., "Newly identified pathogens associated with periodontitis: a systematic review," *Journal of Dental Research*, vol. 93, no. 9, pp. 846–858, 2014.

[2] A. D. Haffajee and S. S. Socransky, "Introduction to microbial aspects of periodontal biofilm communities, development and treatment," *Periodontology 2000*, vol. 42, no. 1, pp. 7–12, 2006.

[3] A. Cekici, A. Kantarci, H. Hasturk, and T. E. Van Dyke, "Inflammatory and immune pathways in the pathogenesis of periodontal disease," *Periodontology 2000*, vol. 64, no. 1, pp. 57–80, 2014.

[4] L. Wolff, G. Dahlén, and D. Aeppli, "Bacteria as risk markers for periodontitis," *Journal of Periodontology*, vol. 65, no. 5s, pp. 498–510, 1994.

[5] G. C. Armitage, "Development of a classification system for periodontal diseases and conditions," *Annals of Periodontology*, vol. 4, no. 1, pp. 1–6, 1999.

[6] N. J. Kassebaum, E. Bernabé, M. Dahiya, B. Bhandari, C. J. L. Murray, and W. Marcenes, "Global burden of severe periodontitis in 1990-2010: a systematic review and meta-regression," *Journal of Dental Research*, vol. 93, no. 11, pp. 1045–1053, 2014.

[7] L. J. A. Heitz-Mayfield, "Peri-implant diseases: diagnosis and risk indicators," *Journal of Clinical Periodontology*, vol. 35, 8 Suppl, pp. 292–304, 2008.

[8] C. R. E. Hardt, K. Grondahl, U. Lekholm, and J. L. Wennstrom, "Outcome of implant therapy in relation to experienced loss of periodontal bone support. a retrospective 5-year study," *Clinical Oral Implants Research*, vol. 13, no. 5, pp. 488–494, 2002.

[9] M. Brezavšček, U. Lamott, and W. Att, "Treatment planning and dental rehabilitation of a periodontally compromised partially edentulous patient: a case report - part I," *The International Journal of Esthetic Dentistry*, vol. 9, no. 3, pp. 402–411, 2014.

[10] M. Brezavšcek, U. Lamott, and W. Att, "Treatment planning and dental rehabilitation of periodontally compromised partially edentulous patient: a case report-part II," *The International Journal of Esthetic Dentistry*, vol. 9, no. 4, pp. 506–515, 2014.

[11] G. G. K. Zafiropoulos, M. O. di Prisco, G. Deli, and O. Hoffmann, "Maintenance of class III trifurcated molars versus implant placement in regenerated extraction sockets: long-term results of 2 cases," *Journal of Oral Implantology*, vol. 37, no. sp1, pp. 141–155, 2011.

[12] G. G. Zafiropoulos and J. Rebbe, "Comprehensive treatment in a case with advanced chronic periodontitis: a 15-year follow-up," *General Dentistry*, vol. 58, no. 4, pp. e149–e155, 2010.

[13] I. Naert and M. Quirynen, "Surgical periodontal interventions: long-term outcomes," *International Journal of Prosthodontics*, vol. 20, no. 4, pp. 345–348, 2007.

[14] M. E. Kreissl, "Complex dental rehabilitation in a periodontally compromised patient. Part 1: diagnosis and treatment planning," *European Journal of Esthetic Dentistry: official journal of the European Academy of Esthetic Dentistry*, vol. 2, no. 2, pp. 222–235, 2007.

[15] M. E. Kreissl, "Complex dental rehabilitation in a periodontally compromised patient. Part 2: treatment and discussion," *European Journal of Esthetic Dentistry: official journal of the European Academy of Esthetic Dentistry*, vol. 2, no. 3, pp. 322–335, 2007.

[16] D. Hofer, C. H. Hämmerle, and N. P. Lang, "Comprehensive treatment concept in a young adult patient with severe periodontal disease: a case report," *Quintessence International*, vol. 33, no. 8, pp. 567–578, 2002.

[17] N. P. L. NP and M. S. Tonetti, "Periodontal risk assessment (PRA) for patients in supportive periodontal therapy (SPT)," *Oral Health & Preventive Dentistry*, vol. 1, no. 1, pp. 7–16, 2003.

[18] J. A. Martin, R. C. Page, C. F. Loeb, and E. K. Kaye, "Reduction of tooth loss associated with periodontal treatment," *International Journal of Periodontics & Restorative Dentistry*, vol. 31, no. 5, pp. 471–479, 2011.

[19] L. Hirschfeld and B. Wasserman, "A long-term survey of tooth loss in 600 treated periodontal patients," *Journal of Periodontology*, vol. 49, no. 5, pp. 225–237, 1978.

[20] W. T. McFall Jr., "Tooth loss in 100 treated patients with periodontal disease, a long-term study," *Journal of Periodontology*, vol. 53, no. 9, pp. 539–549, 1982.

[21] M. J. Goldman, I. F. Ross, and D. Goteiner, "Effect of periodontal therapy on patients maintained for 15 years or longer. A retrospective study," *Journal of Periodontology*, vol. 57, no. 6, pp. 347–353, 1986.

[22] A. Monje, L. Aranda, K. T. Diaz et al., "Impact of maintenance therapy for the prevention of peri-implant Diseases," *Journal of Dental Research*, vol. 95, no. 4, pp. 372–379, 2016.

[23] M. Esposito, J. M. Hirsch, U. Lekholm, and P. Thomsen, "Biological factors contributing to failures of osseointegrated oral implants. (I) Success criteria and epidemiology," *European Journal of Oral Sciences*, vol. 106, no. 1, pp. 527–551, 1998.

[24] J. Slots and T. E. Rams, "New views on periodontal microbiota in special patient categories," *Journal of Clinical Periodontology*, vol. 18, no. 6, pp. 411–420, 1991.

[25] T. Shiba, T. Watanabe, H. Kachi et al., "Distinct interacting core taxa in co-occurrence networks enable discrimination of polymicrobial oral diseases with similar symptoms," *Scientific Reports*, vol. 6, no. 1, 2016.

[26] W. Papaioannou, M. Quirynen, and D. Van Steenberghe, "The influence of periodontitis on the subgingival flora around implants in partially edentulous patients," *Clinical Oral Implants Research*, vol. 7, no. 4, pp. 405–409, 1996.

[27] L. J. A. Heitz-Mayfield and N. P. Lang, "Comparative biology of chronic and aggressive periodontitis vs. peri-implantitis," *Periodontology 2000*, vol. 53, no. 1, pp. 167–181, 2010.

[28] T. Berglundh, N. U. Zitzmann, and M. Donati, "Are peri-implantitis lesions different from periodontitis lesions?," *Journal of Clinical Periodontology*, vol. 38, no. s11, pp. 188–202, 2011.

[29] P. R. Klokkevold and T. J. Han, "How do smoking, diabetes, and periodontitis affect outcomes of implant treatment?," *Internattional Journal of Oral Maxillofacial Implants*, vol. 22, no. 7, pp. 173–202, 2007.

[30] J. Cho-Yan Lee, N. Mattheos, K. C. Nixon, and S. Ivanovski, "Residual periodontal pockets are a risk indicator for peri-implantitis in patients treated for periodontitis," *Clinical Oral Implants Research*, vol. 23, no. 3, pp. 325–333, 2012.

[31] G. Greenstein, J. Caton, and A. M. Polson, "Histologic characteristics associated with bleeding after probing and visual signs of inflammation," *Journal of Periodontology*, vol. 52, no. 8, pp. 420–425, 1981.

[32] S. Luterbacher, L. Mayfield, U. Bragger, and N. P. Lang, "Diagnostic characteristics of clinical and microbiological tests for monitoring periodontal and peri-implant mucosal tissue conditions during supportive periodontal therapy (SPT)," *Clinical Oral Implants Research*, vol. 11, no. 6, pp. 521–529, 2000.

[33] K. Seki, S. Nakabayashi, N. Tanabe, A. Kamimoto, and Y. Hagiwara, "Correlations between clinical parameters in implant maintenance patients: analysis among healthy and history-of-periodontitis groups," *International Journal of Implant Dentistry*, vol. 3, no. 1, p. 45, 2017.

18

The "One Piece" Autologous Tuberosity Graft: A Contemporary Concept in Ridge Preservation

Ronald Younes[1,2] **and Carla Maria Khairallah**[1]

[1]*Department of Oral Surgery, Faculty of Dental Medicine, Saint Joseph University of Beirut, Beirut, Lebanon*
[2]*Craniofacial Research Laboratory-Division of Oral Biology, Saint Joseph University of Beirut, Faculty of Dental Medicine, Beirut, Lebanon*

Correspondence should be addressed to Ronald Younes; ronald.younes@hotmail.com

Academic Editor: Jose López-López

Tooth extraction causes major changes to the ridge, rendering implant placement a more challenging procedure. Proper management of the socket is necessary to ensure sufficient bone and soft tissue for a successful implant-supported prosthesis. This article presents a practical approach for autologous hard and soft tissue grafting. A soft and hard tissue graft is harvested in one piece from the maxillary tuberosity and stabilized in the extraction socket.

1. Background

Placing an implant in the aesthetic zone is a challenging procedure. Following a tooth extraction, dimensional changes to the ridge occur, as a result of the healing process. In fact, based on a systematic review in 2012, 29 to 63% of horizontal bone loss and 11 to 22% of vertical bone loss, corresponding to 3.79 ± 0.23 mm and 1.24 ± 0.11 mm, respectively, occur 6 months after an extraction [1]. And at 12 months, as much as 50% reduction in width of the alveolar ridge occurs [2].

Several treatments following tooth extraction are available: immediate or delayed implant placement with or without bone and/or soft tissue augmentation, and socket preservation followed by a delayed implant placement.

In order to facilitate the choice of treatment, a new classification in 2016 divided single-rooted tooth extraction sockets into three grades, depending on the buccal plate morphology, the apical bone topography, and the interproximal bone available. Thus, a treatment is chosen according to the socket's classification. Therefore, grades I and II with thick biotype are eligible for immediate implant placement, while grade II with thin biotype and grade III, a socket preservation is advisable [3].

While a number of publications showed a significantly lower survival rate of immediately placed implants compared to delayed implants inserted into healed sockets [4–7], socket preservation techniques have been used frequently to idealize the delayed implant placement in sufficient amounts of bone, with an ideal implant position, providing a proper emergence profile for an esthetic and functional prosthesis. Several biomaterials have been applied in alveolar ridge preservation, alone or in combination. They included xenografts [8, 9], allografts [10, 11], alloplastic material, synthetic magnesium-enriched hydroxyapatite [12], recombinant morphogenetic protein-2 (rh-BMP2) [13], autologous bone marrow [14], autologous bone particles [15], and autologous blood-derived products (PRF, PRP) [16, 17]. Those grafting materials were used as socket fillers with or without collagen membrane [8, 10], and/or free gingival grafts [18] as socket sealers.

In general, bone substitutes show complete osseous integration, but they seem to decelerate bone regeneration in the early healing phases and reduce the proportion of vital bone when compared to autologous grafts [19, 20]. Xenografts are known to require long periods of healing and resorption, leading usually to high numbers of residual graft particles at early reentries [21–23]. To the contrary, alloplastic material

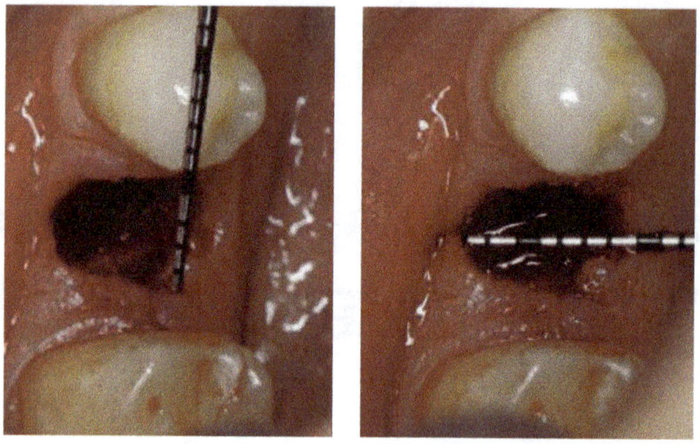

(a) (b)

FIGURE 1: Measurements of the socket with a periodontal probe: (a) mesio-distal; (b) bucco-lingual.

usually has the highest amount of vital bone and the smaller amount of residual graft material [19]. But, xenografts and allografts show more favorable results when compared to alloplastic materials, in preserving socket dimensions [19, 24]. And when attempts were made to use autologous bone chips in socket preservation, they failed to promote healing or stimulate hard tissue formation in the socket [15].

Unfortunately, to this date, no clear consensus was reached on the ideal biomaterial to be used in socket preservation.

The purpose of this article is to present a socket preservation approach using a "one-piece" autologous bone and soft tissue graft harvested from the maxillary tuberosity.

2. Rationale for "One-Piece" Ridge Preservation Technique

This technique is limited to sockets of single-rooted teeth.

2.1. Medications

(i) Amoxicillin with clavulanic acid (Augmentin) 1 g BID for 7 days, starting the morning of the extraction day

(ii) Ibuprofen (Brufen) 400 TID in case of pain

(iii) Chlorhexidine mouthwash 0.12% TID for 21 days (starting the day after the extraction)

2.2. Surgical Technique. Step 1: the patient is asked to rinse for 1 minute a solution of 0.2% chlorhexidine. Afterwards, local anesthesia is administrated. Atraumatic extraction of the tooth, preserving the alveolar bone and the surrounding soft tissue, is performed, followed by a thorough curettage of the socket in order to remove any infected tissue. Deepithelialization of the inner part of the free gingiva surrounding the socket is made using a 15C blade or a diamond bur.

Step 2: a periodontal probe is used to measure the dimensions of the socket in order to determine the size of the tissue punch and trephine bur to be used (Figure 1).

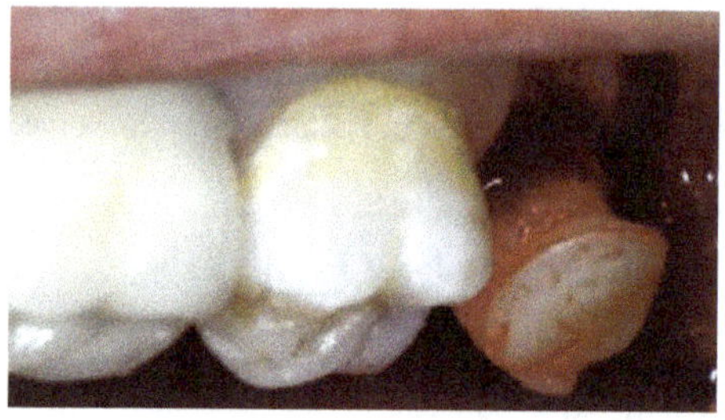

FIGURE 2: The "one-piece" tuberosity graft harvest.

A tuberosity block together with a greater palatine nerve block is performed. Using a soft tissue punch, the gingiva is demarcated. Then, the bone is perforated with a smaller trephine bur, to finally remove the gingivoosseous graft in one piece (Figure 2).

Step 3: the graft should fit adequately in the extraction socket without being compressive to the socket walls or too loose (Figure 3). Occasionally, shaping of the graft is needed, using a rongeur. The soft tissue can also be trimmed, thus avoiding overfilling of the socket.

Step 4: the composite graft is stabilized in the fresh extraction socket with simple interrupted sutures using 6/0 absorbable sutures (Figure 4).

Step 5: maintaining good oral hygiene and avoiding any removable prosthesis over the treated site (Figure 5). Duration of the healing period is 4 months, correlating with autologous bone regeneration principles.

Step 6: implants could be placed at 4 months postextraction (Figures 6 and 7).

A Cone-Beam Computed Tomography (CBCT) scan was taken before the extraction and 4 months after. A superimposition of both CBCTs was made to measure the socket's modifications following tooth extraction and preservation using the "one-piece" technique (Figure 8). Limited vertical and horizontal bone losses were detected. The vertical resorption was 0.71 mm. The horizontal resorption was measured at 3 different levels: 2, 4, and 6 mm from the most coronal bone peak preoperatively. The respective values were 2.71 mm, 1.29 mm, and 0.72 mm. As for the soft tissue on the buccal side, an increase of 1.23 mm in thickness was marked.

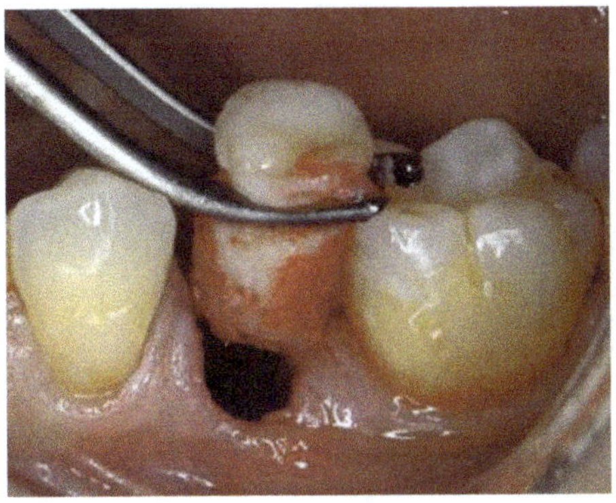

FIGURE 3: Fitting of the graft.

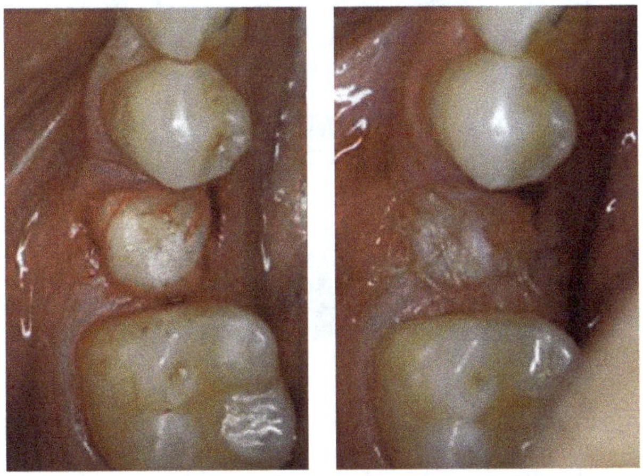

(a) (b)

FIGURE 4: (a) Placement of the graft in the socket; (b) graft stabilized with 6/0 absorbable sutures.

3. Discussion

Alveolar ridge preservation was proven to be an effective approach to decrease dimensional changes after tooth extraction [25–29].

The "one piece" technique we used satisfies the alveolar ridge preservation requirements, such as atraumatic extraction [30], flapless procedure [31], usage of bone as a filler and soft tissue as a sealer of the socket, while providing healing by primary intention.

When a mucoperiosteal flap is elevated, the blood vessels attached to the bone are severed. This will reduce the blood supply and lead to the death of local osteocytes. Hence, the surrounding mineralized tissue of the bone walls necrotize and eventually be eliminated through surface resorption [32]. This is not the case with this technique, since the graft is inserted without flap elevation, keeping the periosteum intact and the mucogingival junction (MGJ) in its original position.

Moreover, the form of the graft mimicking the root anatomy seems to prevent the ridge collapse during the healing phase. This is not the case when bone chips are used.

We have chosen to use autogenous bone and soft tissue graft. In fact, the use of autologous bone in bone regeneration is still considered the "gold standard" due to its osteogenic, osteoinductive, and osteoconductive properties [33, 34]. It has a unique advantage of retaining cell viability and containing osteoblasts and osteoprogenitor stem cells which provides true osteogenesis [34]. In this technique, the maxillary tuberosity showed no complications and better accessibility, an advantage when we know that other intraoral donor sites such as the chin and the ramus present significant postoperative bleeding, swelling, discomfort, and risk of nerve injury [35]. A limitation to its usage is the reduced available amount of bone that makes it an indication in small or medium-sized defects [36, 37]. But furthermore, the tuberosity region usually consists of a thin cortical layer and a mixture of marrow spaces, adipose tissue, and vital osteogenic cells, necessary for bone formation. The type of graft described in this case report is an inlay type of graft.

A paradigm shift in the dynamics of bone grafting has taken place in the recent decades, favoring inlay-type grafts as the one used in this case for alveolar ridge preservation techniques. Whether cortical or cancellous bone of endochondral or membranous origin, bone growth is predictable when the graft is well contained in the socket [38]. Interestingly, and fairly recently (2013), studies by Rosenthal, Buchman, and Kristoffer demonstrated that inlay-type bone grafts maintained a higher volume over the years than onlay-type bone grafts, regardless of their embryological or microarchitecture origin. Furthermore, bone grafts in the inlay position have a higher potential for revascularization, osteogenesis, osteoinduction, and osteoconduction, due to the increased bone-to-bone contact. At these sites, no resorption is noted, but on the contrary, bone growth and real expansion of the site are observed. In addition, cancellous bone results in much greater growth, regardless of its embryological origin. Afterwards, the presence of functional forces creates a favorable biomechanical matrix in which the phenotype of the grafted material is closer to that of the recipient, rather than retaining its native structural tissue. The cortical bone placed in the inlay position becomes more porous over time, while the cancellous bone becomes less and less porous.

In 1989, Whitaker demonstrated that bone grafts retain their volume significantly better in the inlay position than in the onlay position because fewer changes are caused in the overlying soft tissue. While describing the concept of biological boundaries, Whitaker emphasized the importance of the overlying soft tissue envelope. In our technique, soft tissue coverage is maintained attached to the underlying bone and stabilized in situ.

The soft tissue in the tuberosity area is formed of dense collagen fibers covered by a well-keratinized layer. This might positively affect the dimensional stability of the graft and the process of graft revascularization [39, 40]. Additionally, tuberosity grafts are known to heal fast with superior color and contour blending and a reduced pain perception by the patient [39].

To our knowledge, in 2009, Tolstunov was the first to describe the maxillary tuberosity block bone graft [36].

In 2013, da Rosa et al. have introduced a new immediate dentoalveolar restoration (IDR) technique. The IDR consists of an immediate implant placement associated with a

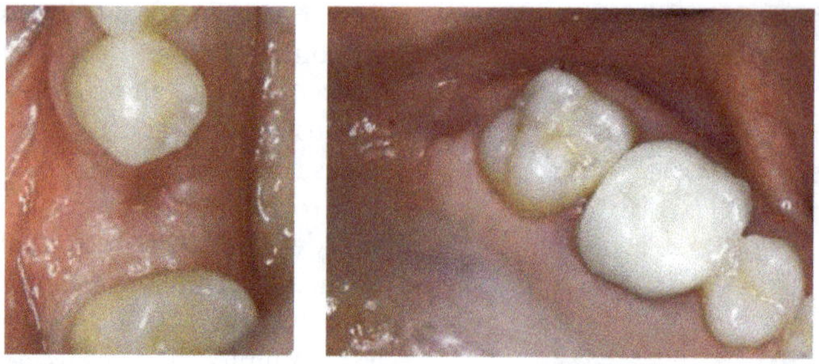

(a) (b)

FIGURE 5: Follow-up 3 weeks post-op: (a) grafted site; (b) donor site.

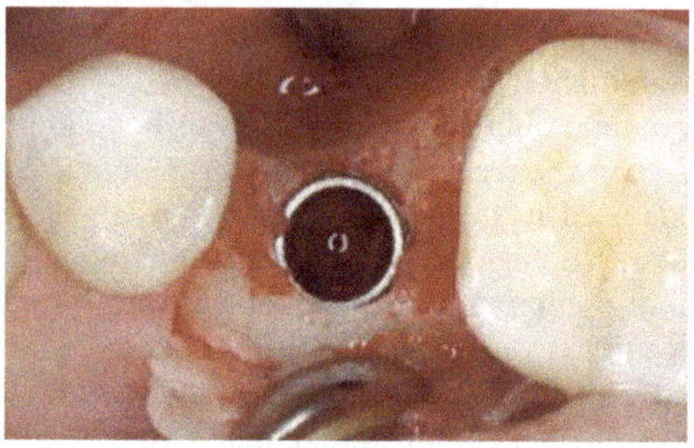

FIGURE 6: Implant placement after 4 months.

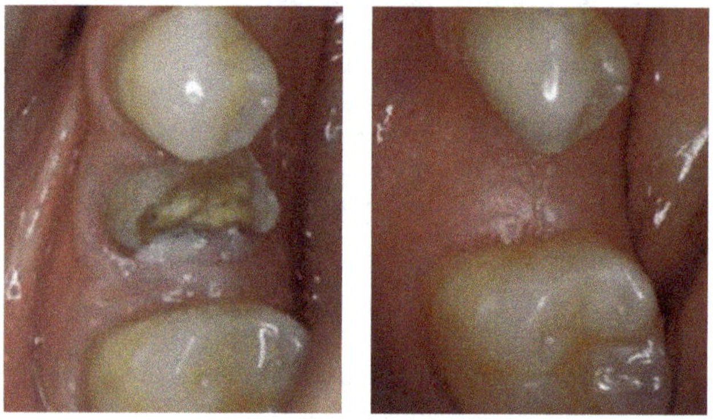

(a) (b)

FIGURE 7: Occlusal view of the lower left second premolar site: (a) before the extraction; (b) 4 months post-op.

corticocancellous block graft harvested from the tuberosity and placed in the gap between the implant and the buccal mucosa (in the absence of buccal bone wall) [41].

In 2014, the same team modified the IDR technique by adding a layer of connective tissue to the corticocancellous block, resulting in a triple graft, reserved for sockets with severe buccal bone wall damage and gingival recession. From a clinical and radiological point of view, hard and soft tissue gain had been demonstrated, leading to a satisfactory, aesthetic, and functional result [42].

Applying the "one-piece" technique for alveolar ridge preservation in this case showed a reduced hard tissue resorption and a gain of soft tissue following tooth extraction, an encouraging result when compared to previous studies reporting on dimensional changes of nontreated extraction sockets [1, 2].

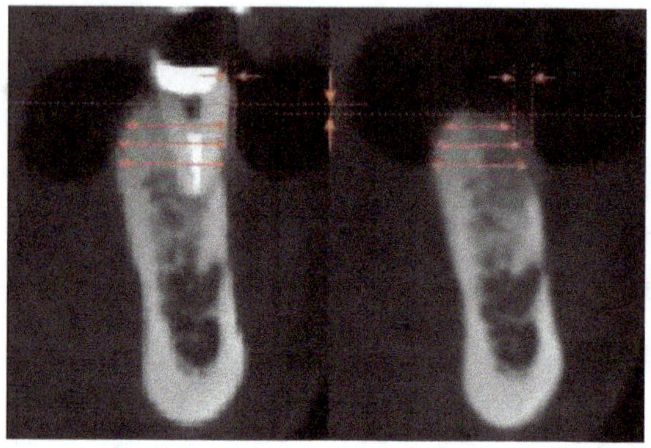

(a) (b)

FIGURE 8: CBCT sagittal view with an illustration of radiological measurements: (a) Before the extraction; (b) 4 months post-op (vertical difference of bone levels; horizontal bone width at 2, 4, and 6 mm; soft tissue thickness at the buccal side).

This technique also contributed to a proper bone and soft tissue formation in the extraction site thus providing sufficient bone and soft tissue for a successful implant-supported prosthesis without the need of complimentary grafts.

4. Conclusion

The "one-piece" tuberosity graft seems to be a safe alveolar ridge preservation technique, integrating soft and hard tissue in one simple approach. It may represent a feasible, user-friendly, low-cost solution for minimizing soft and hard tissue collapse and dimensional loss following single-rooted tooth extraction.

It would be interesting to conduct future RCT studies on this technique in order to present a safe and simple approach to alveolar ridge preservation.

References

[1] W. L. Tan, T. L. T. Wong, M. C. M. Wong, and N. P. Lang, "A systematic review of post-extractional alveolar hard and soft tissue dimensional changes in humans," *Clinical Oral Implants Research*, vol. 23, pp. 1–21, 2012.

[2] L. Schropp, A. Wenzel, L. Kostopoulos, and T. Karring, "Bone healing and soft tissue contour changes following single-tooth extraction: a clinical and radiographic 12-month prospective study," *The International Journal of Periodontics & Restorative Dentistry*, vol. 23, no. 4, pp. 313–323, 2003.

[3] E. El Chaar, S. Oshman, and A. P. Fallah, "Single-rooted extraction sockets: classification and treatment protocol," *Compendium of continuing education in dentistry (Jamesburg, N.J.: 1995)*, vol. 37, no. 8, pp. 537–541, 2016.

[4] C. C. Mello, C. A. A. Lemos, F. R. Verri, D. M. dos Santos, M. C. Goiato, and E. P. Pellizzer, "Immediate implant placement into fresh extraction sockets versus delayed implants into healed sockets: a systematic review and meta-analysis," *International Journal of Oral and Maxillofacial Surgery*, vol. 46, no. 9, pp. 1162–1177, 2017.

[5] M. S. Tonetti, P. Cortellini, F. Graziani et al., "Immediate *versus* delayed implant placement after anterior single tooth extraction: the timing randomized controlled clinical trial," *Journal of Clinical Periodontology*, vol. 44, no. 2, pp. 215–224, 2017.

[6] J. Antetomaso and S. Kumar, "Survival rate of delayed implants placed in healed extraction sockets is significantly higher than that of immediate implants placed in fresh extraction sockets," *The Journal of Evidence-Based Dental Practice*, vol. 18, no. 1, pp. 76–78, 2018.

[7] B. R. Chrcanovic, T. Albrektsson, and A. Wennerberg, "Dental implants inserted in fresh extraction sockets versus healed sites: a systematic review and meta-analysis," *Journal of Dentistry*, vol. 43, no. 1, pp. 16–41, 2015.

[8] V. Iorio-Siciliano, A. Blasi, M. Nicolò, A. Iorio-Siciliano, F. Riccitiello, and L. Ramaglia, "Clinical outcomes of socket preservation using bovine-derived xenograft collagen and collagen membrane post-tooth extraction: a 6-month randomized controlled clinical trial," *The International Journal of Periodontics & Restorative Dentistry*, vol. 37, no. 5, pp. e290–e296, 2017.

[9] A. Barone, M. Ricci, P. Tonelli, S. Santini, and U. Covani, "Tissue changes of extraction sockets in humans: a comparison of spontaneous healing vs. ridge preservation with secondary soft tissue healing," *Clinical Oral Implants Research*, vol. 24, no. 11, pp. 1231–1237, 2013.

[10] J. M. Iasella, H. Greenwell, R. L. Miller et al., "Ridge preservation with freeze-dried bone allograft and a collagen membrane compared to extraction alone for implant site development: a clinical and histologic study in humans," *Journal of Periodontology*, vol. 74, no. 7, pp. 990–999, 2003.

[11] S. Spinato, P. Galindo-Moreno, D. Zaffe, F. Bernardello, and C. M. Soardi, "Is socket healing conditioned by buccal plate thickness? A clinical and histologic study 4 months after mineralized human bone allografting," *Clinical Oral Implants Research*, vol. 25, no. 2, pp. e120–e126, 2014.

[12] R. Crespi, P. Capparè, and E. Gherlone, "Comparison of magnesium-enriched hydroxyapatite and porcine bone in human extraction socket healing: a histologic and histomorphometric evaluation," *International Journal of Oral & Maxillofacial Implants*, vol. 26, no. 5, pp. 1057–1062, 2011.

[13] J. P. Fiorellini, T. H. Howell, D. Cochran et al., "Randomized study evaluating recombinant human bone morphogenetic protein-2 for extraction socket augmentation," *Journal of Periodontology*, vol. 76, no. 4, pp. 605–613, 2005.

[14] A. A. Pelegrine, C. E. S. da Costa, M. E. P. Correa, and J. F. C. Marques, "Clinical and histomorphometric evaluation of extraction sockets treated with an autologous bone marrow graft," *Clinical Oral Implants Research*, vol. 21, no. 5, pp. 535-542, 2010.

[15] M. G. Araújo and J. Lindhe, "Socket grafting with the use of autologous bone: an experimental study in the dog," *Clinical Oral Implants Research*, vol. 22, no. 1, pp. 9–13, 2011.

[16] R. Alissa, M. Esposito, K. Horner, and R. Oliver, "The influence of platelet-rich plasma on the healing of extraction sockets: an explorative randomised clinical trial," *European Journal of Oral Implantology*, vol. 3, no. 2, pp. 121–134, 2010.

[17] A. Temmerman, J. Vandessel, A. Castro et al., "The use of leucocyte and platelet-rich fibrin in socket management and ridge preservation: a split-mouth, randomized, controlled clinical trial," *Journal of Clinical Periodontology*, vol. 43, no. 11, pp. 990–999, 2016.

[18] Ç. Karaca, N. Er, A. Gülşahı, and O. T. Köseoğlu, "Alveolar ridge preservation with a free gingival graft in the anterior maxilla: volumetric evaluation in a randomized clinical trial," *International Journal of Oral and Maxillofacial Surgery*, vol. 44, no. 6, pp. 774–780, 2015.

[19] S. Jambhekar, F. Kernen, and A. S. Bidra, "Clinical and histologic outcomes of socket grafting after flapless tooth extraction: a systematic review of randomized controlled clinical trials," *The Journal of Prosthetic Dentistry*, vol. 113, no. 5, pp. 371–382, 2015.

[20] H.-L. Chan, G.-H. Lin, J.-H. Fu, and H.-L. Wang, "Alterations in bone quality after socket preservation with grafting materials: a systematic review," *The International Journal of Oral & Maxillofacial Implants*, vol. 28, no. 3, pp. 710–720, 2013.

[21] T. Traini, P. Valentini, G. Iezzi, and A. Piattelli, "A histologic and histomorphometric evaluation of anorganic bovine bone retrieved 9 years after a sinus augmentation procedure," *Journal of Periodontology*, vol. 78, no. 5, pp. 955–961, 2007.

[22] J. Bassil, K. Senni, S. Changotade et al., "Expression of MMP-2, 9 and 13 in newly formed bone after sinus augmentation using inorganic bovine bone in human," *Journal of Periodontal Research*, vol. 46, no. 6, pp. 756–762, 2011.

[23] M. Ayna, Y. Açil, and A. Gulses, "Fate of a bovine-derived xenograft in maxillary sinus floor elevation after 14 years: histologic and radiologic analysis," *The International Journal of Periodontics & Restorative Dentistry*, vol. 35, no. 4, pp. 541–547, 2015.

[24] S. S. Jensen, N. Broggini, E. Hjorting-Hansen, R. Schenk, and D. Buser, "Bone healing and graft resorption of autograft, anorganic bovine bone and beta-tricalcium phosphate. A histologic and histomorphometric study in the mandibles of minipigs," *Clinical Oral Implants Research*, vol. 17, no. 3, pp. 237–243, 2006.

[25] G. Avila-Ortiz, L. Chambrone, and F. Vignoletti, "Effect of alveolar ridge preservation interventions following tooth extraction: a systematic review and meta-analysis," *Journal of Clinical Periodontology*, vol. 46, pp. 195–223, 2019.

[26] F. Vignoletti, P. Matesanz, D. Rodrigo, E. Figuero, C. Martin, and M. Sanz, "Surgical protocols for ridge preservation after tooth extraction. A systematic review," *Clinical Oral Implants Research*, vol. 23, pp. 22–38, 2012.

[27] O. Iocca, A. Farcomeni, S. Pardiñas Lopez, and H. S. Talib, "Alveolar ridge preservation after tooth extraction: a Bayesian network meta-analysis of grafting materials efficacy on prevention of bone height and width reduction," *Journal of Clinical Periodontology*, vol. 44, no. 1, pp. 104–114, 2017.

[28] N. MacBeth, A. Trullenque-Eriksson, N. Donos, and N. Mardas, "Hard and soft tissue changes following alveolar ridge preservation: a systematic review," *Clinical Oral Implants Research*, vol. 28, no. 8, pp. 982–1004, 2017.

[29] G. Vittorini Orgeas, M. Clementini, V. De Risi, and M. de Sanctis, "Surgical techniques for alveolar socket preservation: a systematic review," *The International Journal of Oral & Maxillofacial Implants*, vol. 28, no. 4, pp. 1049–1061, 2013.

[30] M. Kubilius, R. Kubilius, and A. Gleiznys, "The preservation of alveolar bone ridge during tooth extraction," *Stomatologija*, vol. 14, no. 1, pp. 3–11, 2012.

[31] J. Lee, J.-B. Lee, K.-T. Koo, Y.-J. Seol, and Y.-M. Lee, "Flap management in alveolar ridge preservation: a systematic review and meta-analysis," *The International Journal of Oral & Maxillofacial Implants*, vol. 33, no. 3, pp. 613–621, 2018.

[32] M. G. Araujo and J. Lindhe, "Dimensional ridge alterations following tooth extraction. An experimental study in the dog," *Journal of Clinical Periodontology*, vol. 32, no. 2, pp. 212–218, 2005.

[33] G. D. Rabelo, P. M. de Paula, F. S. Rocha, C. Jordão Silva, and D. Zanetta-Barbosa, "Retrospective study of bone grafting procedures before implant placement," *Implant Dentistry*, vol. 19, no. 4, pp. 342–350, 2010.

[34] R. Gapski, K. Satheesh, and C. M. Cobb, "Histomorphometric analysis of bone density in the maxillary tuberosity of cadavers: a pilot study," *Journal of Periodontology*, vol. 77, no. 6, pp. 1085–1090, 2006.

[35] D. Reininger, C. Cobo-Vazquez, B. Rosenberg, and J. Lopez-Quiles, "Alternative intraoral donor sites to the chin and mandibular body-ramus," *Journal of Clinical and Experimental Dentistry*, vol. 9, no. 12, pp. e1474–e1481, 2017.

[36] L. Tolstunov, "Maxillary tuberosity block bone graft: innovative technique and case report," *Journal of Oral and Maxillofacial Surgery*, vol. 67, no. 8, pp. 1723–1729, 2009.

[37] A. Khojasteh, P. Nazeman, and L. Tolstunov, "Tuberosity-alveolar block as a donor site for localised augmentation of the maxilla: a retrospective clinical study," *The British Journal of Oral & Maxillofacial Surgery*, vol. 54, no. 8, pp. 950–955, 2016.

[38] K. B. Sugg, A. H. Rosenthal, and W. Ozaki, "Quantitative comparison of volume maintenance between inlay and onlay bone grafts in the craniofacial skeleton," *Plastic and Reconstructive Surgery*, vol. 131, no. 5, pp. 1014–1021, 2013.

[39] P. Amin, "Tuberosity versus palatal donor sites for soft tissue grafting: a split-mouth clinical study," *Quintessence International*, vol. 7, pp. 589–598, 2018.

[40] R. J. Harris, "Histologic evaluation of connective tissue grafts in humans," *The International Journal of Periodontics & Restorative Dentistry*, vol. 23, no. 6, pp. 575–583, 2003.

[41] J. C. M. da Rosa, A. C. Rosa, D. M. da Rosa, and C. M. Zardo, "Immediate dentoalveolar restoration of compromised sockets: a novel technique," *The European Journal of Esthetic Dentistry*, vol. 8, no. 3, pp. 432–443, 2013.

[42] J. C. M. da Rosa, A. C. Rosa, M. A. Fadanelli, and B. S. Sotto-Maior, "Immediate implant placement, reconstruction of compromised sockets, and repair of gingival recession with a triple graft from the maxillary tuberosity: a variation of the immediate dentoalveolar restoration technique," *The Journal of Prosthetic Dentistry*, vol. 112, no. 4, pp. 717–722, 2014.

19

Postextraction Alveolar Preservation and use of the Crown of the Extracted Tooth as a Temporary Restoration

Andrea Rodríguez Moreno,[1] Mariné Ortiz Magdaleno,[1] Marissa Muñoz Islas,[1] Jorge Armando Villar Mercado,[2] María del Pilar Goldaracena Azuara,[1] Everardo Ruiz Cruz,[1] and Gabriel Fernando Romo Ramírez[1]

[1]*Autonomous University of San Luis Potosí, Specialty in Aesthetic, Cosmetic, Restorative, and Implantological Dentistry, Faculty of Stomatology, Av. Dr. Manuel Nava #2, Zona Universitaria, 78290 San Luis Potosí, Mexico*
[2]*Autonomous University of San Luis Potosí, Specialty in Periodontics, Faculty of Stomatology, Av. Dr. Manuel Nava #2, Zona Universitaria, 78290 San Luis Potosí, Mexico*

Correspondence should be addressed to Mariné Ortiz Magdaleno; marine.ortiz@uaslp.mx

Academic Editor: Sukumaran Anil

Ranging from the extraction of teeth from anterior sector commitment to the loss of bone and soft tissues, alveolar preservation is a regenerative technique that employs biomaterials that induce the preservation of bone tissue and minimize resorption. Placement of provisional restorations at the defect site maintains the stability of the soft tissues and aesthetics at which the definitive restoration is found. The objective of this clinical case was alveolar preservation postextraction of the anterior tooth that presented a coronal fracture, placing the clinical crown of the extracted tooth as the provisional restoration to maintain stability and to avoid soft tissue collapse and compromise to an aesthetic area.

1. Introduction

Losing a tooth involves surgical, periodontal, restorative, and aesthetic procedures. The surgical procedure for the extraction of a tooth with a poor prognosis, due either to caries, periodontal conditions, or trauma in the anterior sector, causes a series of dimensional and morphological changes in the soft and hard tissues [1]. The loss of bone volume is a factor that affects the placement of implants: if placement of an implant at the extraction site is desired, then ideally, at the time of surgery, tissue regeneration should be performed by placement of grafts or biomaterials with osteoinductive properties and use of osteogenics, which regenerate the lost tissue for later implant placement [2]. When a tooth is extracted, a process of bone resorption usually occurs, causing atrophy of the alveolar ridge. To prevent this type of defect, therapeutic treatments have emerged that preserve the alveolar tissue and maintain the soft tissue and the emerging dimensions of the alveolar contours [3–5].

After dental surgery, the soft tissue collapses, and the bone tissue that makes up the alveolus undergoes biological healing processes that affect its dimensions both in volume and in morphology. In addition, it is not possible to predict the morphology of the defect site because the width of the reabsorbed bone (vestibular-palatal) is increased; it is related to the thickness of the alveolar external crest of the maxilla in vertical terms (apico-coronal) [6, 7]. Techniques of alveolar preservation are the set of techniques aimed at the preservation of the ridge volume determined at the time of tooth extraction, minimizing reabsorption of the alveolar ridge [8, 9]. This is intended to decrease; however, it does not completely eliminate its resorption horizontally, since its objective is to maintain bone volume [10]. The alveolar ridge has been reported to lose 50% of its height and width during

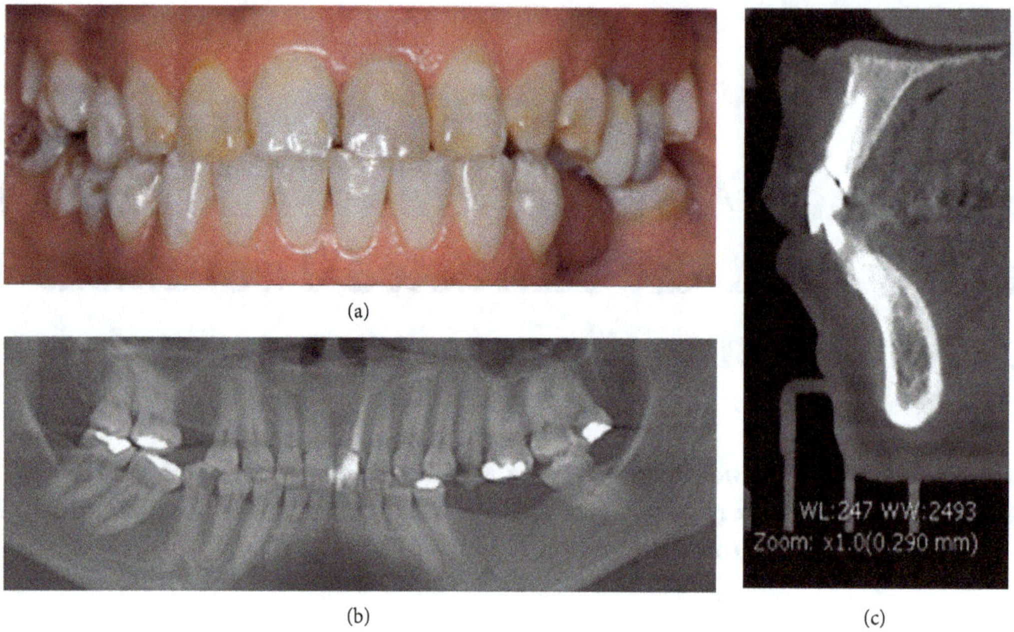

(a) (b) (c)

Figure 1: Anterosuperior sector: the clinical crown fracture of tooth #21 is clinically not observed (a); panoramic x-ray (b) and computerized axial tomography (c).

the first 6 months; therefore, studies have reported that socket-sealing surgery minimizes the loss of alveolar bone and soft tissues [11, 12].

Alveolar preservation is indicated when, for surgical reasons, there is a contraindication to placing a postextraction implant, when the desire is to improve and restore the loss of bone tissue and soft tissue that have been lost by a traumatic dental extraction and the presence of dehiscence and fenestration [13–15]. The bone morphology of the maxilla in the anterior sector compromises the aesthetics of the soft tissues; thus, planning the definitive restoration will depend on the design of the provisional restoration. Once alveolar preservation has been carried out, provisionalization of the edentulous sector should be considered with the use of a provisional restoration that does not affect the regeneration of bone and soft tissues. An accurate diagnosis and appropriate management of postextraction alveolar preservation techniques allow us to succeed in the predictability of the clinical case.

This case report will show a clinical case in which a fracture of coronal tooth #21 was diagnosed without the possibility of prosthetic rehabilitation. Dental extraction and alveolar preservation were indicated, while placement of the postextraction implant was contraindicated due to the lack of sufficient thickness in the buccal vestibular crest, and the provisional restoration consisted of the same fractured autologous clinical crown of tooth #21. This case report presents a step-by-step alveolar preservation protocol and provisional restoration.

2. Case Description

A 41-year-old female patient attended the Specialty in Cosmetic Dentistry, Cosmetic, Restorative, and Implantology Clinic of the Faculty of Stomatology, Autonomous University of San Luis Potosí, Mexico, for consultation due to the mobility of the clinical crown of tooth #21 because of a trauma The patient did not have relevant medical records, and thus, we requested a computerized axial tomography (CT) scan to assess the thickness of the buccal bone table and the coronal fracture.

2.1. Clinical Examination. In the intraoral clinical evaluation (Figure 1(a)), mobility grade 3 of the clinical crown of tooth #21 was diagnosed. A panoramic X-ray was taken to assess the root morphology of tooth #21 (Figure 1(b)). The CT revealed that tooth #21 was fractured at the cervical level of the clinical crown (Figure 1(c)) and that dental extraction was indicated without the possibility of placing a postextraction implant, since there was insufficient thickness of the external vestibular table and the available remnants would lead to a fenestration or lack of primary stability.

2.2. Treatment Plan. Atraumatic extraction of tooth #21 was planned, along with alveolar preservation to minimize bone reabsorption, placing a provisional restoration with the same autologous clinical crown of extracted tooth #21, which would maintain the same gingival level as that of the natural tooth.

2.3. Dental Extraction and Alveolar Preservation. The tooth extraction procedure for tooth #21 consisted of first separating the fractured clinical crown (Figure 2(a)) to subsequently and atraumatically extracting the root remnant with #65 forceps. The alveolus was curetted to eliminate any remaining granulation tissue and periodontal ligament, and to induce bleeding, an InterOss® alveolus was placed in the 0.5 g bone xenograft (Anorganic Cancellous Bone Graft Granules) (Figure 2(b)) to subsequently seal the alveolus

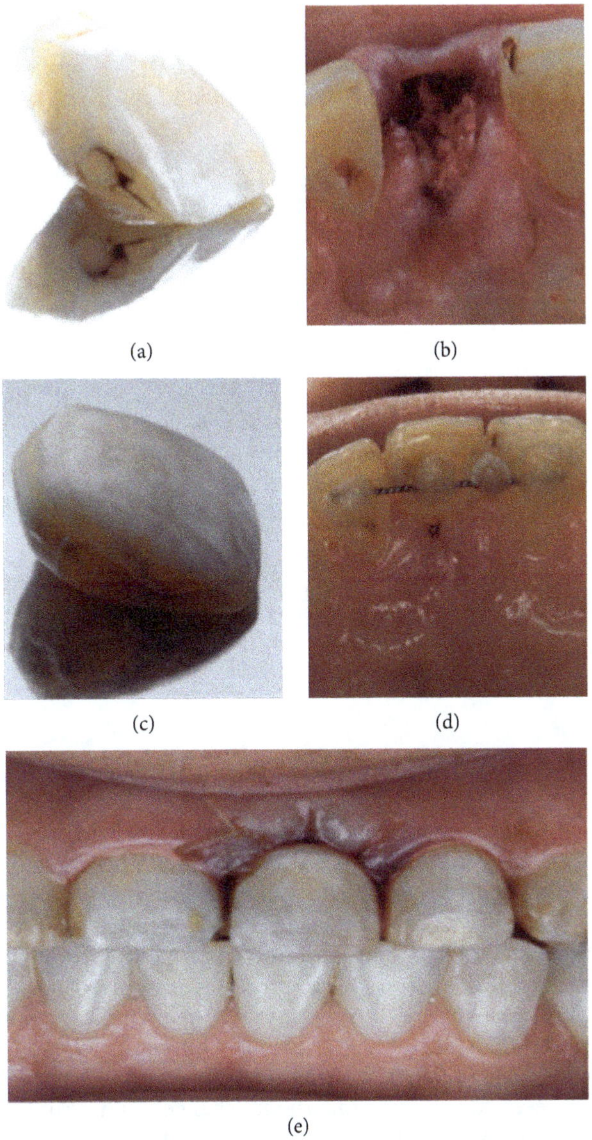

FIGURE 2: Extracted autologous clinical crown (a); filling of the alveolus with InterOss® (b); formation of the ovoid pontic in the cervical part of the clinical crown (c); adherence with conventional composite and orthodontic wire in the palatal sides of teeth #11 and #22 (d); the provisional restoration is left out of occlusion in intercuspid position (e).

surface with a collagen membrane of 8 mm × 12 mm (Colla Tape, Zimmer) sutured with Vicryl 4-0.

2.4. Provisionalization. Once the clinical crown was separated from the root of tooth #21, it was washed with physiological serum and disinfected with 2% chlorhexidine, and a pulpotomy of the crown was performed to eliminate the pulp tissue and to seal the pulp chamber with a conventional composite and the ovoid pontic (Figure 2(c)). The crown was fused with a metal ligature and conventional composite on the palatal surfaces of teeth #11 and #22 (Figure 2(d)). The cervical part of the provisional crown should exert slight pressure in the area of the extraction, thus beginning to create a natural emergence profile for at least 3 months after this alveolar preservation to set the implant in place. The provisional restoration was omitted from the occlusion in the opening-closing and mandibular eccentric movements (Figure 2(e)).

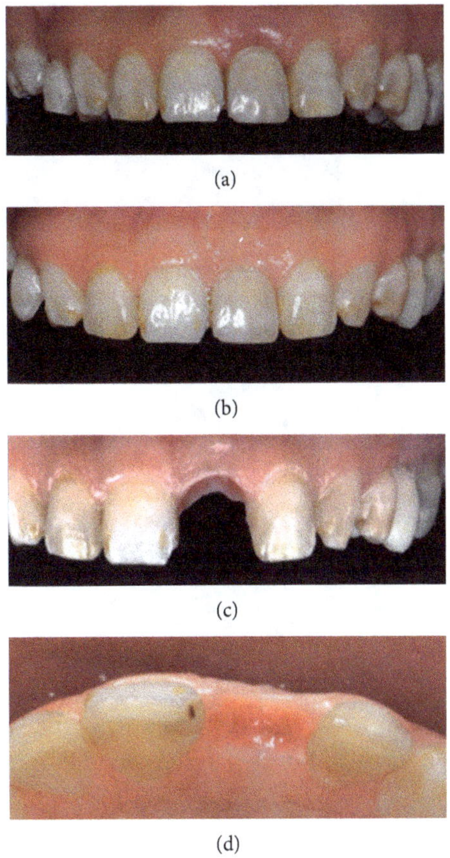

FIGURE 3: The patient is scheduled for a weekly appointment for the removal of the sutures (a); good aesthetic after 1 month with papilla preservation (b); the provisional restoration is removed (c–d).

2.5. Postoperative Follow-Up. The patient was scheduled for an appointment 1 week after the tooth extraction to remove the sutures (Figure 3(a)) and to evaluate possible inflammation after extraction. Nevertheless, a healthy gum was observed, including a coral pink color, and the dental papilla had maintained its dimensions. At 1 month after surgery, the soft tissue was evaluated and was not collapsed, did not present gingival inflammation, and demonstrated a maintained confirmation of the volume and dimension of the papillae (Figure 3(b)). The autologous clinical crown was removed to evaluate the edentulous flange. Next, we evaluated the conformation of the ovoid pontic, and we decided to add a small amount of the conventional composite on the pontic to provide a natural emergence profile (Figures 3(c) and 3(d)). At 3 months after the extraction, the level of the soft tissue was observed (Figures 4(a) and 4(b)). An intraoral scanner (3Shape) was applied for dental implant placement and surgical guidance (Figures 5(a) and 5(b)).

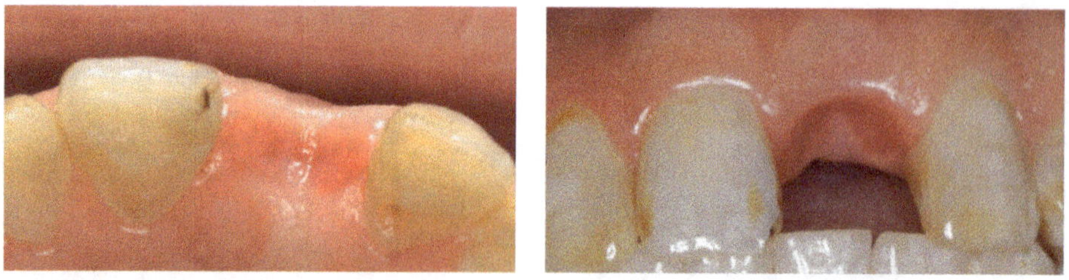

(a) (b)

FIGURE 4: Final result after 3 months with the autologous clinical crown as a provisional restoration (a); emerging dimensions of the alveolar contours (b).

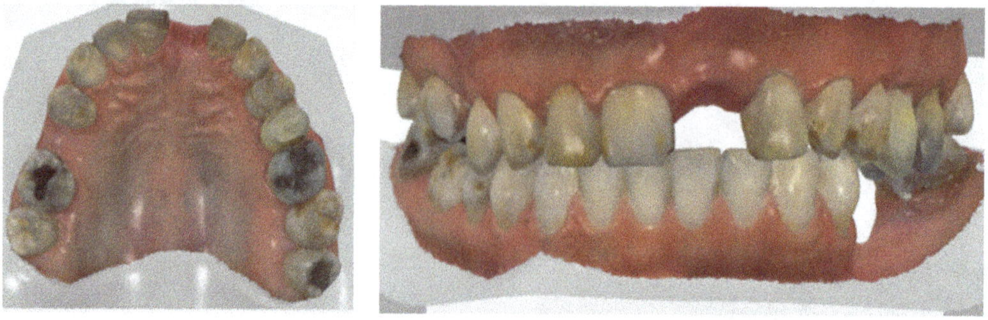

(a) (b)

FIGURE 5: Images obtained from an intraoral scanner to plan the placement of the implant.

3. Discussion

The objective of this clinical case was to maintain the biological parameters of bone and soft tissues by performing postextraction alveolar preservation and using the complete crown of the extracted tooth as a provisional restoration; the results revealed success in the contouring and festooning of the gum without a loss of gingival papillae, as well as preservation of the integrity and architecture of the soft tissues. Advantages obtained in this manner of provisionalization reduce the probability of soft tissue collapse, and alveolar preservation after extraction limits the loss of bone tissue. Further scope of this research was to disseminate information concerning the importance of an adequate way to provisionalize edentulous spaces in an aesthetically and functionally compromised area such as the anterior superior sector of the maxilla and the preservation of an alveolus postextraction that minimizes bone resorption to the greatest extent possible.

The loss of a tooth in the anterior maxilla gives rise to a series of problems that, if not resolved at the correct time, can be detrimental to the implant and restorative features. However, loss of a tooth from an aesthetic zone also has an impact on the patient, both in his or her manner of speaking and masticatory function, and it can even affect socialization due to sensing the absence of the tooth [16].

In this clinical case, an adequate diagnosis and treatment plan was shown to successfully predict the definitive restoration by the placement of an adequate provisional restoration, due to the fracture of the clinical crown of tooth #21. Alveolar preservation postextraction was proposed to maintain the morphology and dimensions of the alveolus and to decrease the process of bone resorption after the dental extraction, as well as the time required for bone healing, in this manner avoiding the collapse of soft tissues.

Studies have shown that the loss of alveolar ridge volume postextraction consists of an irreversible process that forms part of the biological processes and alveolar bone changes due to the loss of a tooth, involving horizontal and vertical reductions [17, 18]. The effects of filling with bone-grafting materials and of not filling with any material have revealed variable dimensional changes, and a superior impact of alveolar preservation can be clearly observed [19]. However, resorption after tooth extraction may be limited, but it cannot be eliminated with alveolar preservation, since the formation of new bone is not always promoted at the histological level [8].

In vivo and *in vitro* studies have revealed the study of a wide variety of materials as substitutes for the regeneration of bone tissue, including autografts, allografts, xenografts, and alloplasts, maintaining the bone volume after extraction, compensating for the degree of bone resorption, and accelerating the formation of bone tissue [20, 21]. In this clinical case, we decided to use a natural hydroxyapatite bone-grafting material derived from bovine bone, which acts as a guide for body fluids, growth factors, and cells. In contrast, the wound dressing consisted of a resorbable regenerative membrane, which is indicated for inducing hemostasis and coating of surgical beds [22]. Prior to filling of the alveolus with the regenerative material in this clinical case, a collagen membrane was placed; this membrane functions as a dressing that controls bleeding by stabilizing the blood clot and accelerating the healing process [23]. These membranes have been shown to be effective at protecting the alveolus and graft material from the oral environment through a barrier effect, preventing the rapid growth of soft tissues [24].

The placement of a provisional restoration should be scheduled as soon as possible after the final restoration, regarding the shape and dimensions of the tooth, as well as the emergence profile and axial inclination following positioning of the root of the missing tooth. At the level of the soft tissues after dental extraction, the entrance to the alveolus is empty, and healing occurs by secondary intention, such that subsequent cell proliferation causes an increase in the volume in the outer part of the alveolus, and the behavior of the soft tissues depends on the dimensional changes in the bone tissue [17].

An advantage of this clinical case was that the margin of the fracture occurred at the cervical level of the tooth without compromising the clinical crown. Therefore, it could be utilized as a provisional restoration. The postoperative images at 1 week and 1 month demonstrated no collapse of the soft tissues or loss of the volume and dimensions of the papillae, since the crown maintained the contact points.

Alveolar preservation is a key factor for minimizing bone loss; however, the fabrication of a suitable provisional restoration will help to maintain soft tissue integrity without necessarily being interrelated. The options for provisionalizing unitary edentulous spaces postextraction with alveolar preservation include fixed partial prostheses in the case of multiple restorations or a Maryland-type restoration, which is an adhesive prosthesis. Importantly, the provisional restoration should not exert a strong pressure at the defect site to avoid compromising the vascularization and healing processes. After it has healed, it is recommended to remove the provisional restoration, add a conventional composite for the formation of the ovoid pontic, and configure the crest profile in the desired manner [20].

4. Conclusion

In this case report, we showed a successful outcome in terms of the integrity, margin, and architecture of the soft tissues after extraction of a superior central tooth, demonstrating that placement of the patient's autologous clinical crown as a provisional crown provides stability to the soft tissues and offers the creation and modeling of an emergence profile as natural as the extracted tooth itself. It also offers aesthetics that provide the patient with assurance to speak and smile without the need for placement of a temporary removable restoration.

Acknowledgments

This work was supported by a grant to Andrea Rodríguez--Moreno, a CONACYT fellow (Grant 663536-575404).

References

[1] M. A. Atieh, N. H. M. Alsabeeha, A. G. T. Payne et al., "Interventions for replacing missing teeth: alveolar ridge preservation techniques for dental implant site development," *Cochrane Database of Systematic Reviews*, vol. 28, no. 5, article CD010176, 2015.

[2] T. Irinakis, "Rationale for socket preservation after extraction of a single-rooted tooth when planning for future implant placement," *Journal Canadian Dental Association*, vol. 72, no. 10, pp. 917–922, 2006.

[3] B. K. Bartee, "Extraction site reconstruction for alveolar ridge preservation. Part 1: rationale and materials selection," *Journal of Oral Implantology*, vol. 27, no. 4, pp. 187–193, 2001.

[4] S. H. Bassir, M. Alhareky, B. Wangsrimongkol, Y. Jia, and N. Karimbux, "Systematic review and meta-analysis of hard tissue outcomes of alveolar ridge preservation," *The International Journal of Oral & Maxillofacial Implants*, vol. 55, no. 33, pp. 979–994, 2018.

[5] G. Avila-Ortiz, S. Elangovan, K. W. O. Kramer, D. Blanchette, and D. V. Dawson, "Effect of alveolar ridge preservation after tooth extraction: a systematic review and meta-analysis," *Journal of Dental Research*, vol. 93, no. 10, pp. 950–958, 2014.

[6] C. H. F. Hämmerle, M. G. Araújo, M. Simion, and On Behalf of the Osteology Consensus Group 2011, "Evidence-based knowledge on the biology and treatment of extraction sockets," *Clinical Oral Implants Research*, vol. 23, Supplement 5, pp. 80–82, 2012.

[7] F. Vignoletti, P. Matesanz, D. Rodrigo, E. Figuero, C. Martin, and M. Sanz, "Surgical protocols for ridge preservation after tooth extraction. A systematic review," *Clinical Oral Implants Research*, vol. 23, Supplement 5, pp. 22–38, 2012.

[8] A. Horváth, N. Mardas, L. A. Mezzomo, I. G. Needleman, and N. Donos, "Alveolar ridge preservation, a systematic review," *Clinical Oral Investigations*, vol. 17, no. 2, pp. 341–363, 2013.

[9] J. M. Iasella, H. Greenwell, R. L. Miller et al., "Ridge preservation with freeze-dried bone allograft and a collagen membrane compared to extraction alone for implant site development: a clinical and histologic study in humans," *Journal of Periodontology*, vol. 74, no. 7, pp. 990–999, 2003.

[10] S. T. Chen, T. G. Wilson Jr, and C. H. Hämmerle, "Immediate or early placement of implants following tooth extraction: review of biologic basis, clinical procedures, and outcomes," *The International Journal of Oral & Maxillofacial Implants*, vol. 19, pp. 12–25, 2004.

[11] S. Y. Kim, Y. K. Kim, H. S. Kim, P. Y. Yun, S. G. Kim, and Y. H. Choi, "Extraction socket sealing using palatal gingival grafts and resorbable collagen membranes," *Maxillofacial plastic and reconstructive surgery*, vol. 39, no. 1, 2017.

[12] C. Masaki, T. Nakamoto, T. Mukaibo, Y. Kondo, and R. Hosokawa, "Strategies for alveolar ridge reconstruction and preservation for implant therapy," *Journal of Prosthodontic Research*, vol. 59, no. 4, pp. 220–228, 2015.

[13] W. L. Tan, T. L. T. Wong, M. C. M. Wong, and N. P. Lang, "A systematic review of post-extractional alveolar hard and soft tissue dimensional changes in humans," *Clinical Oral Implants Research*, vol. 23, Supplement 5, pp. 1–21, 2012.

[14] F. Van der Weijden, F. Dell'Acqua, and D. E. Slot, "Alveolar bone dimensional changes of post-extraction sockets in humans: a systematic review," *Journal of Clinical Periodontology*, vol. 36, no. 12, pp. 1048–1058, 2009.

[15] V. Lekovic, P. M. Camargo, P. R. Klokkevold et al., "Preservation of alveolar bone in extraction sockets using bioabsorbable membranes," *Journal of Periodontology*, vol. 69, no. 9, pp. 1044–1049, 1998.

[16] A. E. Gerritsen, P. F. Allen, D. J. Witter, E. M. Bronkhorst, and N. H. Creugers, "Tooth loss and oral health-related quality of life: a systematic review and meta-analysis," *Health and Quality of Life Outcomes*, vol. 8, no. 1, p. 126, 2010.

[17] L. Schropp, A. Wenzel, L. Kostopoulos, and T. Karring, "Bone healing and soft tissue contour changes following single-tooth extraction: a clinical and radiographic 12-month prospective study," *The International Journal of Periodontics & Restorative Dentistry*, vol. 23, no. 4, pp. 313–323, 2003.

[18] M. G. Araújo and J. Lindhe, "Ridge alterations following tooth extraction with and without flap elevation: an experimental study in the dog," *Clinical Oral Implants Research*, vol. 20, no. 6, pp. 545–549, 2009.

[19] J. G. De Buitrago, G. Avila-Ortiz, and S. Elangovan, "Quality assessment of systematic reviews on alveolar ridge preservation," *The Journal of the American Dental Association*, vol. 144, no. 12, pp. 1349–1357, 2013.

[20] M. G. Gargallo, S. Y. García, and A. B. Martínez, "Ridge preservation and ridge augmentation procedures: a literatura review," *Av Periodon Implantol*, vol. 28, no. 2, pp. 71–81, 2016.

[21] L. Fee, "Socket preservation," *British Dental Journal*, vol. 222, no. 8, pp. 579–582, 2017.

[22] S. Kesmas, S. Swasdison, S. Yodsanga, S. Sessirisombat, and P. Jansisyanont, "Esthetic alveolar ridge preservation with calcium phosphate and collagen membrane: preliminary report," *Oral Surgery, Oral Medicine, Oral Pathology, Oral Radiology, and Endodontology*, vol. 110, no. 5, pp. e24–e36, 2010.

[23] O. Catanzano, V. D'Esposito, P. Formisano, J. S. Boateng, and F. Quaglia, "Composite alginate-hyaluronan sponges for the delivery of tranexamic acid in postextractive alveolar wounds," *Pharmaceutics, Drug Delivery and Pharmaceutical Technology*, vol. 107, no. 2, pp. 654–661, 2018.

[24] V. L. Ford-Martinelli, G. Hanly, J. Valenzuela, L. M. Herrera-Orozco, and S. Muñoz-Zapata, "Alveolar ridge preservation?: Decision making for dental implant placement," *Revista CES Odontologia*, vol. 25, no. 2, pp. 44–53, 2012.

20

Mandibular Full-Arch Rehabilitation over 3 Straight Immediately Loaded Implants: 8 Years of Follow-Up

Márcio de Carvalho Formiga, Magda Nagasawa, and Jamil Awad Shibli

Department of Periodontology and Oral Implantology, Dental Research Division, University of Guarulhos, Sao Paulo, Brazil

Correspondence should be addressed to Márcio de Carvalho Formiga; marciocformiga@gmail.com

Academic Editor: Konstantinos Michalakis

Mandibular full-arch restoration is a good and successful treatment option for totally edentulous patients. In the past years, several studies have described the placement of 4 to 6 implants to restore this type of case; however, an option using 3 dental implants placed in strategic and specific positions could also be an alternative. Therefore, this case report describes a full-arch rehabilitation on 3 straight, immediately loaded implants after 8 years of follow-up. The restoration presented no biological or technical complications during this follow-up period, showing that an adequate treatment plan was able to allow good results using this treatment option.

1. Introduction

Full-arch implant-supported fixed restoration is a very reliable option for completely edentulous patients. According to the original Bränemark protocol, four to six implants should be inserted in the interforaminal area to support a fixed, screw-retained restoration using an immediate or delayed loading protocol [1, 2]. A complementary treatment option for totally edentulous subjects is the All-on-4 concept. In this technique, two anterior implants are placed in parallel position and two distally tilted implants are placed in the most distal position, between molar and premolar areas [3]. With this configuration, the distal cantilever length can be reduced, decreasing peri-implant bone stress and consequently bone loss [4].

There are several clinical and *in vitro* studies that have concluded that both situations have similar stress distribution on the surrounding bone of the distal implants, leaving the choice of choosing one or other depending on the preference of the operator and anatomical situation [5, 6]. Early studies have proposed that in specific and well-indicated cases, full-arch rehabilitation on 3 straight immediate-loaded implants should be performed [7]. This configuration could simplify the treatment and reduce costs to the patients, in spite of the scarcity of studies with long-term follow-up periods [8, 9].

Therefore, the aim of this case report was to present the case of a patient, submitted to a mandibular fixed rehabilitation on 3 straight immediate-loaded implants, with a follow-up period of 8 years.

2. Case Report

The patient, a 65-year-old woman, came to our private practice in 2010, with the complaint that she could not eat without discomfort in the mental foramen region due to the use of a mandibular complete denture. The patient had been using the same dentures for 30 years (Figures 1 and 2). On clinical examination, it was possible to feel the alveolar nerve on the crest of the mandible, and its compression during clenching usually caused the patient to feel pain. After imaging analysis (Figure 3), a fixed full-arch rehabilitation on 3 straight immediately loaded implants was planned because the interforaminal distance limited the placement of four implants, according to the surgeon's experience.

Before the surgery, a new complete denture had to be made, with better and adequate vertical dimension, centric relation, harmonious tooth positioning, and lip support.

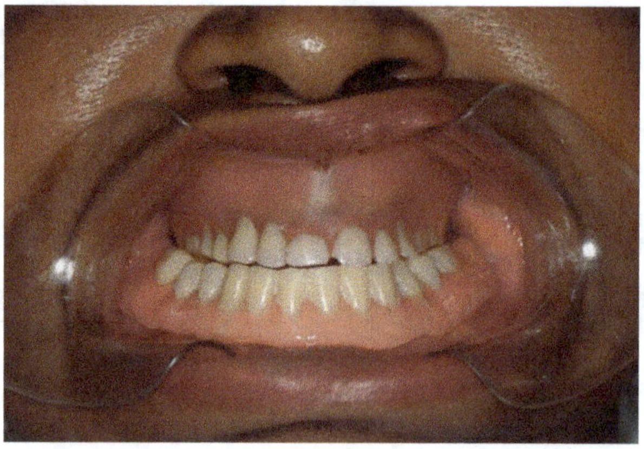

Figure 1: Clinical aspect of the removable complete dentures: note the absence of occlusal contact and marginal adaptation to the jaws.

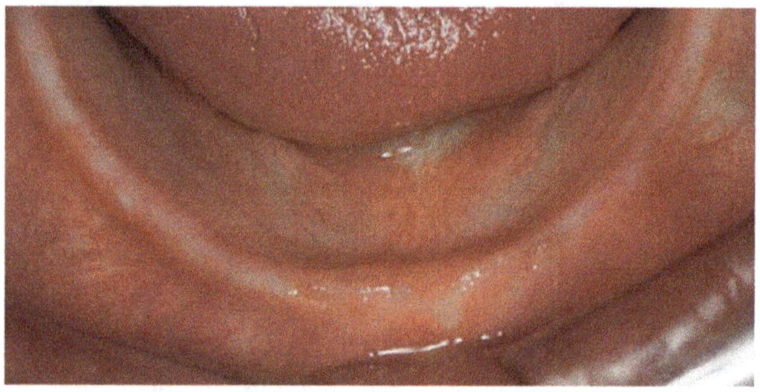

Figure 2: Preoperative intraoral clinical view.

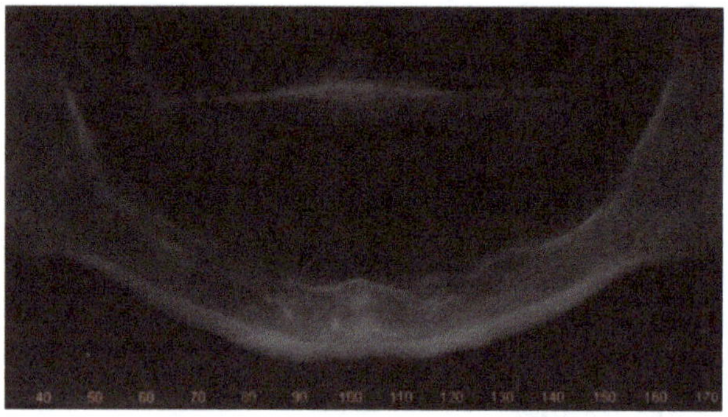

Figure 3: Preoperative panoramic radiograph.

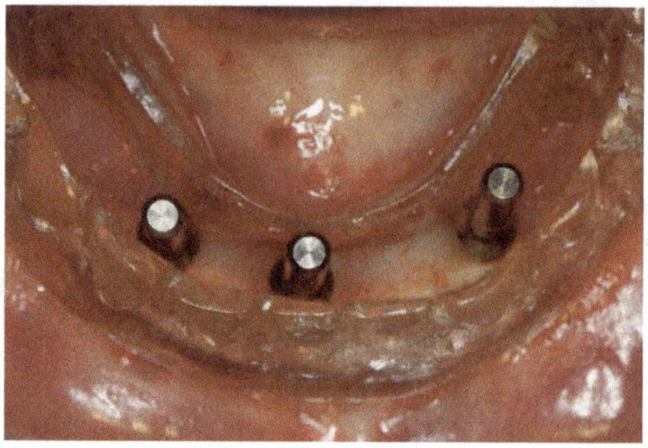

Figure 4: Intraoperative intraoral view of the surgical guide showing parallelism pins.

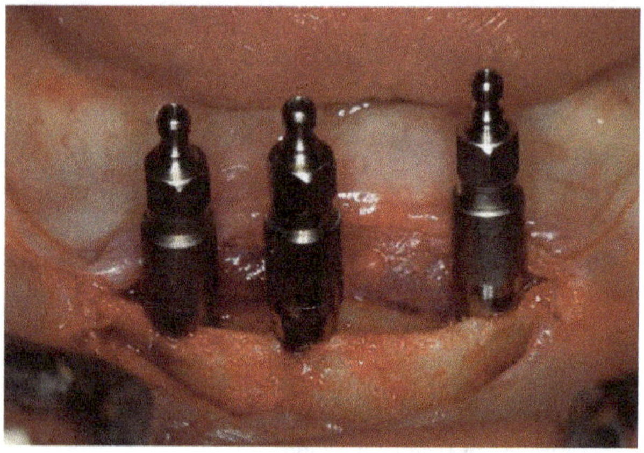

Figure 5: Intraoperative intraoral view of the 3 implants inserted in the jaw.

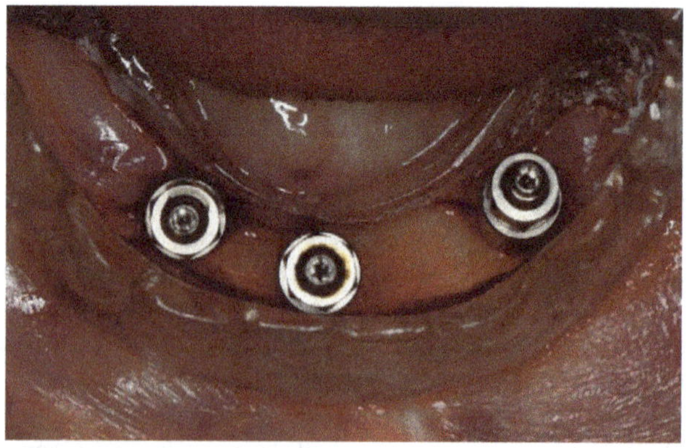

Figure 6: Intraoperative intraoral view of the surgical guide showing good positioning of the 3 implants.

With these parameters tested and approved by the patient and the operator, the surgical procedures were planned, using a multifunctional surgical guide to determine the best implant placement positions. After anesthesia with Articaine 4% 1 : 100,000 (DFL, Rio de Janeiro, Brazil), a crestal incision was made next to the emergence of the alveolar nerve, which we could feel by touch, to avoid any nerve damage caused by the scalpel. A full thickness incision flap was performed to expose the alveolar ridge; then, with the help of the surgical guide, the implant osteotomies were performed. The implant positions were tested with the parallel pins and the surgical guide before completing the osteotomies (Figure 4). Three Titamax GT 3.75 × 11 mm implants (Neodent, Curitiba, Brazil) were inserted in the interforaminal region (Figures 5 and 6), with an insertion torque ranging between 60 and 80 N/cm.

The multifunctional surgical guide was used to help transfer the implant positions and register the vertical dimension and positions of the teeth. The day after surgery,

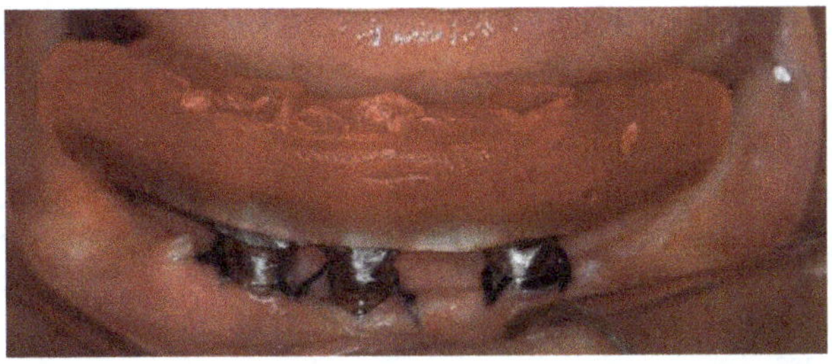

FIGURE 7: Intraoral view of the bar proof with occlusion vertical dimension wax block registration.

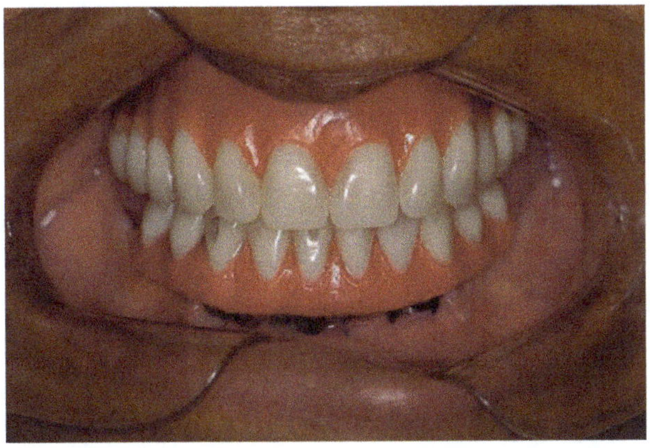

FIGURE 8: Intraoral view of the wax mounted teeth try-in.

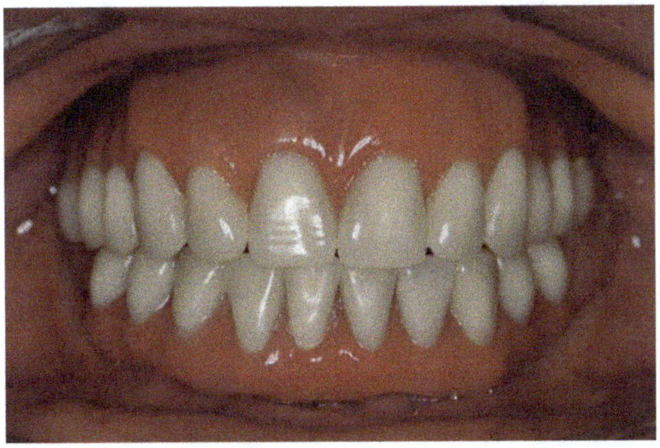

FIGURE 9: Clinical aspects of the new maxillary denture and mandibular fixed prosthetic restoration on 3 implants on the delivery day.

the nickel-chromium metal bar, which had been made according to the position in the wax-up of the future teeth, was tried and sent for mounting the teeth, after being approved by the patient (Figure 7). On the next day, the esthetic appearance, which provided adequate lip support, smile line, positioning of the teeth, and occlusal guidelines (Figure 8), was approved. After patient and dentist approval, the prostheses were sent for full laboratory processing with acrylic. Finally, on the third day after surgery, the screw-retained full-arch rehabilitation on the three implants was installed (Figures 9 and 10).

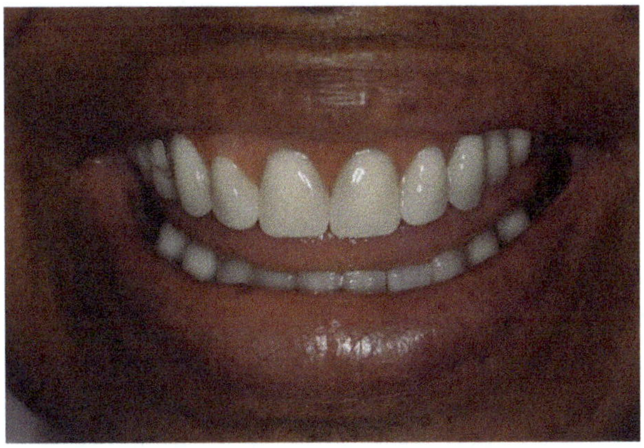

FIGURE 10: Extraoral view of the patient with the new oral rehabilitation.

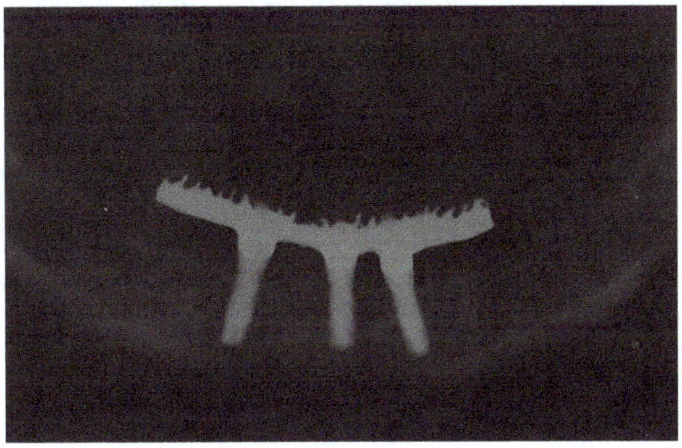

FIGURE 11: One-year postoperative follow-up panoramic radiograph.

The patient was instructed not to sleep with the opposing complete denture for 7 days, eat only soft foods, put ice bags on the surgical area for 48 hours, and take analgesic medication if necessary. The sutures were removed after seven days. The patient was recommended to return after 3, 6, and 12 months. The patient returned after one year for a clinical and radiographic evaluation (Figure 11). After this, the patient returned seven years later, for the second follow-up. This clinical evaluation showed that the fixed restoration, screw-retained on 3 implants, did not show any type of failure in the teeth or the acrylic denture base. There was no bleeding on probing (2 mm probing depths around all implants), the appearance of the gingival tissue around the implants was very good, and there were no complaints about the fixed rehabilitation. In the evaluation by panoramic radiograph, there were no aspects of bone loss or bone remodeling around the implants (Figure 12). Only a few adjustments on the complete dentures of the opposite arch were made to address minor discomfort and mucosal injuries.

3. Discussion

Although the full-arch fixed rehabilitation on 3 implants is not a new alternative for the treatment of completely

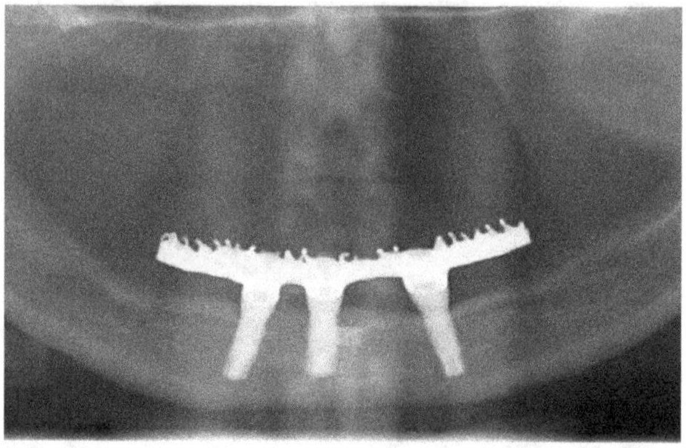

Figure 12: Eight-year follow-up panoramic radiograph: note that there is no bone loss around the implants.

edentulous patients [6], there are very few articles about it in the literature and even fewer articles with follow-up periods of over 3 years [9, 10]. Because of the reduced costs of this treatment modality and the simpler surgical procedure for the placement of only 3 implants for a fixed rehabilitation, the authors consider that there should be more studies about it. Furthermore, these studies should have longer follow-up periods to prove whether or not this treatment is effective or not so that it could be offered as an equivalent treatment alternative, especially for those who cannot afford the regular implant treatment options. The case presented here, with anatomical limitations for the placement of 4 implants, was taken from the files of a private practice and agreed with the conditions for the placement of 3 straight implants and an immediately loaded full-arch fixed rehabilitation.

The patient had a complete denture on the opposite arch, which could help with the success of the treatment [8]; however, in the literature, there are studies in which both arches were rehabilitated with All-on-4 or other treatment modalities, even with zirconia prostheses [10]. Immediate loading was the preference for this case, since there were no systemic or local contraindications, and the follow-up visits showed a 100% success rate, for the prosthetic components and the implants. There are studies with similar results for rehabilitation on 3 implants but with delayed load [10] and others with survival rates similar to those of the All-on-4 immediate load concept [8, 9]—a more than well documented treatment alternative for patients with an edentulous mandible [3, 10]. The implants used in this case were Neodent GT, which are one-stage single-body implants, with the only indication for use being in immediate loading mandibular protocols. Therefore, the microgap would remain above the bone crest [11], decreasing the possibility of bone remodeling around the implant neck usually seen in external and internal hexagon implants [12]. This was evident in the 1- and 8-year control panoramic radiographs of the patient, in which almost no bone loss could be seen. The result of this particular case is in agreement with one cited in a recent systematic review that assessed complications in the All-on-4 protocol, with tilted or not tilted implants [13]. The implant configuration used in this case differed from the one proposed by Costa et al. [14], but during the 8 years of follow-up, there were no failures or complications related to the implants or the metal-acrylic resin complete fixed prostheses, as reported by Bozini et al. [15]. In addition, the patient reported greater confidence in relating to other people in public because she no longer experienced discomfort while chewing, and her appearance had improved. These long-term results indicated that this could be a good option for improving the quality of life of patients who had lost their teeth, irrespective of the cause [16].

4. Conclusion

Within the limitations of this report, this type of rehabilitation with 3 implants in immediate function seems to be a feasible treatment option in the long term for patients with a completely edentulous mandible, when the anatomy is unfavorable or the patients cannot afford the conventional and more well-documented treatment options.

Acknowledgments

The references used to support the findings of this case report are listed in References and can be found at PubMed.

References

[1] P. I. Brånemark, B. O. Hansson, R. Adell et al., "Osseointegrated implants in the treatment of the edentulous jaw. Experience from a 10-year period," *Scandinavian Journal of Plastic and Reconstructive Surgery*, vol. 16, pp. 1–132, 1977.

[2] P. I. Branemark, B. Svensson, and D. van Steenberghe, "Ten-year survival rates of fixed prostheses on four or six implants ad modum Branemark in full edentulism," *Clinical Oral Implants Research*, vol. 6, no. 4, pp. 227–231, 1995.

[3] P. Maló, M. de Araújo Nobre, A. Lopes, A. Ferro, and I. Gravito, "All-on-4 treatment concept for the rehabilitation of the completely edentulous mandible: a 7-year clinical and 5-year radiographic retrospective case series with risk assessment for implant failure and marginal bone level," *Clinical Implant Dentistry and Related Research*, vol. 17, Supplement 2, pp. e531–e541, 2015.

[4] L. Baggi, S. Pastore, M. di Girolamo, and G. Vairo, "Implant-bone load transfer mechanisms in complete-arch prostheses supported by four implants: a three-dimensional finite element approach," *The Journal of Prosthetic Dentistry*, vol. 109, no. 1, pp. 9–21, 2013.

[5] T. Takahashi, I. Shimamura, and K. Sakurai, "Influence of number and inclination angle of implants on stress distribution in mandibular cortical bone with All-on-4 concept," *Journal of Prosthodontic Research*, vol. 54, no. 4, pp. 179–184, 2010.

[6] A. Agnini, A. M. Agnini, D. Romeo, M. Chiesi, L. Pariente, and C. F. J. Stappert, "Clinical investigation on axial versus tilted implants for immediate fixed rehabilitation of edentulous arches: preliminary results of a single cohort study," *Clinical Implant Dentistry and Related Research*, vol. 16, no. 4, pp. 527–539, 2014.

[7] P.-I. Brånemark, P. Engstrand, L.-O. Öhrnell et al., "Brånemark Novum®: A new treatment concept for rehabilitation of the edentulous mandible. Preliminary results from a prospective clinical follow-up study," *Clinical Implant Dentistry and Related Research*, vol. 1, no. 1, pp. 2–16, 1999.

[8] E. G. Rivaldo, A. Montagner, H. Nary, L. C. da Fontoura Frasca, and P. I. Branemark, "Assessment of rehabilitation in edentulous patients treated with an immediately loaded complete fixed mandibular prosthesis supported by three implants," *The International Journal of Oral & Maxillofacial Implants*, vol. 27, no. 3, pp. 695–702, 2012.

[9] F. Gualini, G. Gualini, R. Cominelli, and U. Lekholm, "Outcome of Brånemark Novum® Implant treatment in edentulous mandibles: a retrospective 5-year follow-up study," *Clinical Implant Dentistry and Related Research*, vol. 11, no. 4, pp. 330–337, 2009.

[10] J. Oliva, X. Oliva, and J. D. Oliva, "All-on-three delayed implant loading concept for the completely edentulous maxilla and mandible: a retrospective 5-year follow-up study," *The International journal of oral & maxillofacial implants*, vol. 27, no. 6, pp. 1584–1592, 2012.

[11] D. A. Garber, H. Salama, and M. A. Salama, "Two-stage versus one-stage. Is there really a controversy?," *Journal of Periodontology*, vol. 72, no. 3, pp. 417–421, 2001.

[12] R. Judgar, G. Giro, E. Zenobio et al., "Biological width around one- and two-piece implants retrieved from human jaws," *BioMed Research International*, vol. 2014, Article ID 850120, 5 pages, 2014.

[13] K. A. Apaza Alccayhuaman, D. Soto-Peñaloza, Y. Nakajima, S. N. Papageorgiou, D. Botticelli, and N. P. Lang, "Biological and technical complications of tilted implants in comparison with straight implants supporting fixed dental prostheses. A systematic review and meta-analysis," *Clinical Oral Implants Research*, vol. 29, Supplement 18, pp. 295–308, 2018.

[14] R. Costa, P. Filho, H. Filho, and P.-I. Brånemark, "Key Biomechanical Characteristics of Complete-Arch Fixed Mandibular Prostheses Supported by Three Implants Developed at P-I Brånemark Institute, Bauru," *The International Journal of Oral & Maxillofacial Implants*, vol. 30, no. 6, pp. 1400–1404, 2015.

[15] T. Bozini, H. Petridis, K. Tzanas, and P. Garefis, "A meta-analysis of prosthodontic complication rates of implant-supported fixed dental prostheses in edentulous patients after an observation period of at least 5 years," *The International Journal of Oral & Maxillofacial Implants*, vol. 26, no. 2, pp. 304–318, 2011.

[16] F. Berton, C. Stacchi, T. Lombardi, A. Rapani, R. Rizzo, and R. Di Lenarda, "How does immediately loaded implant-supported fixed rehabilitation influence the oral health-related quality of life?," *Global Journal of Oral Science*, vol. 4, no. 1, pp. 1–7, 2018.

21

Digital Workflow for Immediate Implant Placement and Chairside Provisionalization in the Esthetic Zone

Vincent J. J. Donker[1] **Gerry M. Raghoebar**[1] **Arjan Vissink**[1] **and Henny J. A. Meijer**[1,2]

[1]*University of Groningen, University Medical Center Groningen, Department of Oral and Maxillofacial Surgery, Groningen, Netherlands*
[2]*University of Groningen, University Medical Center Groningen, Department of Implant Dentistry, Groningen, Netherlands*

Correspondence should be addressed to Vincent J. J. Donker; v.j.j.donker@umcg.nl

Academic Editor: Konstantinos Michalakis

Introduction. Immediate implant placement and immediate chairside provisionalization in the esthetic zone require meticulous treatment planning. A digital workflow that combines intraoral scans and a cone beam computed tomography scan can be used to visualize the surgical and restorative aspects of the treatment and to plan a prosthetically driven implant position. A digital workflow in implant dentistry enables the prefabrication of an individualized CAD/CAM temporary restoration, based on the planned implant position. This could be a predictable method to deliver a screw-retained temporary restoration, directly after static computer-assisted immediate implant surgery. *Interventions*. Three patients with a failing tooth in the maxillary esthetic zone were treated with immediate implant placement and chairside provisionalization using this digital workflow. After 3 months, a final restoration was placed. Clinical, radiographic, and patient-reported outcome measures were collected prior to implant treatment, 6 weeks after placing the temporary restoration and then 1 month and 1 year after placing the final restoration. *Outcomes*. At the 1-year follow-up, healthy soft tissues were observed, and peri-implant bone levels were stable. Patient satisfaction after the treatment was high. *Conclusion*. The three reported cases demonstrate the potential for predictable immediate implant placement and chairside provisionalization using a digital workflow.

1. Introduction

When a failing tooth in the esthetic zone needs to be removed, it can be replaced with an implant-supported restoration. There is a growing tendency towards immediate implant placement after tooth extraction. This reduces treatment time because implant osseointegration and extraction socket healing occur simultaneously, while also preserving the hard and soft peri-implant tissues [1]. When immediate implant placement is combined with buccal socket grafting, a stable bone layer can be maintained buccally of the implant, regardless of the presence of a preoperative buccal bone defect [2, 3]. To achieve an optimal esthetic outcome, the peri-implant soft tissues must be conditioned during the socket healing. This requires customization of the emergence profile by contouring it with a temporary restoration [4, 5]. Good clinical outcomes can be achieved with immediate implant placement and immediate provisionalization, resulting in high patient satisfaction [6, 7].

However, immediate implant placement and immediate provisionalization require meticulous treatment planning. To assist the clinician with this, a digital workflow can be used [8]. Such a digital workflow combines the information of the patients' hard and soft tissues by integrating intraoral scans and a cone beam computed tomography (CBCT) scan. This allows the clinician to visualize the surgical and restorative aspects of the treatment and to plan a prosthetically driven implant position. Consequently, an individualized temporary restoration can be designed and prefabricated.

Using static computer-assisted implant surgery with a surgical template, the implant can then be placed in the correct three-dimensional position and the individualized screw-retained temporary restoration can be delivered. The whole digital workflow could be a predictable method for immediate implant placement and chairside provisionalization.

The objective of this case report is to describe a treatment with this digital workflow for immediate implant placement and chairside provisionalization in the esthetic zone and to report the clinical, radiographic, and patient-reported outcome measures of three cases with a 1-year follow-up after placing the final restoration.

2. Study Design

Recruitment of patients, treatment, and follow-up took place in the Department of Oral and Maxillofacial Surgery at the University Medical Center Groningen (UMCG), the Netherlands, between August 2020 and December 2021. The research protocol was approved by the Medical Ethics Review Board of the UMCG (METc 2020/014). This manuscript was written following the CARE guidelines for case reports [9].

3. Patient Information and Clinical Findings

Patients were eligible for inclusion if they met the following criteria: at least 18 years of age when being treated, in need of a single tooth implant-supported restoration in a postextraction site in the anterior region of the maxilla, the bone height of the planned implant site apicopalatal of the extraction socket was sufficient (≥4 mm, measured on a CBCT scan) to allow immediate implant placement, suitable anatomical conditions (mesial-distal, buccal-palatal, and interocclusal space) to place an anatomically designed screw-retained restoration, and complies with good oral hygiene practices. Patients with medical and general contraindications for the surgical procedure, smoking habits exceeding 10 units a day, severe bruxism with dysfunctional tendencies, the presence of acute untreated periodontitis in the implant site or adjacent tissue, acute infections in the planned implant site or adjacent tissue, and a history of local radiotherapy to the head and neck region were excluded.

Three consecutively recruited patients agreed to participate in the study (Table 1). An explanation of the costs, benefits, and risks of an implant-supported restoration, and possible alternative treatment options was given. Written informed consent was obtained from all the patients before being enrolled for implant treatment.

4. Timeline

The patients underwent immediate implant placement and chairside provisionalization according to the treatment procedures described in Table 2. One case is presented for illustrative purposes.

5. Diagnostic and Planning Procedures

Prior to the implant treatment, intraoral scans (TRIOS 3, 3Shape, Copenhagen, Denmark) of the upper jaw, lower jaw, and occlusion were made, as well as intraoral photographs (Figure 1) and a CBCT scan (ProMax 3D Max ProFace, Planmeca, Helsinki, Finland). The voxel size of the CBCT scan was 0.2 mm, and the field of view was 130 × 55 mm. The intraoral scans and CBCT Digital Imaging and Communications in Medicine (DICOM) file were superimposed with an implant planning software (DTX Studio Implant, Version 3.5, Medicim, Mechelen, Belgium) to create an individualized digital set-up of the failing tooth (Figure 2). The prosthetically driven implant position was planned in a palatal position with ≥2 mm distance between the implant and the buccal crest [10] and at a depth of 3-4 mm apical of the prospective restorative zenith point [11]. The implant length was chosen based on the available bone height apicopalatal of the extraction socket (Figure 3).

A pilot-drill surgical template to facilitate static computer-assisted implant surgery was designed with the implant planning software (Figure 4) and manufactured by a dental laboratory (Dental LT Clear Resin, Formlabs, Somerville, MA, United States) (Figure 5). Furthermore, the dental laboratory milled a multilayered polymethyl methacrylate (PMMA) (Vipi Block Trilux, Vipi Odonto Products, Pirassununga, Brazil) temporary shell restoration based on the individualized digital set-up (Figure 6) using a dental computer-aided design (CAD) software (DTX Studio Lab, Version 1.10, Medicim).

6. Surgical Procedures

The patient was instructed to start oral disinfection with a 0.12% chlorhexidine mouthwash twice daily on the day before surgery and to continue for seven days. One hour prior to surgery, the patient took a prophylactic antibiotic (amoxicillin 2 g or clindamycin 600 mg in case of penicillin allergy). The surgical procedure was performed using local anesthesia (Ultracain D-S forte, Sanofi-Aventis Deutschland GmbH, Frankfurt am Main, Germany).

The periodontal ligament was detached by careful intrasulcular incision. A periotome and forceps (rotational movement only) were used to remove the failing tooth as minimally traumatic as possible (Figure 7). Any periodontal ligament remnants and granulation tissue were cleaned away with a bone curette and sterile gauze pads. The implant site was prepared flapless using the surgical template. With the last drill placed in the prepared implant site to prevent congestion, the jumping gap between the buccal crest and the implant site was grafted with a 1 : 1 mixture of bovine bone (Geistlich Bio-Oss, Geistlich Pharma AG, Wolhusen, Switzerland) and autogenous bone (Figure 8). After removing the drill from the grafted alveolar socket, a tapered implant with a conical connection (NobelActive TiUltra, Nobel Biocare AB, Gothenburg, Sweden) was inserted according to the manufacturer's instructions (Figure 9). Primary implant stability was attained with an insertion torque of ≥45 Ncm, verified with a manual torque controller (NobelActive Manual

TABLE 1: Patient information.

	Case 1	Case 2	Case 3
Sex	Male	Male	Male
Age in years	22	63	29
Reason for treatment	Root fracture	Endodontic failure	Root fracture
Implant position	Upper left central incisor	Upper right central incisor	Upper left central incisor
Implant diameter	4.3 mm	4.3 mm	4.3 mm
Implant length	15 mm	15 mm	18 mm

TABLE 2: Timeline of the immediate implant placement, provisionalization, and final restoration treatment.

Treatment phase	Procedures
Diagnostic	Intraoral scans Cone beam computed tomography scan
Planning	Digital set-up Digital prosthetically driven implant planning Computer-aided design and milling of the temporary shell restoration Manufacturing of the surgical template
Surgical	Tooth extraction Buccal socket grafting Flapless static computer-assisted immediate implant surgery
Restorative	Chairside provisionalization
Restorative	Intraoral scans with a scanbody Computer-aided design and milling of the final abutment Porcelain veneering of the final restoration Placement of the final restoration

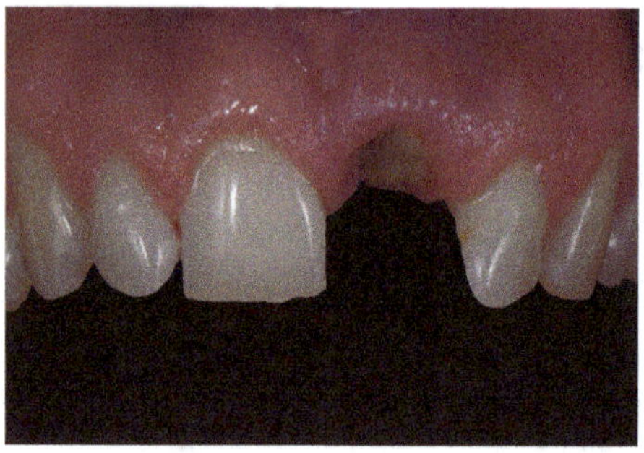

FIGURE 1: Clinical view of the patient with a root fracture of the upper left central incisor. The root is still in situ.

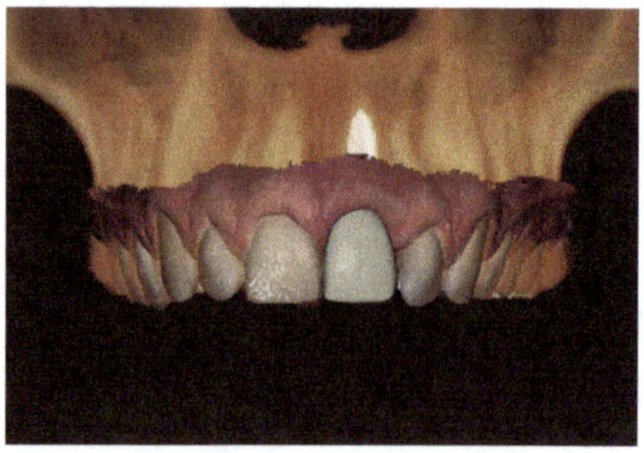

FIGURE 2: Digital set-up of the upper left central incisor, based on a superimposed intraoral scan and CBCT scan.

Torque Wrench Surgical, Nobel Biocare AB). The surgical procedures were performed by one oral and maxillofacial surgeon (GMR).

7. Restorative Procedures

The implant was restored chairside with a temporary restoration, immediately after implant placement. A temporary abutment (Temporary Snap Abutment Engaging CC, Nobel Biocare AB) trimmed to the correct length was snapped onto the implant (Figure 10). The temporary shell restoration was placed in position with the lateral wings seated on the adjacent teeth (Figure 11) and was connected to the temporary abutment with a dentine shaded composite resin (Filtek Supreme XTE, 3 M, Saint Paul, MN, United States). After light curing, the temporary restoration was removed with the abutment from the implant. The lateral wings were trimmed, and a screw-access hole was prepared in the restoration (Apical Drill, Nobel Biocare AB). The cervical part of the restoration was contoured with composite resin to create an emergence profile to support the adjacent papillae [12] (Figure 12). The restoration was polished using polishing rubbers (Diacomp Plus Twist, EVE Ernst Vetter GmbH, Keltern, Germany) and tightened on the implant with a torque value of 35 Ncm using a manual torque controller (Manual Torque Wrench Prosthetic, Nobel Biocare AB). The screw access hole was sealed with polytetrafluoroethylene (PTFE) tape and composite resin (Figure 13). The temporary

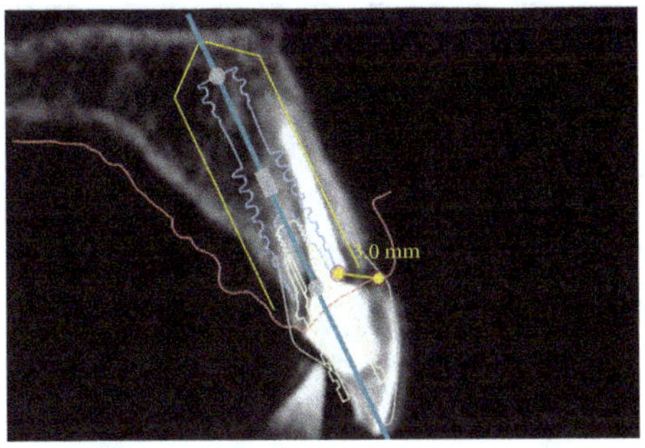

Figure 3: Sagittal view of the CBCT scan showing the prosthetically and biologically driven implant planning.

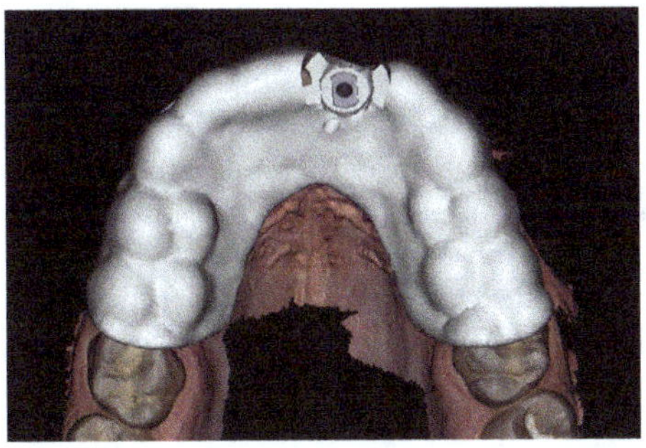

Figure 4: CAD surgical template based on the intraoral scan and the implant planning.

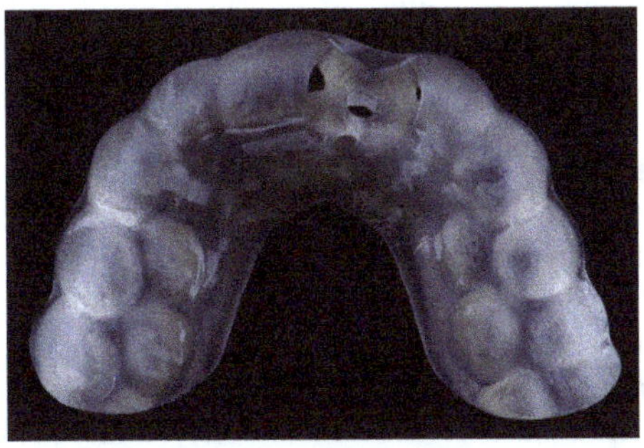

Figure 5: Printed surgical template.

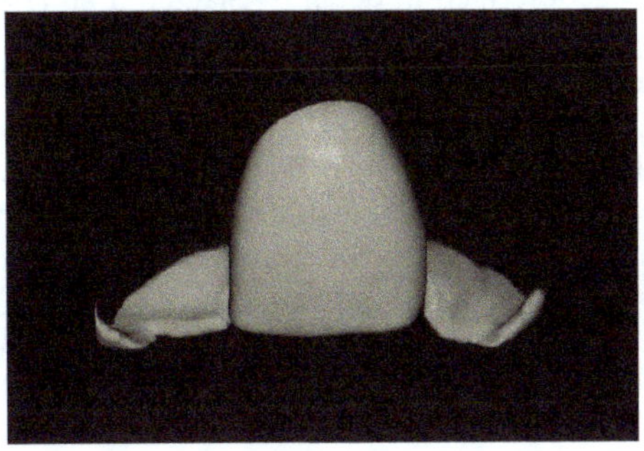

Figure 6: CAD temporary shell restoration with two lateral wings to aid seating.

restoration was free from centric and eccentric movements and the patient was instructed to avoid excess force during the healing period. Oral hygiene instructions were given.

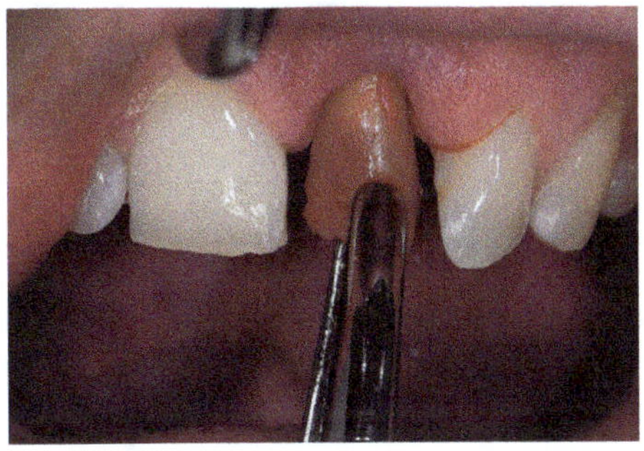

Figure 7: Minimally traumatic removal of the failing tooth using forceps with rotational movement.

After 3 months, an intraoral scan was made directly after removing the temporary restoration to capture the emergence profile. Furthermore, an intraoral scan was made with a scanbody (Elos Accurate Scan Body, Elos Medtech, Gothenburg, Sweden) after screwing it onto the implant (Figure 14). The dental laboratory designed a final restoration using a dental CAD software (DTX Studio Lab). The restoration was screw-retained with a CAD/CAM angulated screw-channel zirconia abutment, mechanically attached to a titanium base (NobelProcera ASC Abutment, Nobel Biocare AB), and buccally veneered with porcelain. The final restoration was tightened onto the implant with a torque value of 35 Ncm (Figure 15). The screw access hole was sealed with PTFE tape and composite resin. After placing the final restoration, oral hygiene instructions were given. All the laboratory procedures were carried out by one dental laboratory. The restorative procedures were performed by two dentists (HJAM, VJJD).

8. Follow-Up and Case Outcomes

Clinical, radiographic, and patient-reported outcome measures were collected prior to the treatment (Tpre), 6 weeks after placing the temporary restoration (Ttemp), and then 1 month (T1) and 1 year (T12) after placing the final restoration. No implants or restorations had been lost, and no technical or biologic complications had occurred at T12 resulting in a survival rate and success rate of 100% for the implants and the restorations according to the modified United States Public Health Service criteria for evaluating implant-supported restorations [13].

The soft tissue outcomes were assessed at T12 with the modified Plaque Index [14], the modified Sulcus Bleeding Index [14], the Gingival Index [15], keratinized mucosa width (KMW) measured to the nearest 1 mm with a periodontal probe [16], the Papilla Index [17], and the pocket probing depth at four sites (mesial, distal, buccal, and palatal) measured to the nearest mm (the highest value is reported). Midbuccal mucosal level (MBML) changes were assessed at Tpre and T12 on intraoral photographs (Nikon D750, Nikon Corporation, Tokyo, Japan) taken with a periodontal probe held close to and parallel to the tooth for calibration purposes (Figure 16). MBML changes were measured with a raster graphics editing software (Adobe Photoshop, Version

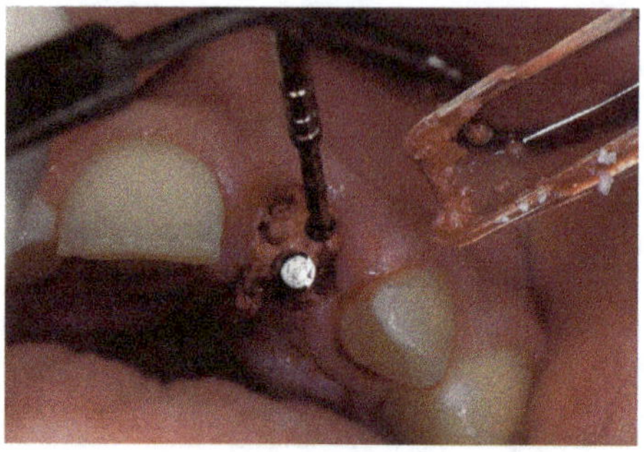

FIGURE 8: Buccal socket grafting with the last used drill placed in the implant site.

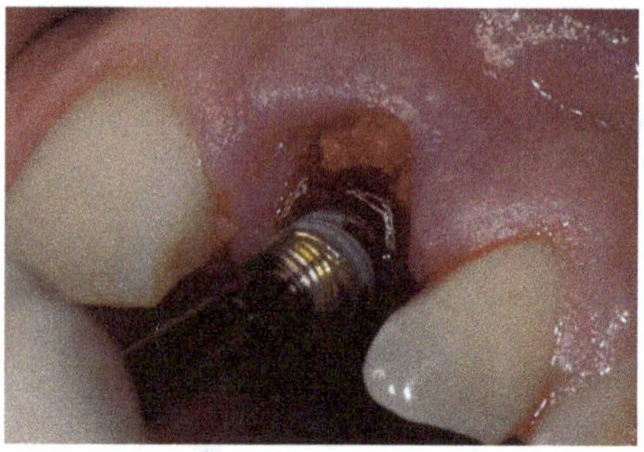

FIGURE 9: Insertion of the implant in the grafted alveolar socket.

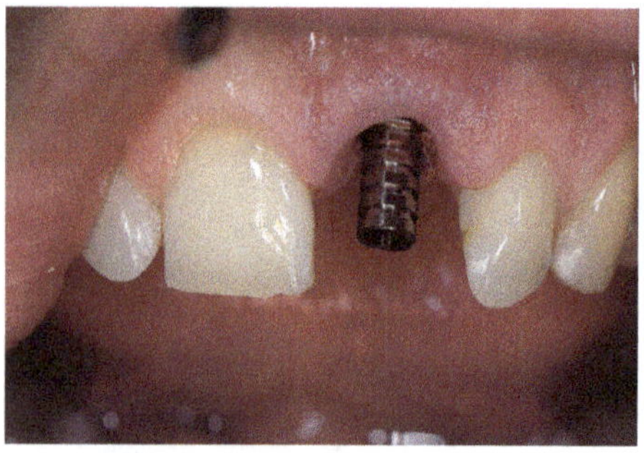

FIGURE 10: Temporary abutment snapped onto the implant.

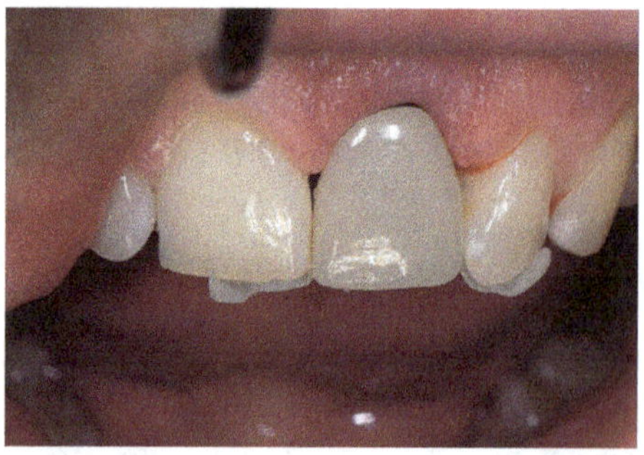

FIGURE 11: Temporary shell restoration with the lateral wings seated on the adjacent teeth.

23.0, Adobe Inc. San Jose, CA, Unites States), and were defined as a change in the vertical distance in mm measured from the zenith point to a reference line drawn between the incisal edges of the two adjacent teeth [7].

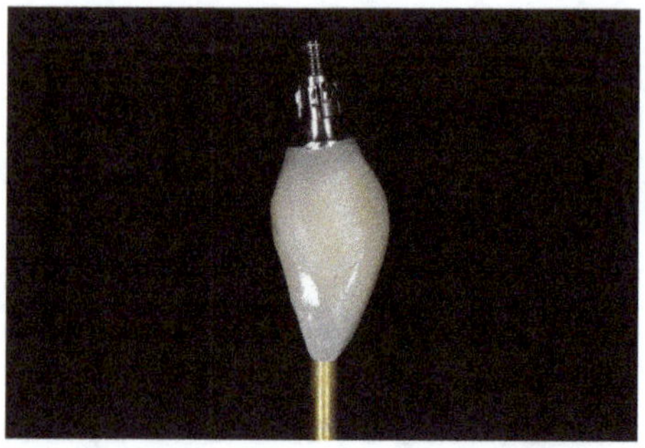

FIGURE 12: Emergence profile of the finished and polished temporary restoration.

The esthetic outcome at Tpre, Ttemp, and T12 was assessed with the modified Pink Esthetic and White Esthetic Score (PES/WES) [18] from intraoral photographs with a contrastor (Flexipalette, Smile Line SA, Saint-Imier, Switzerland). The WES at Tpre was not assessed for one case due to the absence of a clinical crown.

Marginal bone level (MBL) changes from T1 to T12 were assessed on calibrated intraoral radiographs with a long cone paralleling technique. The MBL change was measured by a dedicated software (DicomWorks, Biomedical Engineering, UMCG, The Netherlands), and was defined as a change in the vertical distance in mm measured from the implant shoulder to the first bone to implant contact on the mesial and distal site of the implant [6] (Figure 17). Buccal bone thickness (BBT) at T12 was assessed on a CBCT scan. The exact implant position in the CBCT DICOM file was determined with multimodality image registration using information theory (MIRIT) in a medical imaging software (Maxilim, Version 2.3, Medicim). The BBT was measured by an implant planning software with a dedicated research add-on for the measurements (NobelClinician, version 2.1, Nobel Biocare Belgium NV, Mechelen, Belgium) and was defined as the horizontal distance in mm measured from the implant outline to the buccal bone outline. The area of interest was the upper 5 mm of the implant, starting at the implant neck (Figure 18). This validated BBT measurement method was described in detail by Slagter et al. [19].

The patient-reported outcome at Tpre, Ttemp, and T12 was assessed with a questionnaire on overall satisfaction based on a 10-point rating scale. All the data were collected by one observer (VJJD). The mean values and standard deviations were calculated using statistical software (IBM SPSS Statistics, Version 23.0. Armonk, NY, United States). The outcome measures of all cases are shown in Table 3.

9. Discussion

This case report described a treatment with a digital workflow for immediate implant placement and chairside provisionalization in three patients with a failing tooth in the maxillary esthetic zone. The clinical, radiographic, and patient-reported outcome measures up to 1 year after placing the final restoration were favorable, which is similar to the 1-year results of immediate implant placement and

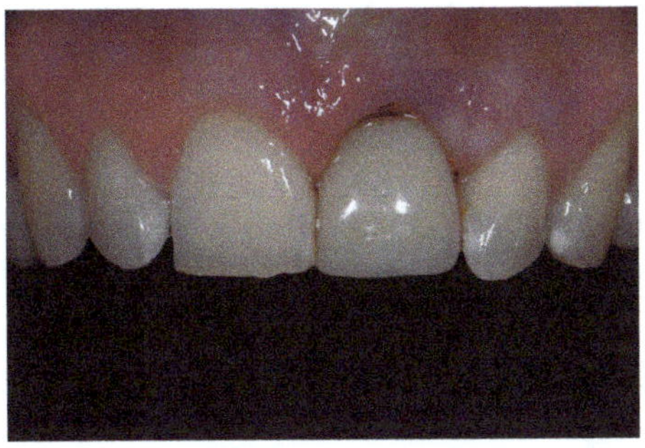

FIGURE 13: Clinical view after immediate implant placement and immediate provisionalization.

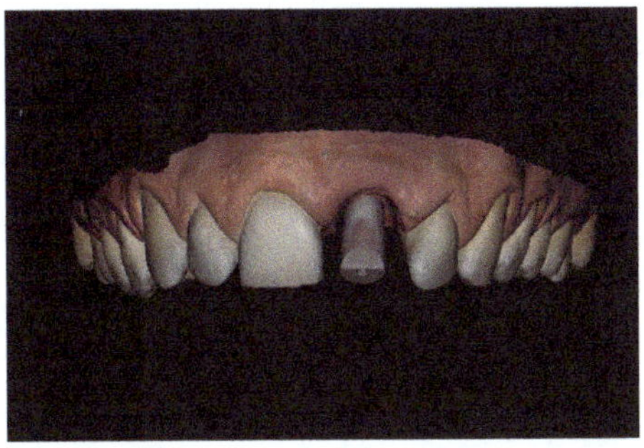

FIGURE 14: Intraoral scan with a scanbody screwed onto the implant.

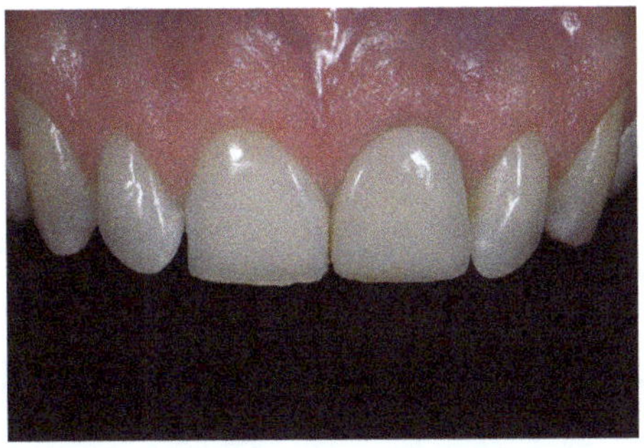

FIGURE 15: Final upper left central incisor restoration after 1 year in function.

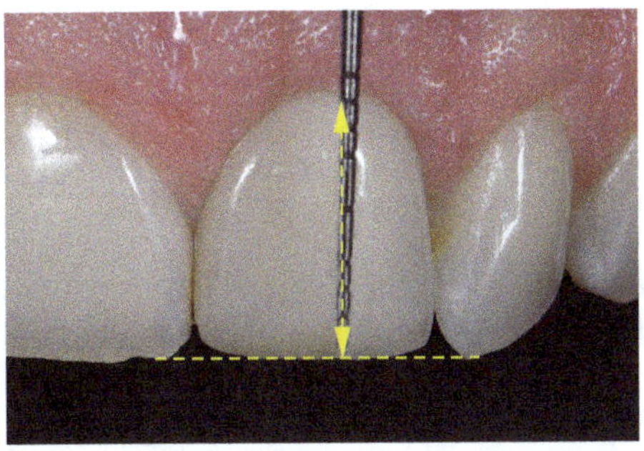

FIGURE 16: MBML measurement on a calibrated intraoral photograph with reference lines.

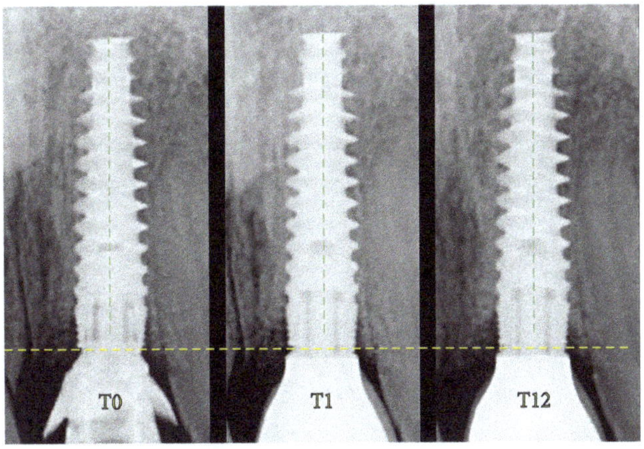

FIGURE 17: MBL measurement on calibrated intraoral radiographs at T0, T1, and T12.

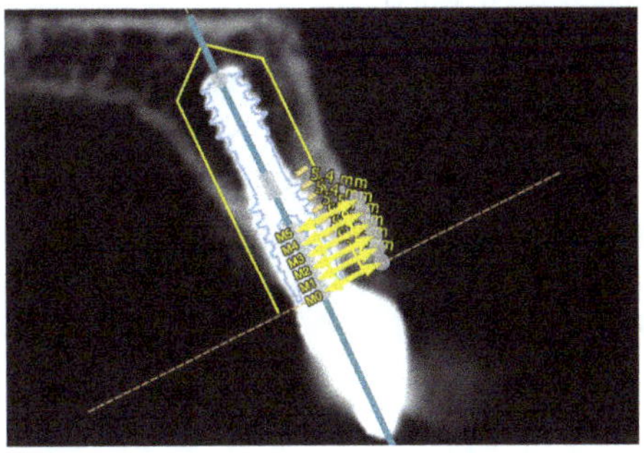

FIGURE 18: BBT measurement at the upper 5 mm of the implant on a CBCT scan at T12.

provisionalization studies with a conventional workflow, conducted in the same center [6, 7]. However, the digital workflow used in this case report offered several advantages over a conventional treatment.

In the diagnostic and planning phase, the superimposed intraoral scans and CBCT scan yielded simultaneous visualization of the hard and soft tissues with a digital set-up of the failing tooth. This facilitated the planning of a prosthetically driven implant position and, at the same time, a priori assessment of the available bone height at the implant site, apicopalatal of the extraction socket. It is suggested that at least 4 mm of bone is needed to attain primary implant stability during immediate implant placement [20]. Hence the inclusion criterion for the present case report. Primary stability of the implant was indeed reached in all three cases, which allowed immediate provisionalization. The digital planning also aided in selecting an implant diameter and length that fit within the biologic boundaries. The planned distance of ≥ 2 mm between the implant and the buccal crest and the subsequent buccal socket grafting resulted in a mean BBT ranging from 2.35 ± 1.02 mm to 2.88 ± 0.66 mm at the 1-year follow-up. These findings differ from another study that evaluated the BBT 1 year after immediate implant placement and provisionalization combined with buccal socket grafting [2]. The mean BBT in the present cases was 0.62 mm to 0.92 mm thicker in the upper 5 mm along the axis of the implant. In the previously mentioned study, the

TABLE 3: Modified Plaque Index, modified Sulcus Bleeding Index, and Gingival Index (scores 0-3), keratinized mucosa width, Papilla Index (scores 0-4), and pocket probing depth at T12. Midbuccal mucosal level changes from Tpre to T12. Modified Pink Esthetic Score and White Esthetic Score (scores 0-10). Marginal bone level changes from T1 to T12. Buccal bone thickness at T12. Patient-reported satisfaction (scores 1-10).

	Case 1	Case 2	Case 3	Mean (SD)
Modified Plaque Index	Score 0	Score 0	Score 0	0.0 ± 0.0
Modified Sulcus Bleeding Index	Score 0	Score 1	Score 0	0.3 ± 0.6
Gingival Index	Score 0	Score 0	Score 0	0.0 ± 0.0
Keratinized mucosa width (mm)	≥2	≥2	≥2	≥2
Papilla Index				
Tpre mesial	Score 3	Score 1	Score 3	2.3 ± 1.2
Tpre distal	Score 3	Score 0	Score 2	1.7 ± 1.5
T12 mesial	Score 3	Score 1	Score 3	2.3 ± 1.2
T12 distal	Score 3	Score 0	Score 2	1.7 ± 1.5
Pocket probing depth (mm)	5	3	5	4.3 ± 1.2
Mid-buccal mucosal level changes (mm)*	-0.51	-0.56	1.45	0.13 ± 1.5
Pink Esthetic Score				
Tpre	8	6	8	7.3 ± 1.2
Ttemp	8	6	8	7.3 ± 1.2
T12	9	7	9	8.3 ± 1.2
White Esthetic Score				
Tpre	4	7	N/A	5.5 ± 2.1
Ttemp	6	7	6	6.3 ± 0.6
T12	8	9	9	8.7 ± 0.6
Marginal bone level changes (mm)*	0.06	0.02	0.11	0.06 ± 0.05
Buccal bone thickness (mm)				
M0 (at neck)	2.34	1.84	3.14	2.44 ± 0.66
M1	2.46	1.86	3.36	2.56 ± 0.76
M2	2.98	2.18	3.48	2.88 ± 0.66
M3	2.95	1.85	3.35	2.71 ± 0.78
M4	2.75	1.65	3.25	2.55 ± 0.82
M5	2.55	1.25	3.25	2.35 ± 1.02
Patient-reported satisfaction				
Tpre	5	5	5	5.0 ± 0.0
Ttemp	8	9	8	8.3 ± 0.6
T12	8	10	9	9.0 ± 1.0

Tpre: prior to the treatment; Ttemp: 6 weeks after temporary restoration placement; T1: 1 month after final restoration placement; T12: 1 year after final restoration placement; N/A: not applicable. *A positive value indicates tissue/bone level gain, and a negative value indicates loss.

implant planning and ensuing pilot-drill surgical template fabrication was based on a stone cast with a conventional wax set-up. Possibly, the combined visualization of the hard and soft tissues in the digital workflow used in this case report enabled to plan the implant in a more palatal position, resulting in a thicker BBT.

In the surgical phase, static computer-assisted immediate implant surgery with the pilot-drill surgical template resulted in correct three-dimensional implant placement. It must be acknowledged that a fully guided surgical technique can offer more accuracy and that a certain degree of deviation from the digital planning should be taken into consideration when using a pilot-drill surgical template [21, 22]. In the present case report, the temporary shell restorations were connected to the temporary abutment after immediate implant placement. This compensated for any deviations while still resulting in temporary restorations with screw-access holes on the palatal side in all cases, indicating that this method for immediate single-implant provisionalization can be used when a fully guided technique is not feasible.

In the restorative phase, the temporary restorations could be delivered in the same appointment as the implant placement. Whereas in the studies with a conventional workflow mentioned earlier [6, 7], impression taking after the surgery was necessary to design and manufacture a customized temporary restoration afterwards in the dental laboratory, as well as an extra appointment for the temporary restoration placement. Thus, chair time was reduced by using the digital workflow. Other advantages of a digital workflow for implant restoration procedures are that intraoral scanning lowers the procedure time and patient discomfort compared to conventional impression taking [23] and that CAD and computer-aided manufacturing (CAM) can lower the production time and fabrication costs of the restorations [24]. These are all possible arguments for choosing a digital workflow over a conventional workflow.

A downside of the temporary shell restorations used in these cases is the grayish discoloration of the metal temporary abutment through the composite and the PMMA. Due to this discoloration, the mean WES for the temporary restorations was just above the threshold of clinical acceptance (6.3 ± 0.6 on a scale of 0-10) [18]. However, this was not reflected by the patient-reported satisfaction for the provisional restorations (8.3 ± 0.6 on a scale of 1-10). It must be mentioned that the satisfaction score of the patient that started the treatment without a clinical crown might be biased. But aside from that, it can be assumed that patients are easily satisfied with a fixed temporary restoration, even when the color does not match the adjacent teeth. The fact that patients are more satisfied with the treatment outcome than the professional observers has been recorded before [7, 25], thus, further underlining the importance of including both parameters when evaluating esthetic outcomes.

Although the initial results of immediate implant placement and chairside provisionalization using a digital workflow are successful, the number of cases is limited. Clinical studies with a larger sample size are required to further evaluate the treatment outcomes. In conclusion, the three reported cases demonstrate the potential for predictable immediate implant placement and chairside provisionalization using a digital workflow.

Consent

Written informed consent for publication of photographs and radiographs was obtained from the patients.

Authors' Contributions

V.J.J. Donker contributed to the conceptualization, data curation, formal analysis, investigation, methodology, project administration, and writing—original draft. G.M. Raghoebar contributed to the conceptualization, investigation, methodology, supervision, project administration, and writing—review and editing. A. Vissink contributed to the conceptualization, methodology, supervision, project administration, and writing—review and editing. H.J.A. Meijer contributed to the conceptualization, data curation, investigation, methodology, supervision, project administration, and writing—review and editing.

Acknowledgments

Implant materials for the clinical study were provided by Nobel Biocare Services AG, Zürich, Switzerland (study code: 2019-1627).

References

[1] H. Francisco, D. Marques, C. Pinto, L. Aiquel, and J. Caramês, "Is the timing of implant placement and loading influencing esthetic outcomes in single-tooth implants?—A systematic review," *Clinical Oral Implants Research*, vol. 32, no. S21, pp. 28–55, 2021.

[2] K. W. Slagter, G. M. Raghoebar, N. A. Bakker, A. Vissink, and H. J. A. Meijer, "Buccal bone thickness at dental implants in the aesthetic zone: A 1-year follow-up cone beam computed tomography study," *Journal of Cranio-Maxillofacial Surgerys*, vol. 45, no. 1, pp. 13–19, 2017.

[3] H. J. A. Meijer, K. W. Slagter, A. Vissink, and G. M. Raghoebar, "Buccal bone thickness at dental implants in the maxillary anterior region with large bony defects at time of immediate implant placement: A 1-year cohort study," *Clinical Implant Dentistry and Related Research*, vol. 21, no. 1, pp. 73–79, 2019.

[4] M. Steigmann, A. Monje, H.-L. Chan, and H.-L. Wang, "Emergence Profile Design Based on Implant Position in the Esthetic Zone," *International Journal of Periodontics & Restorative Dentistrys*, vol. 34, no. 4, pp. 559–563, 2014.

[5] T. De Rouck, K. Collys, I. Wyn, and J. Cosyn, "Instant provisionalization of immediate single-tooth implants is essential to optimize esthetic treatment outcome," *Clinical Oral Implants Research*, vol. 20, no. 6, pp. 566–570, 2009.

[6] K. W. Slagter, H. J. A. Meijer, N. A. Bakker, A. Vissink, and G. M. Raghoebar, "Feasibility of immediate placement of single-tooth implants in the aesthetic zone: A 1-year randomized controlled trial," *Journal of Clinical Periodontology*, vol. 42, no. 8, pp. 773–782, 2015.

[7] E. G. Zuiderveld, H. J. A. Meijer, L. den Hartog, A. Vissink, and G. M. Raghoebar, "Effect of connective tissue grafting on peri-implant tissue in single immediate implant sites: A RCT," *Journal of Clinical Periodontology*, vol. 45, no. 2, pp. 253–264, 2018.

[8] I. Gamborena, Y. Sasaki, and M. B. Blatz, "Predictable immediate implant placement and restoration in the esthetic zone," *Journal of Esthetic and Restorative Dentistry*, vol. 33, no. 1, pp. 158–172, 2021.

[9] D. S. Riley, M. S. Barber, G. S. Kienle et al., "CARE guidelines for case reports: explanation and elaboration document," *Journal of Clinical Epidemiology*, vol. 89, pp. 218–235, 2017.

[10] E. Groenendijk, T. A. Staas, F. E. J. Graauwmans et al., "Immediate implant placement: the fate of the buccal crest. A retrospective cone beam computed tomography study," *International Journal of Oral and Maxillofacial Surgery*, vol. 46, no. 12, pp. 1600–1606, 2017.

[11] J. Esquivel, R. Meda, and M. Blatz, "The Impact of 3D Implant Position on Emergence Profile Design," *International Journal of Periodontics & Restorative Dentistry*, vol. 41, no. 1, pp. 79–86, 2021.

[12] R. Gomez-Meda, J. Esquivel, and M. B. Blatz, "The esthetic biological contour concept for implant restoration emergence profile design," *Journal of Esthetic and Restorative Dentistry*, vol. 33, no. 1, pp. 173–184, 2021.

[13] S. C. Bayne and G. Schmalz, "Reprinting the classic article on USPHS evaluation methods for measuring the clinical research performance of restorative materials," *Clinical Oral Investigations*, vol. 9, no. 4, pp. 209–214, 2005.

[14] A. Mombelli, M. A. C. van Oosten, E. Schürch, and N. P. Lang, "The microbiota associated with successful or failing osseointegrated titanium implants," *Oral Microbiology and Immunology*, vol. 2, no. 4, pp. 145–151, 1987.

[15] H. Löe, "The Gingival Index, the Plaque Index and the Retention Index Systems," *Journal of Periodontology*, vol. 38, no. 6, pp. 610–616, 1967.

[16] G. Avila-Ortiz, O. Gonzalez-Martin, E. Couso-Queiruga, and H. L. Wang, "The peri-implant phenotype," *Journal of Periodontology*, vol. 91, no. 3, pp. 283–288, 2020.

[17] T. Jemt, "Regeneration of gingival papillae after single-implant treatment," *International Journal of Periodontics & Restorative Dentistry*, vol. 17, no. 4, pp. 326–333, 1997.

[18] U. C. Belser, L. Grütter, F. Vailati, M. M. Bornstein, H.-P. Weber, and D. Buser, "Outcome Evaluation of Early Placed Maxillary Anterior Single-Tooth Implants Using Objective Esthetic Criteria: A Cross-Sectional, Retrospective Study in 45 Patients With a 2- to 4-Year Follow-Up Using Pink and White Esthetic Scores," *Journal of Periodontology*, vol. 80, no. 1, pp. 140–151, 2009.

[19] K. W. Slagter, G. M. Raghoebar, A. Vissink, and H. J. A. Meijer, "Inter- and intraobserver reproducibility of buccal bone measurements at dental implants with cone beam computed tomography in the esthetic region," *International Journal of Implant Dentistry*, vol. 1, no. 1, pp. 1–5, 2015.

[20] G. Juodzbalys, D. Sakavicius, and H.-L. Wang, "Classification of Extraction Sockets Based Upon Soft and Hard Tissue Components," *Journal of Periodontology*, vol. 79, no. 3, pp. 413–424, 2008.

[21] F. Younes, J. Cosyn, T. De Bruyckere, R. Cleymaet, E. Bouckaert, and A. Eghbali, "A randomized controlled study on the accuracy of free-handed, pilot-drill guided and fully guided implant surgery in partially edentulous patients," *Journal of Clinical Periodontology*, vol. 45, no. 6, pp. 721–732, 2018.

[22] A. Tahmaseb, V. Wu, D. Wismeijer, W. Coucke, and C. Evans, "The accuracy of static computer-aided implant surgery: A systematic review and meta-analysis," *Clinical Oral Implants Research*, vol. 29, pp. 416–435, 2018.

[23] U. Schepke, H. J. A. Meijer, W. Kerdijk, and M. S. Cune, "Digital versus analog complete-arch impressions for single-unit premolar implant crowns: Operating time and patient preference," *Journal of Prosthetic Dentistry*, vol. 114, no. 3, pp. 403–406, 2015.

[24] S. Mühlemann, R. D. Kraus, C. H. F. Hämmerle, and D. S. Thoma, "Is the use of digital technologies for the fabrication of implant-supported reconstructions more efficient and/or more effective than conventional techniques: A systematic review," *Clinical Oral Implants Research*, vol. 29, pp. 184–195, 2018.

[25] C. M. Meijndert, G. M. Raghoebar, A. Vissink, and H. J. A. Meijer, "Alveolar ridge preservation in defect sockets in the maxillary aesthetic zone followed by single-tooth bone level tapered implants with immediate provisionalization: a 1-year prospective case series," *International Journal of Implant Dentistry*, vol. 7, no. 1, 2021.

22

A Clinical Case Report of a Potential Acute Allergic Reaction with Titanium Dental Implant

Ali Robaian Alqahtani,[1] Khalid Gufran,[2] Fred Silva,[3] Mateus Garcia Rocha,[4] and Jia Chang[5]

[1]*Department of Conservative Dental Sciences, College of Dentistry, Prince Sattam Bin Abdulaziz University, Alkharj, Saudi Arabia*
[2]*Department of Preventive Dental Sciences, College of Dentistry, Prince Sattam Bin Abdulaziz University, Alkharj, Saudi Arabia*
[3]*Department of Periodontics, Texas A & M College of Dentistry, Dallas, TX 75246, USA*
[4]*Center for Dental Biomaterials, Division of Operative Dentistry, Department of Restorative Dental Sciences, College of Dentistry University of Florida, USA*
[5]*Department of Periodontology, College of Dentistry, University of Florida, USA*

Correspondence should be addressed to Khalid Gufran; khalidg08@gmail.com

Academic Editor: Wen Lin Chai

Titanium hypersensitivity is rare, but it may exist among patients who need dental implant treatment. It could contribute to mild or severe peri-implant tissue hypersensitivity reactions and affect patients' oral and general health according to some clinical reports. In extreme cases, it may lead to implant failure or extraction. In this case report, a 64-year-old Caucasian female patient received a titanium implant placement on #5. Right after the implant placement, she reported the symptoms of pain, eczema, and slight extraoral swelling, along with significant burning sensation occurring intra- and extraorally. The symptoms were not released after the systemic intervention of antibiotics for six days. On retrieving her medical history, the patient reported a previous allergic reaction to jewelry-like earrings in her childhood. The diagnosis of titanium hypersensitivity was made based on the rapid onset of symptoms and her metal allergy history. Therefore, the dental implant was removed after diagnosis, and a bone allograft was used to preserve the alveolar bone volume. Immediately after implant extraction, the swelling and burning sensation were receded. A complete recovery was achieved three weeks later. The dimension of the alveolar ridge bone was found well maintained in 10 weeks follow-up visit. *Conclusion.* Rapid onset of peri-implant gingival swelling may indicate a hypersensitivity to titanium implant in the clinic. For patients with a history of allergy to jewelry, the hypersensitivity tests to titanium alloy such as patch test or lymphocyte transformation test should be recommended as part of the dental implant treatment plan.

1. Introduction

Titanium (Ti) and its alloys have been widely used as dental implant material due to high biocompatibility, resistance to corrosion, and mechanical properties [1–3]. However, some clinicians reported their patients may show hypersensitivity to medical or dental titanium implants, which is demonstrated by a temporal association between exposure to titanium and occurrence of tissue reaction proximal to implanted titanium [4–10]. For example, Sicilia et al. reported approximately 0.6% of patients receiving titanium dental implant treatment presented a positive reaction to titanium in the epicutaneous tests [6]. Egusa et al. reported an implant failure case due to suspected severe titanium allergy. The patient exhibited facial eczema following the placement of mandibular titanium dental implants for supporting overdenture. The removal of the implants resulted in a complete remission of symptoms [5]. Pigatto et al. reported a clinical case of exfoliative cheilitis correlated to a titanium dental implant placement in a 41-year-old female

[11]. Clinically, the oral manifestations of hypersensitivity to dental materials and dental implant may present as mucosal erythema, swelling of lips or purpuric patches on hard and soft palate, ulcers in oral cavity, hyperplastic gingivitis, tongue depapillation, angular cheilitis, eczematous eruptions on the face, or lichenoid reactions, etc. [12].

Allergic reactions include immediate humoral response due to antibody/antigen complexes in type I, II, III reactions, or type IV delayed hypersensitivity. In oral cavity, titanium implant-related allergic reactions usually occurred as type IV hypersensitivity reactions [13, 14]. The mechanism of such allergic reactions is commonly related to tribocorrosion, which is a material degradation process due to the combined effect of wear and corrosion. Mechanical wear occurs during implant placement and loading. Corrosion occurs once the oxide layer of titanium implants is disturbed after titanium exposed to fluid media or air. Any disruption of the oxide surface layer will cause corrosion and compromise implant biocompatibility [13]. Mechanical wear and corrosion can generate metal debris or particles from titanium or its alloy components. In animal studies, researchers found the increased presence of titanium ions in peri-implant tissues following implant placement and detected titanium ions in regional lymph nodes and the lungs [15–17]. These metal ions may bind with serum proteins and activate the immune system by inducing the production of specific T lymphocytes, which eventually resulting in type IV hypersensitivity reaction [18, 19]. Usually, an epicutaneous patch test is used to diagnose metal allergies in patients. However, its results could be a false positive reaction because the procedure itself may induce sensitivity or cause a flare-up of symptoms [20]. The lymphocyte transformation test (LTT) becomes a more suitable test to assist in diagnosing metal hypersensitivity, including titanium materials [21, 22]. Its predictive value needs more studies in order to be proven [4].

In this case report, we exhibited a female patient's acute allergic reaction to a titanium implant placed in her maxillary premolar area. Her initial symptoms of hypersensitivity reaction, response to antibiotics intervention, medical history retrieval, implant extraction, and tissue healing outcomes in the short-term and long-term follow-up were recorded. We aim to introduce the process of our clinical diagnosis and management of dental implant hypersensitivity, as well as addressing the importance of retrieving a patient's hypersensitivity history and performing a hypersensitivity test during implant treatment planning for patients with a history of hypersensitivity to jewelry or dental materials.

2. Case Presentation

A 64-year-old Caucasian female patient was referred to the Graduate Periodontics Clinic at the University of Florida College of Dentistry for implant placement in the area of #5 (Figure 1). In the patient's self-report about her medical history, she has known allergies to Codeine/Narcotics and some food products, along with hypertension and hypothyroidism. All of her medical conditions were well monitored and controlled by medications. The extraoral and intraoral examinations were performed, including a full periodontal charting examination, periapical radiography, and cone-beam computed tomography. The implant treatment plan was made after assessing the bone volume as well as its proximity to the vital structures in #5 site (Figure 2). After obtaining the patient's consent, the surgical implant placement was performed at #5 area (4.2 mm × 10 mm Astra Tech EV OsseoSpeed, Dentsply International) (Figures 3 and 4). The placed implant achieved good primary stability. The cover screw was tightened, and the site was sutured using a 4-0 chromic gut absorbable suture. The surgery was completed smoothly. The surgical wound showed no bleeding and swelling after suturing. The patient took Ibuprofen for post-surgical pain management. Four days after implant surgery, the patient called the surgeon and complained of the progressing pain, swelling, and burning sensation intraorally and extraorally on her implant surgery side. The patient was scheduled for a follow-up appointment immediately. In the follow-up visit, this patient claimed that from 2nd day after the implant placement, she felt mild to moderate pain at the implant surgery site, which gradually became severe with a score of 8 out of 10 on the pain scale. There was mild swelling with redness on her right side of the face. No significant lymphadenopathy in the orofacial and neck regions was found. The intraoral examination showed erythema of the oral mucosa around the surgical site with purpuric patches on the palate along with few mouth ulcers. The surgical site and adjacent teeth were tender to palpation with hyperplastic gingival (Figure 5). A periapical radiograph was taken during the appointment, and no apparent abnormality was detected (Figure 6). The patient was reassured, and a prescription of amoxicillin (500 mg every 8 hours for seven days by oral administration) was given. The patient texted the surgeon six days later, claiming the symptoms had not been improved since her last visit. Besides, she wrote, "My mother called and reminded me I am allergic to certain metals. For example, I cannot wear some earrings; my ear lobe swells up then bleeds. Do you think this could be the case with this implant?" Based

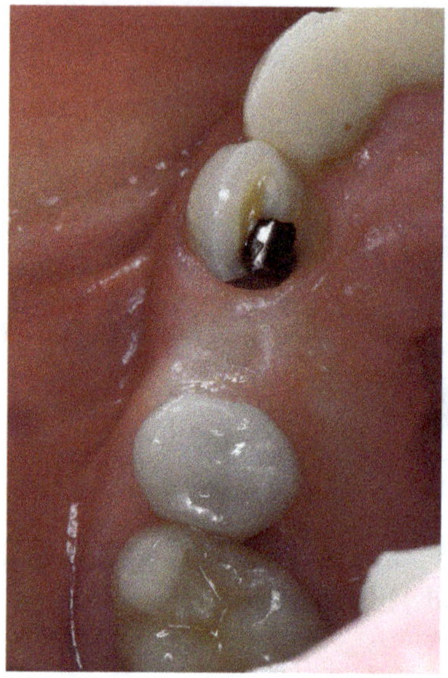

Figure 1: Preimplant surgery photo.

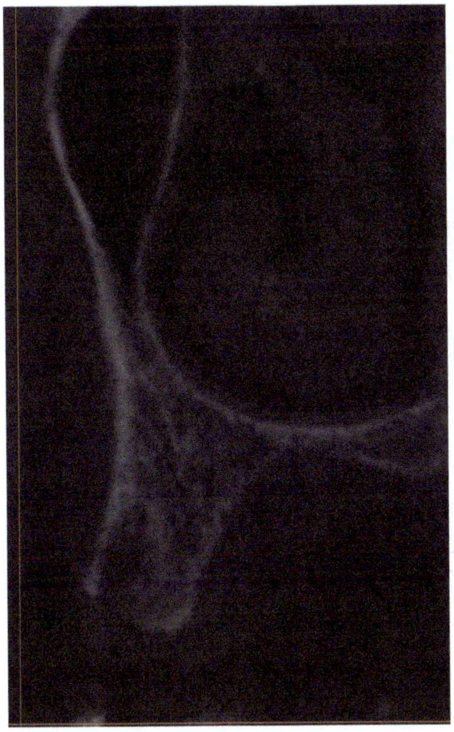

FIGURE 2: CBCT image before implant placement.

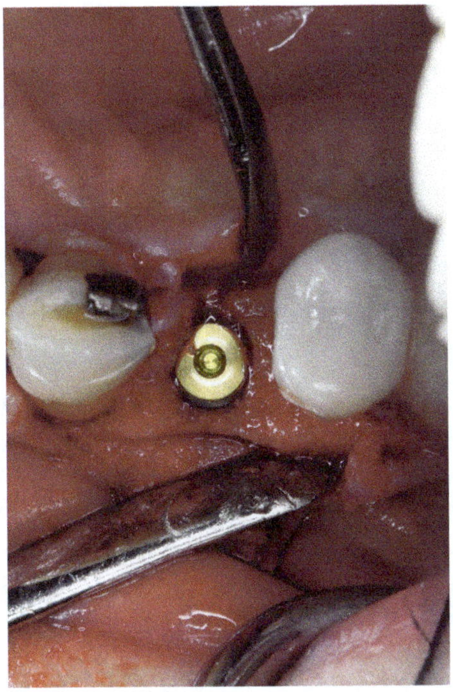

FIGURE 3: Implant placement.

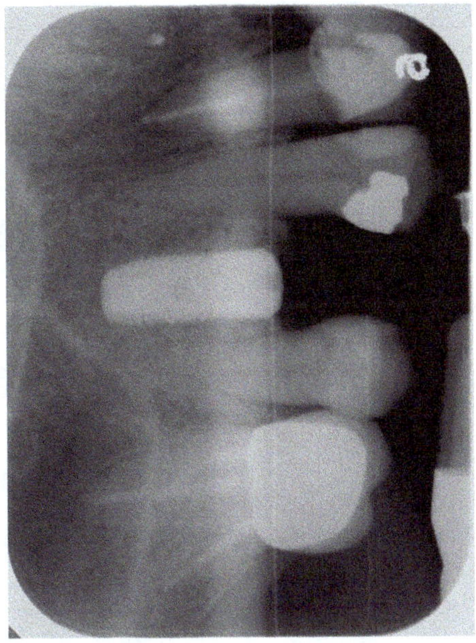

FIGURE 4: X-ray following the implant placement.

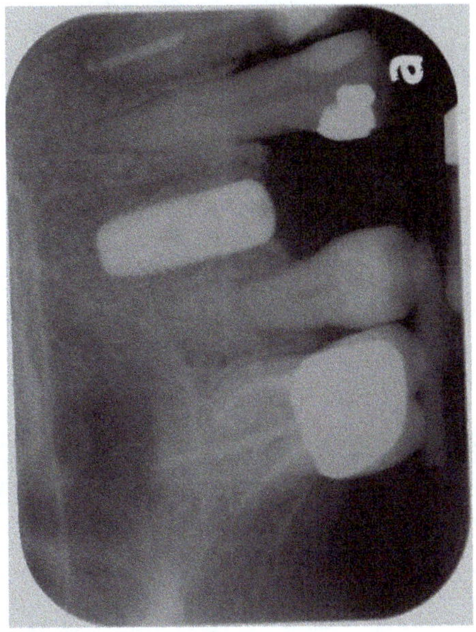

FIGURE 5: 10 days after implant placement. The patient exhibited significant allergy symptoms.

on the patient's history of metal hypersensitivity and her postimplant surgery symptoms, we highly suspected she was allergic to the newly-placed titanium implant on #5. The patient was immediately scheduled for the explant surgery, and the implant on #5 was removed (Figures 7(a) and 7(b)). The extracted site was grafted with freeze-dried bone allograft (Symbios allograft, Dentsply Sirona) and covered with resorbable collagen membrane (Symbios Collagen Membrane pre-hydrated, Dentsply Sirona) (Figure 7(c)). The wound was closed using 3-0 PTFE nonabsorbable suture material. The patient was instructed to continue with her medication. The patient reported that the facial and gum swelling, the burning sensation, and severe pain had subsided soon after the surgery. The patient had 3, 6, and 10-week follow-up visits (Figures 8 and 9). The surgical wound healed very well after the surgery. The ridge bone volume on the site was well-maintained. The patient still interests in implant-supported crown restoration. She will be scheduled for a hypersensitivity test to have the diagnostic analysis. It may

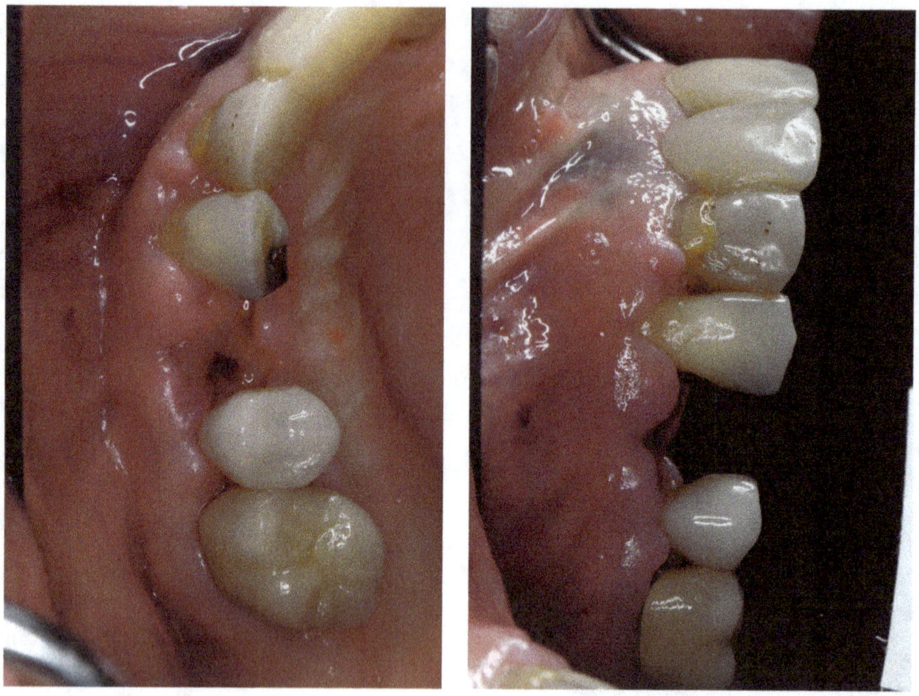

(a) (b)

FIGURE 6: Intraoral photos taken on day 4 after implant placement exhibit significant allergy symptoms. ((a) occlusal view; (b) buccal view).

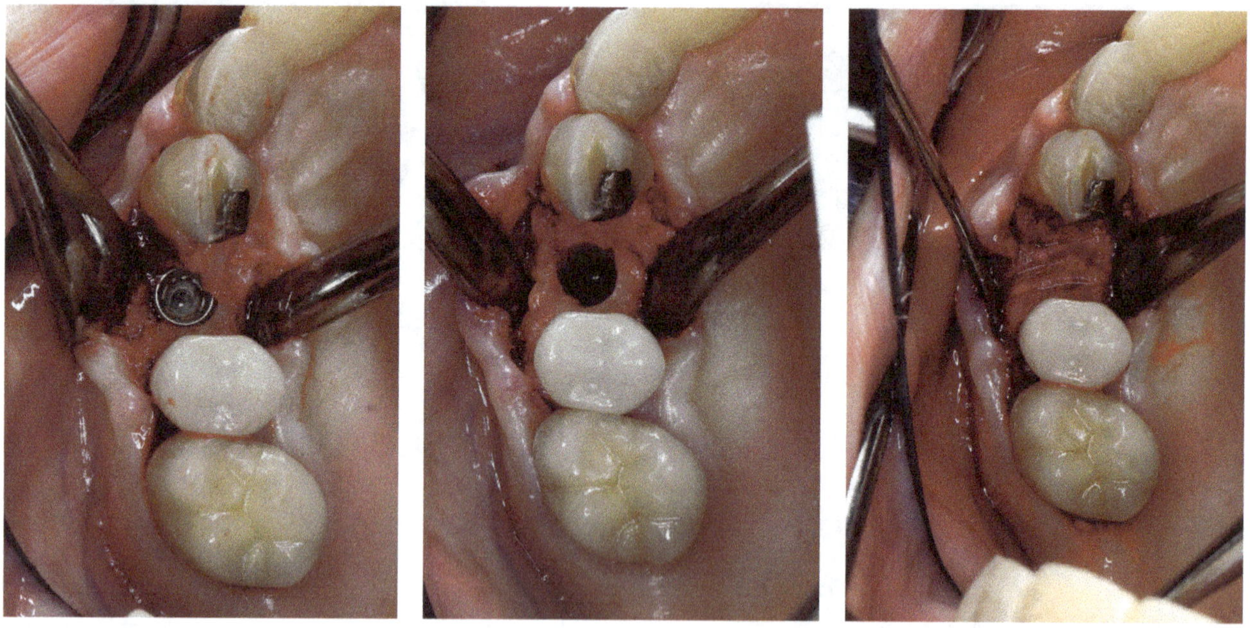

(a) (b) (c)

FIGURE 7: Implant removal surgery. (a) Implant exposure. (b) Implant removal. (c) Bone grafting of implant site.

help to determine whether she is indicated for zirconium implant in the future.

3. Discussion and Conclusions

In this case report, the patient received titanium dental implant surgery and exhibited pain, eczema, slight extraoral swelling, and burning sensation intra- and extraorally within four days after the implant placement. The symptoms got worse and spread to the broader orofacial area even with antibiotic administration, which, in this case, excludes bacterial infection as the etiology. A history of allergy to metal earrings was retrieved according to her communication with her mother. Based on her previous dental treatment record, we

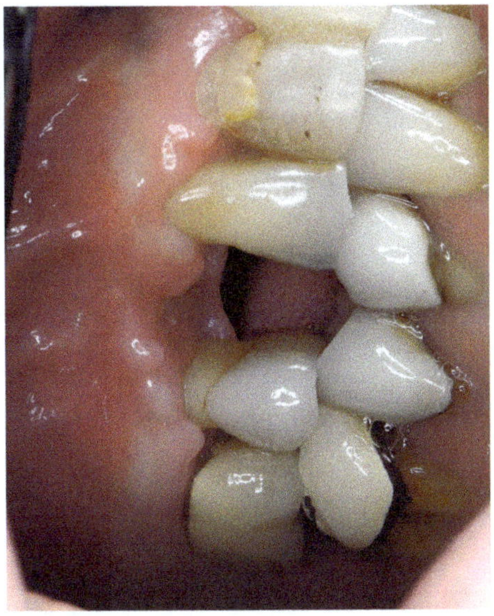

FIGURE 8: Three-week postsurgical follow-up.

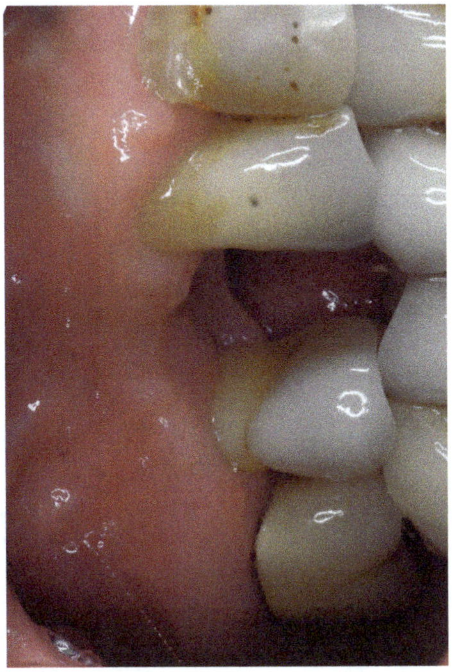

FIGURE 9: Ten-week postsurgical follow-up.

excluded possible allergic reaction to chromic gut absorbable suture placed during her implant surgery and ibuprofen medication for pain management after the implant surgery. Therefore, the initial diagnosis of titanium hypersensitivity was highly suspected. To manage her significant tissue reactions, the titanium implant was extracted, and the drilling site was grafted with allograft bone materials. All intra- and extraoral symptoms receded right after the implant removal, and a complete recovery was achieved three weeks later. Such responses confirmed the initial clinical diagnosis of hypersensitivity to titanium-based dental implants. The patient was referred to an immunology center to have a medical consult about potential allergens before implant treatment plan in the future.

There are 3 types of allergic reactions related to the orofacial region—type I, III, and IV. While type I is an immediate anaphylactic reaction to allergens, type III can occur 2–8 hours after the placement of implants due to the increase in circulatory antibodies. However, it may appear even after fourteen days. Type IV is a delayed reaction, which occurs 24–72 hours after the surgery, and it occurs after recurrent contact of the allergen with the mucosa or skin, but the symptoms may appear up to 14 days postimplant placement. Allergic reaction could appear at some distance from the implant and can cause a systemic reaction, which could be overlooked or misinterpreted [23].

The rapid onset of hypersensitivity reaction proximal to the inserted dental implant as shown in this case report is extremely rare, and most of titanium hypersensitivity reactions are of delayed type [24].

Titanium alloys are preferred as dental implants when compared to pure titanium, owing to their superior strength. It is worth noting that even pure titanium is not free of trace impurities such as aluminum, manganese, iron, beryllium, and nickel, which can cause an allergic reaction. Allergic reaction to metals including titanium occurs due to the ions produced as a result of implant corrosion, which could either come in contact with the mucosa or could be ingested. Although these ions by themselves are not irritating, they can combine with native proteins to form complexes, which could be a potential allergen-inducing hypersensitive reaction [23].

Since titanium is considered a gold standard for dental implants, an allergic reaction is not expected by dental professionals. Literature contains very limited data regarding the incidence and management of allergic reaction arising from titanium dental implants. Therefore, improved guidelines are warranted before the placement of an implant, and if an allergic reaction does occur post implant placement, all possible treatment alternatives must be explained and made available. Carrying out titanium allergy test should be routinely followed, especially in patients with known allergies to metals. If the patient experiences hypersensitive reaction following dental implant placement, the possibility of explanation should be considered depending on the risks and benefits for the patient. Zirconium dioxide implants ($ZrO2$) or yttria-stabilized zirconia can serve as good substitutes as no allergic reactions have been reported yet from zirconium oxide [25]. It can be concluded that although rare, titanium hypersensitivity is a real possibility and should not be overlooked since an allergic reaction could cause various symptoms.

Abbreviations

Ti: Titanium
LTT: Lymphocyte transformation tests.

Consent

A written consent to publish this information was obtained from the study participant for publication of this case report and any accompanying images and photos. The proof of consent to publish from the study participant can be requested at any time.

Authors' Contributions

Dr. A.R.A contributes to patient care, clinical data collection, and manuscript writing; Dr. K.G contributes to the manuscript writing and editing; Dr. F.S contributes to clinical data collection; Dr. M.G.R contributes to the manuscript editing; Dr. J.C contributes to the patient care, clinical data collection, clinical document preparation, manuscript writing, and editing.

References

[1] S. Lugowski, D. C. Smith, H. Bonek, D. Deporter, P. Watson, and A. McHugh, *Systemic metal ion levelsin dental implant patients after five years*, Actualites en Biomateriaux, Paris, France: Romillat, 2000.

[2] D. C. Smith, S. Lugowski, A. McHugh, D. Deporter, P. A. Watson, and M. Chipman, "Systemic metal ion levels in dental implant patients," *The International Journal of Oral & Maxillofacial Implants*, vol. 12, no. 6, pp. 828–834, 1997.

[3] T. Albrektsson, "The response of bone to titanium implants," *CRC Crit Rev Biocompat*, vol. 1, pp. 53–84, 1985.

[4] A. Mombelli, D. Hashim, and N. Cionca, "What is the impact of titanium particles and biocorrosion on implant survival and complications? A critical review," *Clinical Oral Implants Research*, vol. 29, no. 18, pp. 37–53, 2018.

[5] H. Egusa, N. Ko, T. Shimazu, and H. Yatani, "Suspected association of an allergic reaction with titanium dental implants: a clinical report," *The Journal of Prosthetic Dentistry*, vol. 100, no. 5, pp. 344–347, 2008.

[6] A. Sicilia, S. Cuesta, G. Coma et al., "Titanium allergy in dental implant patients: a clinical study on 1500 consecutive patients," *Clinical Oral Implants Research*, vol. 19, no. 8, pp. 823–835, 2008.

[7] A. Siddiqi, A. G. T. Payne, R. K. De Silva, and W. J. Duncan, "Titanium allergy: could it affect dental implant integration?," *Clinical Oral Implants Research*, vol. 22, no. 7, pp. 673–680, 2011.

[8] L. A. du Preez, K. W. Butow, and T. J. Swart, "Implant failure due to titanium hypersensitivity/allergy?-Report of a case," *SADJ*, vol. 62, no. 22, pp. 24-25, 2007.

[9] H. P. Lim, K. M. Lee, Y. I. Koh, and S. W. Park, "Allergic contact stomatitis caused by a titanium nitride-coated implant abutment: a clinical report," *The Journal of Prosthetic Dentistry*, vol. 108, no. 4, pp. 209–213, 2012.

[10] M. Hosoki, K. Nishigawa, Y. Miyamoto, G. Ohe, and Y. Matsuka, "Allergic contact dermatitis caused by titanium screws and dental implants," *Journal of Prosthodontic Research*, vol. 60, no. 3, pp. 213–219, 2016.

[11] P. D. Pigatto, E. Berti, F. Spadari, G. P. Bombeccari, and G. Guzzi, "Photoletter to the editor: exfoliative cheilitis associated with titanium dental implants and mercury amalgam," *J Dermatol Case Rep*, vol. 5, no. 4, pp. 89-90, 2011.

[12] J. S. Vamnes, G. B. Lygre, A. G. Gronningsaeter, and N. R. Gjerdet, "Four years of clinical experience with an adverse reaction unit for dental biomaterials," *Community Dentistry and Oral Epidemiology*, vol. 32, no. 2, pp. 150–157, 2004.

[13] T. P. Chaturvedi, "An overview of the corrosion aspect of dental implants (titanium and its alloys)," *Indian Journal of Dental Research*, vol. 20, no. 1, pp. 91–98, 2009.

[14] D. Williams, *Definations in Biomaterials, Proceedings of concensus conference of European Society for Biomaterials, Chester, England, March 3-5, 1986*, Elsevier Science Limited, Amsterdam, 1987.

[15] D. Brune, "Metal release from dental biomaterials," *Biomaterials*, vol. 7, no. 3, pp. 163–175, 1986.

[16] K. W. Frisken, G. W. Dandie, S. Lugowski, and G. Jordan, "A study of titanium release into body organs following the insertion of single threaded screw implants into the mandibles of sheep," *Australian Dental Journal*, vol. 47, no. 3, pp. 214–217, 2002.

[17] H. Schliephake, G. Reiss, R. Urban, F. W. Neukam, and S. Guckel, "Metal release from titanium fixtures during placement in the mandible: an experimental study," *The International Journal of Oral & Maxillofacial Implants*, vol. 8, no. 5, pp. 502–511, 1993.

[18] N. J. Hallab, M. Caicedo, R. Epstein, K. McAllister, and J. J. Jacobs, "In vitro reactivity to implant metals demonstrates a person-dependent association with both T-cell and B-cell activation," *Journal of Biomedical Materials Research. Part A*, vol. 92, pp. 667–682, 2009.

[19] N. J. Hallab, M. Caicedo, A. Finnegan, and J. J. Jacobs, "Th1 type lymphocyte reactivity to metals in patients with total hip arthroplasty," *Journal of Orthopaedic Surgery and Research*, vol. 3, no. 1, p. 6, 2008.

[20] M. Hannuksela, "Epicutaneous testing," *Allergy*, vol. 34, no. 1, pp. 5–10, 1979.

[21] K. Muller and E. Valentine-Thon, "Hypersensitivity to titanium: clinical and laboratory evidence," *Neuroendocrinology Letters*, vol. 27, no. 1, pp. 31–35, 2006.

[22] E. Valentine-Thon, K. Muller, G. Guzzi, S. Kreisel, P. Ohnsorge, and M. Sandkamp, "LTT-MELISA is clinically relevant for detecting and monitoring metal sensitivity," *Neuroendocrinology Letters*, vol. 27, no. 1, pp. 17–24, 2006.

[23] R. Comino-Garayoa, B. B. Jorge Cortés, J. Peláez, L. S. Carlos, M. G. Jose, and J. S. María, "Allergies to titanium dental implants: what do we really know about them? A scoping review," *Biology*, vol. 9, no. 11, p. 404, 2020.

[24] S. W. Fage, J. Muris, S. S. Jakobsen, and J. P. Thyssen, "Titanium: a review on exposure, release, penetration, allergy, epidemiology, and clinical reactivity," *Contact Dermatitis*, vol. 74, no. 6, pp. 323–345, 2016.

[25] N. Cionca, D. Hashim, and A. Mombelli, "Zirconia dental implants: where are we now, and where are we heading?," *Periodontology*, vol. 73, no. 1, pp. 241–258, 2017.

23

Hard and Soft Tissue Augmentation with Single-Implant Restoration in the Esthetic Zone

Igor Ashurko, Nataliia Blagushina, Anisa Borodiy, and Mary Magdalyanova

Department of Oral Surgery, E.V. Borovsky Institute of Dentistry of I.M. Sechenov First Moscow State Medical University (Sechenov University), Mozhaisky Val, 11 Moscow, Russia

Correspondence should be addressed to Igor Ashurko; ashurko@yandex.ru

Academic Editor: Rui Amaral Mendes

The removal of the central incisor of the upper jaw is a challenging process, since the restoration of a single implant in the esthetic zone is of great responsibility. When tooth extraction with immediate implant placement is not possible, modern protocols imply the use of the socket preservation technique. This method of preserving socket properties significantly reduces changes that occur during the healing process of the postextracted area and along with soft tissue augmentation allows to achieve a satisfying aesthetic result. The aim of present case report is to assess capabilities of socket preservation concept and application of soft tissue augmentation in the anterior maxillary region. The treatment steps of a 35-year-old woman who needed to remove tooth 11 with further dental implant placement are described. The clinical case is of interest because after socket preservation and soft tissue augmentation, an acceptable aesthetic result was not reached. However, additional soft tissue augmentation made it possible to achieve the desired result, which was stable for 7 years.

1. Introduction

Rehabilitation in an aesthetic zone is often challenging. It is even more complicated when it is necessary to remove one of the teeth and replace it with an implant. There are many factors that influence peri-implant tissue stability in the anterior region. Therefore, several methods have been proposed to prevent bone loss and preserve the volume of soft tissue in the intervention area, including different timing protocols of implant placement and implant loading, specific implant positioning and developing a new implant design, the use of bone graft materials, and soft tissue augmentation procedures [1, 2]. After tooth extraction, the process of atrophy of bone tissue is triggered, which leads to a decrease in the volumetric parameters of the socket and a deterioration of the conditions to obtain a satisfactory aesthetic result of treatment [3]. One of the well-known methods to reduce the degree of alveolar bone loss is a socket preservation technique. The effectiveness of the method has been proven by many clinical and experimental studies [4, 5]. However, according to a number of authors, the use of the socket preservation alone does not fully compensate for the loss of volume of the alveolar ridge [6]. Many authors recommend soft tissue augmentation when working with implants in the anterior region [7–9]. It allows to create the most natural contour of the alveolar ridge and restore the lost aesthetics.

This article describes a clinical case of the removal of an inconsistent tooth with a technique to preserve the parameters of the socket, the subsequent implant installation with a two-stage soft tissue augmentation. This clinical case is interesting in that it not only confirms the need for the above manipulations to achieve a long-term functional and aesthetic result but also shows the problems the clinician may face.

2. Case Presentation

A 35-year-old female patient came to the clinic in order to change old metal-ceramic restorations on the upper and lower jaws. The patient was concerned about the appearance of her teeth. In particular, alignment of the gingival contours of the central incisors on the upper jaw was not sufficient.

According to the patient, the metal-ceramic constructions were made about 7 years ago. Prosthetic treatment was preceded by endodontic preparation of the teeth.

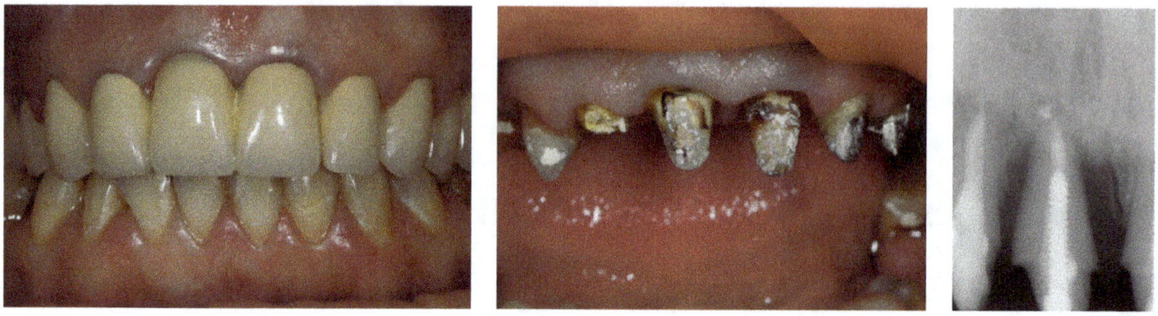

(a) (b) (c)

Figure 1: (a) Frontal area of the upper jaw. (b) After removal of metal-ceramic crowns. (c) Periapical X-ray of the tooth 11.

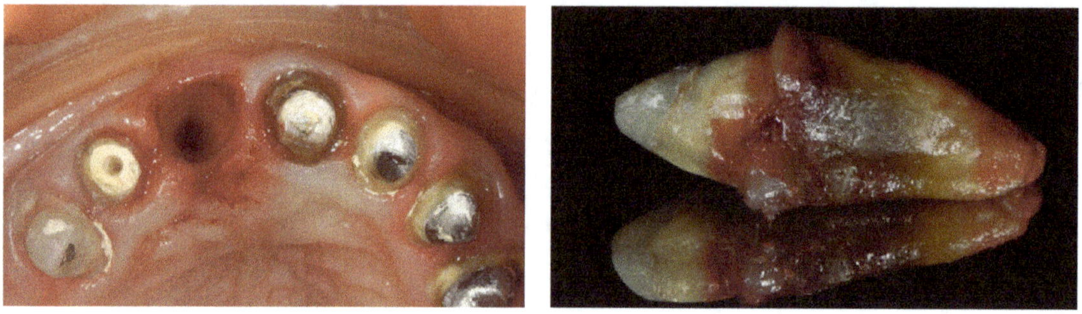

(a) (b)

Figure 2: (a) Situation after tooth extraction. (b) Extracted tooth 11.

The patient is somatically healthy, and no chronic diseases or allergies have been reported.

2.1. Planning. During clinical examination, an asymmetry of the gingival contours of the frontal part of the upper jaw was revealed (apical displacement of the gingival margin of tooth 11).

Periodontal examination revealed a pocket of 12 mm in depth on the mesial side of the tooth root, 9 mm on the distal side, 6-8 mm on the palatal, and 4-5 mm on the vestibular sides.

The intraoral periapical radiograph showed bone resorption in the apical direction in the form of a reduced bone density area in 2/3 of the radiolucent periapical lesion of the root length. An excess of root filling material was detected beyond the apex (Figure 1).

Since immediate implant placement was not possible in this case, we recommended extracting the tooth and performing the method of the socket preservation.

Following the main procedure, dental implantation, soft tissue augmentation, and subsequent prosthetics were planned to be performed.

2.2. Surgical Procedures. The patient received a prophylactic dose of antibiotic (1 g Amoxiclavi, LEK, d.d., Slovenia) 1 hour prior to surgery. Dissection of the circular ligament of tooth 11 was made using surgical blades 15c and 12d under local anaesthesia with 4% articaine hydrochloride (Ubistesin; 3M ESPE). Atraumatic extraction of the tooth was implemented (Figure 2). After curettage of the socket, it was rinsed with 0.05% chlorhexidine solution [10, 11].

The socket was filled with Bio-Oss collagen bone substitute material (Geistlich Pharma AG). In the process of packing the material, it was gradually impregnated with blood. The bone-substitute material was covered with a Bio-Gide native resorbable collagen membrane (Geistlich Pharma AG), which was fixed by Prolene monofilament 6-0 cross suture (Ethicon W8005, Johnson & Johnson) (Figure 3).

For hermetic closure of the socket, we decided to install a temporary bridge construction over the defect.

Postoperative recommendations included rinsing with 0.2% chlorhexidine gluconate mouthwash solution (Corsodyl, GlaxoSmithKline) twice a day for a week and receiving antibiotic (1 g Amoxiclavi, LEK, d.d., Slovenia) twice a day for 5 days. To relieve pain, 100 mg of Nimesulide (Nise; Dr. Reddy's Laboratories Ltd., India) was prescribed. We also recommended to minimize trauma at the site; no special diet was proposed. The sutures were removed 14 days after surgical treatment.

The feasibility of implant placement was carried out at the 4 months postoperative visit. In the area of the previous surgical treatment, complete epithelialization of the socket was evident; the mucosa was pale pink, and no pathological changes were found. However, soft tissue deficiency was found in the area of the 11 tooth socket on the vestibular surface (Figure 4).

At the same time, on the basis of cone-beam computed tomography (CBCT), the adequate height and width of the alveolar ridge (bone volume parameters) for dental implant placement was determined.

The density of newly formed bone tissue in the area of previous socket augmentation corresponded to the normal

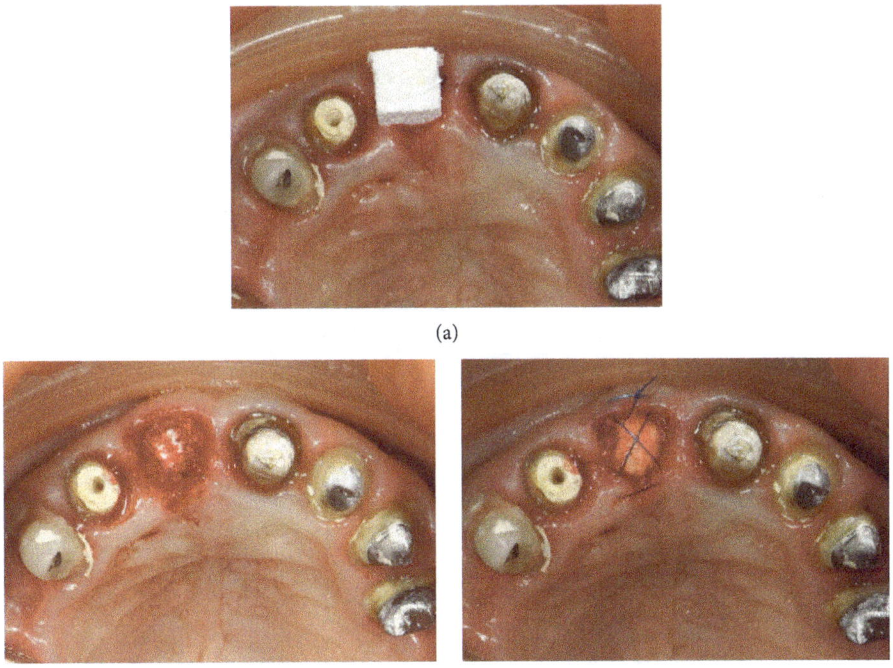

(a)

(b) (c)

FIGURE 3: (a) Insertion of Bio-Oss collagen in a dry form. (b) The alveolus is completely packed with the material. (c) A resorbable membrane is laid, and stabilizing sutures are applied.

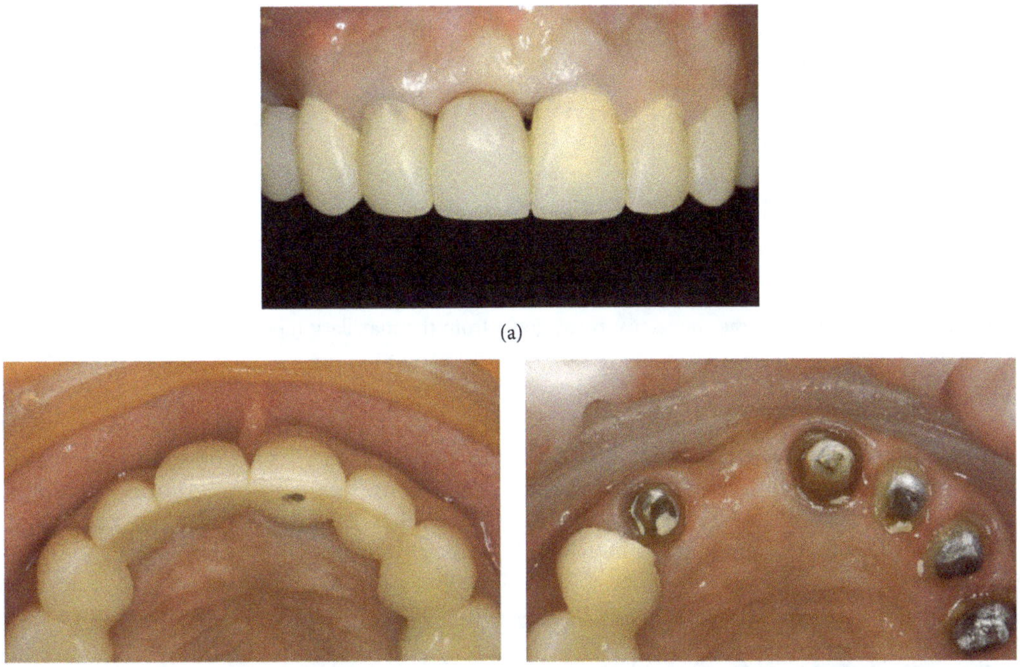

(a)

(b) (c)

FIGURE 4: (a, b) 4 months after the operation. (c) After the removal of the temporary appliance, a change in the contour of the crest in the vestibular-oral direction.

density, without pathological changes. According to this clinical situation, we decided to place a dental implant with soft tissue augmentation using a free connective tissue graft (CTG) from the tuberosity area.

The patient received a prophylactic dose of antibiotic (1 g Amoxiclavi, LEK, d.d., Slovenia) 1 hour prior to surgery. Under local anaesthesia with 4% articaine hydrochloride (Ubistesin; 3M ESPE) using a 15c blade, the mucosa was

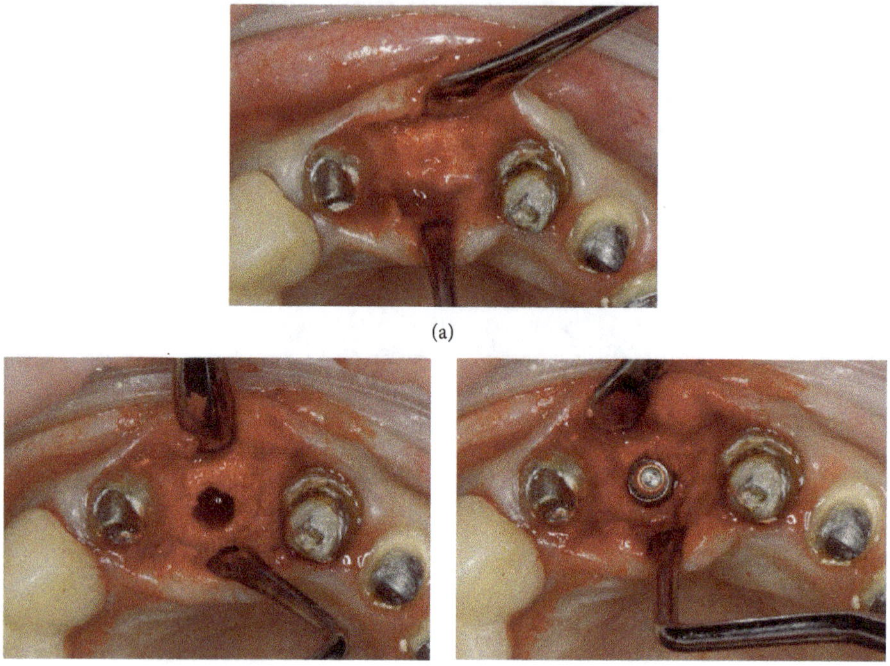

(a) (b) (c)

Figure 5: (a) The mucoperiosteal flap is detached. (b) The implant bed preparation. (c) The implant placement.

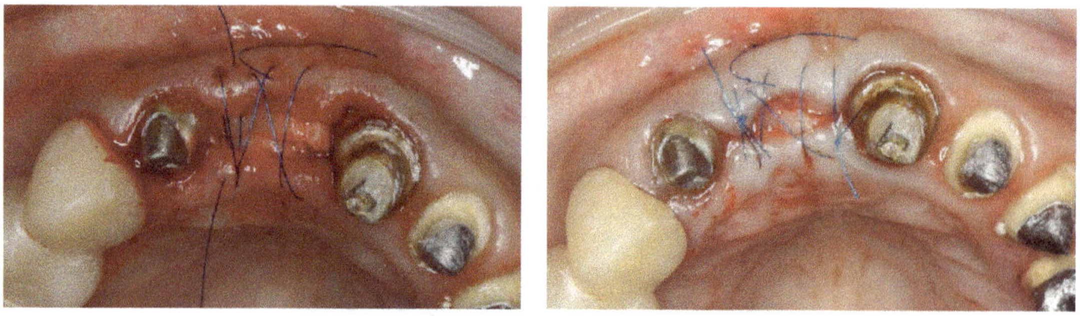

(a) (b)

Figure 6: (a) Fixation of free connective tissue grafts from the maxillary tuberosity. (b) Final suturing.

dissected along the top of the alveolar ridge within teeth 21 and 12.

The mucoperiosteal flap was elevated. According to the following surgical protocol, an Astra Tech dental implant (Dentsply Sirona, York, Pennsylvania) 3.5×11 was placed at the site of the extracted tooth 11. The implant insertion torque was 35 N/cm; the implant stability quotient (ISQ) value was 60 (Figure 5).

Three fragments of CTG were taken from the maxilla tuber region on the right side and fixed to the vestibular flap with Prolene monofilament 6-0 horizontal mattress suture (Ethicon W8005, Johnson & Johnson) (Figure 6).

A temporary bridge construction was installed over the defect, which was modified taking into account the changes in the configuration of the alveolar ridge.

Postoperative therapy included rinsing with 0.2% chlorhexidine gluconate mouthwash solution (Corsodyl, GlaxoSmithKline) twice a day for a week and receiving antibiotic (1 g Amoxiclavi, LEK, d.d., Slovenia) twice a day for 5 days. To relieve pain, 100 mg of Nimesulide (Nise; Dr. Reddy's Laboratories Ltd., India) was prescribed. We advised to minimize trauma at the site; no special diet was recommended. The sutures were removed 14 days after surgical treatment.

Further follow-up evaluations occurred at 2 weeks. A sufficient volume of the alveolar ridge was visualized in the vestibulooral direction. However, at 3 months postsurgery, the soft tissue volume of the vestibular surface was not sufficient (Figure 7).

For a good aesthetic result, we made a decision about implant disclosure with one-stage soft tissue grafting procedure using deepithelialized free gingival graft.

Under local anaesthesia with 4% articaine hydrochloride (Ubistesin; 3M ESPE) using a 15c blade, the mucosa was split along the top of the alveolar ridge within teeth 21 and 12. Splitted flap was stripped away; screw end cap was removed. The tunnel was performed on the vestibular site. Free gingival graft with a size of 12×6 *mm* and thickness of 2 mm was harvested from the palate area on the right side.

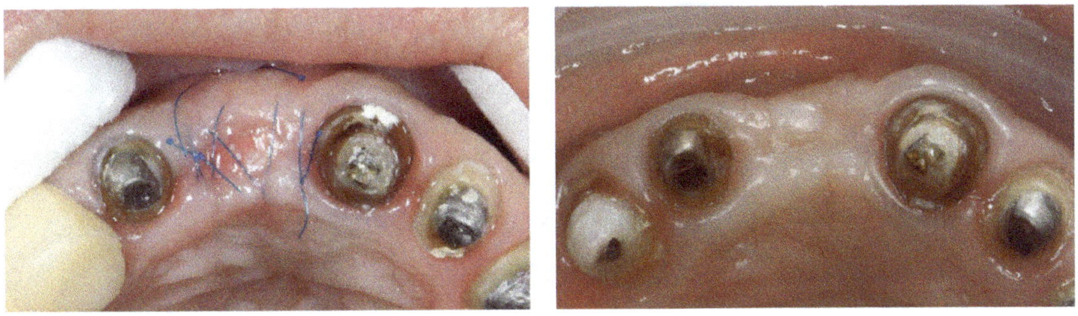

(a) (b)

Figure 7: (a) Appearance of the alveolar crest 14 days after surgery. (b) 3 months after surgery.

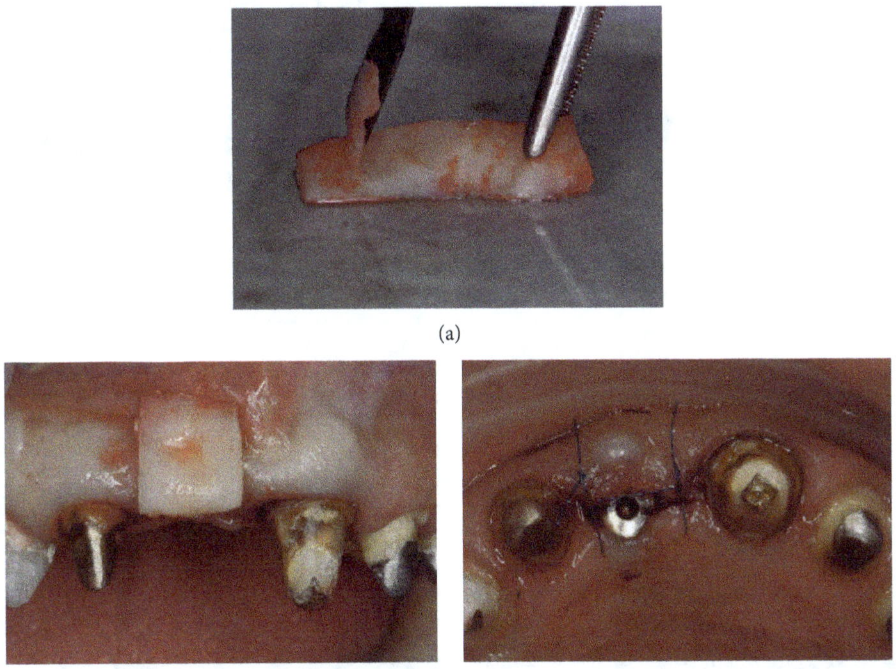

(a)

(b) (c)

Figure 8: (a) Deepithelization of the free connective tissue graft from the hard palate. (b) Projection of the graft on the formed tunnel from the vestibular surface. (c) The graft is placed in the formed bed; the wound is sutured.

The graft was deepithelialized using an 11c blade. Then, it was folded in half, inserted into the tunnel bed, and fixed with a horizontal mattress suture. After that, healing abutment was performed; simple interrupted sutures were applied (Ethicon W8005, Johnson & Johnson) (Figure 8).

Postoperative recommendations included rinsing with 0.2% chlorhexidine gluconate mouthwash solution (Corsodyl, GlaxoSmithKline) twice a day for a week and receiving antibiotic (1 g Amoxiclavi, LEK, d.d., Slovenia) twice a day for 5 days. To relieve pain, 100 mg of Nimesulide (Nise; Dr. Reddy's Laboratories Ltd., India) was prescribed. We also recommended to minimize trauma at the site; no special diet was recommended. The sutures were removed 14 days after surgical treatment.

At 2 months after surgery, sufficient tissue volume in the vestibulooral direction was determined. The patient was referred for prosthetics.

2.3. Prosthetic Procedures. Prosthetic procedures were initiated after 2 months of healing. Visually pathological changes in the area of the installed implant were not determined; the condition and volume of the soft tissue were satisfactory. Additionally, no pathological changes were found on the contact periapical X-ray. The implant stability quotient (ISQ) value was 78.

Considering that tooth 11 restoration was part of a complex rehabilitation, the stage of prosthetics was performed simultaneously on the upper and lower jaws. At the first stage, a temporary crown was made and fixed on the implant, which was corrected 1 time in 2 weeks during 2 months, and then, we proceeded to permanent prosthetics. The impressions were taken with polyvinyl siloxane impression material (Impregum, 3M ESPE, St. Paul, MN, USA).

The individual abutment of the implant was made of zirconium dioxide on a titanium base (Astra Tech-Dentsply

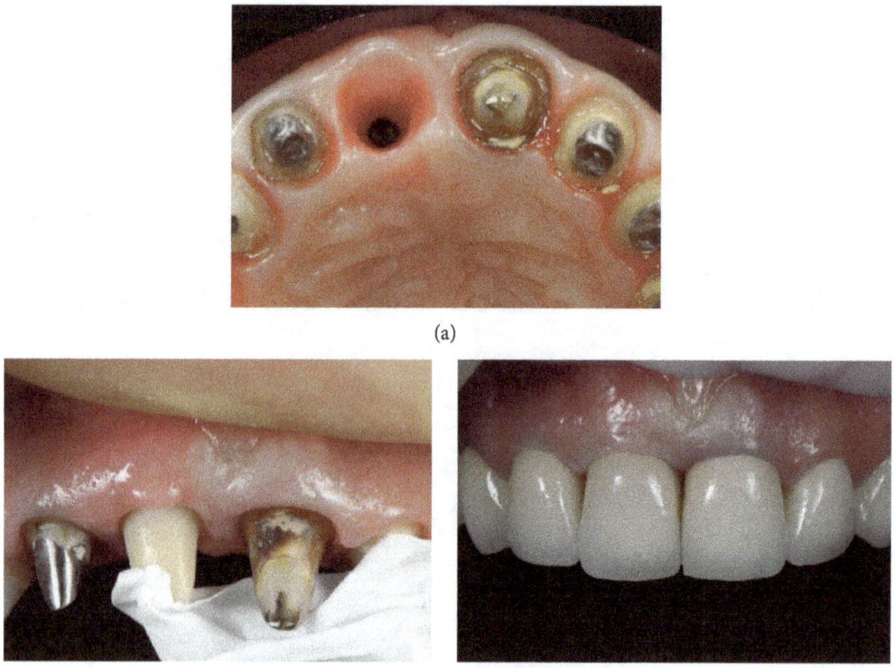

(a)

(b) (c)

FIGURE 9: (a) Condition of soft tissues at the beginning of the prostheses stage. (b) Fixation of the individual zirconium abutment. (c) Final restoration.

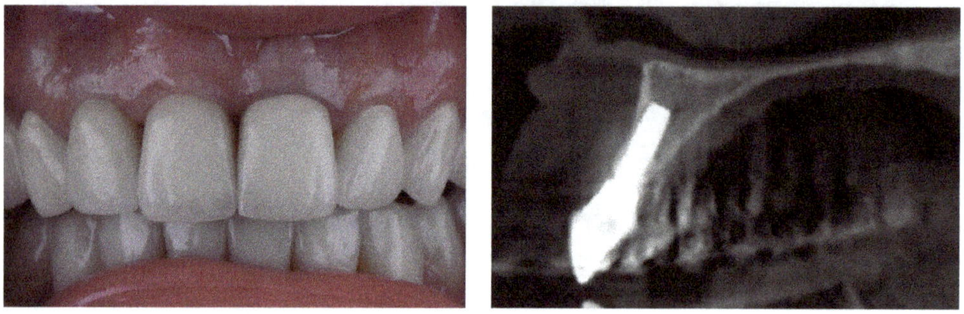

(a) (b)

FIGURE 10: (a) 7 years after the treatment. (b) Stable volume of bone tissue.

Sirona, York, Pennsylvania). Then, the abutment was inserted into the titanium base. Accordingly, each part of the restoration was bonded to the titanium base in the following ways: both surfaces were treated with 50 microns of aluminium oxide particles at 2 bar pressure (0.25 MPa) for 20 s at a distance of 10 mm (RONDOflex Plus 360, KaVo, Germany). After that, a universal single-component priming agent (Monobond Plus, Ivoclar Vivadent, Liechtenstein) was applied to the zirconia and titanium bases accordingly. Dual-curing luting composite for the aesthetic and permanent cementation of ceramic (Variolink Esthetic DC, Ivoclar Vivadent, Liechtenstein) was used to lute the two components extraorally according to the manufacturer's recommendations. Abutment was fixed with torque 25 N/cm. The screw access hole was filled with temporary material. The final E-Max (IVOCLAR Vivadent, Liechtenstein) restoration was fixed on Relyx U200 cement (3M ESPE, St. Paul, MN, USA) using a rubber dam (Figure 9).

Postoperative instructions including hygiene care were advised to the patient.

The multidisciplinary regular check-up was emphasized. The patient was followed at 6 months, 1-7 years postloading. A CBCT scan was taken after 7 years, and no any bone resorption was found around the implant platform. The soft tissues were completely healthy at the follow-up time (Figure 10).

3. Discussion

The restoration of a single implant in the anterior maxillary region is a very complicated and challenging task due to the aesthetic aspect. In addition to the correct position of the implant, the success of the treatment also depends on the quality and quantity of hard and soft tissues [12], especially important to consider the changes that occur in the post extracted socket, which was described by many authors [3,

12–14]. When simultaneous implantation is not possible, the contemporary approach implies carrying out the method of saving the parameters of the socket [15]. For example, a systematic review and meta-analysis by Bassir et al. in 2018 demonstrated that using alveolar ridge preservation techniques after tooth extraction is effective in minimizing loss of horizontal and vertical hard tissue volume. No clear advantages have yet been identified in using bone substitute material or barrier membranes for this procedure [5]. Despite this fact, most scientists conclude on the feasibility of this procedure because it gives possibilities to reduce bone resorption and achieve better conditions for further implant treatment [4, 16–18]. In our clinical case, socket augmentation also allowed us to obtain a sufficient volume of bone for subsequent implant placement, while using a quickly resolvable bone-grafting material Bio-OSS collagen made it possible to carry out implant placement 4 months later.

Despite successful preservation of bone tissue parameters, vestibular collapse of soft tissues was revealed at the time of implant placement. In practice, according to a number of authors, the procedure of saving the socket parameter allows us to save most of the bone volume [19]. Most of the authors suggest combining socket preservation techniques with soft tissue augmentation, which helps to increase soft tissue volume and thickness and allows to prevent a vestibular collapse [7, 12]. The gold standard for this procedure is the use of an autogenous connective tissue graft. However, recently, there have been more and more reports of successful use of soft tissue substitute materials [7, 20]. In our clinical case, we used a free connective tissue graft from the maxilla tuber, which was fixed to the vestibular covering flap.

The healing process was auspicious, and the clinical picture in the early postoperative period was good. Although, 3 months later, soft tissue collapse was detected on the vestibular surface.

This clinical situation could be caused by many factors such as multiple alterations in the alveolar ridge following tooth extraction, partial resorption of the vestibular bone due to mucoperiosteal flap elevation, and connective tissue structure of the donor area.

The last factor is improbable, as the thickness of connective tissue in the tuber area is significantly greater compared to the hard palate, while the maintenance of adipose tissue and glandular tissue is minimal according to current data [21].

Nevertheless, using deepithelialized free connective tissue graft at the second stage of the implant surgery procedure and the healing abutment placement allowed us to reach a stable state of the contour of the alveolar ridge by the time of prosthetics and even after 7 years after complete treatment.

This clinical report demonstrated what changes in parameters of bone are possible after tooth removal and preservation of the socket. The reasons that caused soft tissue collapse after soft tissue augmentation, as well as the question of which stage of treatment is more suitable for soft tissue augmentation in similar cases, remain the subjects of discussion. However, it was concluded that an additional surgery to augment the soft tissues around dental implants may be a good solution for such clinical situations as the one presented.

4. Conclusion

The aim of the present study was to assess the possibilities of socket preservation technique and soft tissue augmentation in the anterior maxillary region. This case showed that these procedures are effective enough to preserve the parameters of the socket after tooth removal, and soft tissue augmentation allows to achieve satisfactory aesthetic outcomes. However, during the rehabilitation process, difficulties occur that clinicians may encounter and that need to be taken into account. For example, it may be the need for additional surgical intervention to achieve long-term stable condition of the soft tissues around dental implants. The scientific significance of this case report is that it has been demonstrated the necessity of further investigations of factors that may affect the success of soft tissue augmentation in the frontal teeth area during implant treatment, in particular when combining a soft tissue augmentation procedure with socket preservation. This study can expand existing knowledge on this topic and help clinicians to achieve favorable results while taking into account the experience that was described.

Abbreviations

CBCT: Cone-beam computed tomography
CTG: Connective tissue graft
ISQ: Implant stability quotient.

References

[1] S. Chen and D. Buser, "Esthetic outcomes following immediate and early implant placement in the anterior maxilla—a systematic review," *The International Journal of Oral & Maxillofacial Implants*, vol. 29, pp. 186–215, 2014.

[2] A. Scarano, B. Assenza, F. Inchingolo, F. Mastrangelo, and F. Lorusso, "New implant design with midcrestal and apical wing thread for increased implant stability in single postextraction maxillary implant," *Case Reports in Dentistry*, vol. 2019, Article ID 9529248, 4 pages, 2019.

[3] M. Farmer and I. Darby, "Ridge dimensional changes following single-tooth extraction in the aesthetic zone," *Clinical Oral Implants Research*, vol. 25, no. 2, pp. 272–277, 2014.

[4] N. MacBeth, A. Trullenque-Eriksson, N. Donos, and N. Mardas, "Hard and soft tissue changes following alveolar ridge preservation: a systematic review," *Clinical Oral Implants Research*, vol. 28, no. 8, pp. 982–1004, 2017.

[5] S. Bassir, M. Alhareky, B. Wangsrimongkol, Y. Jia, and N. Karimbux, "Systematic review and meta-analysis of hard tissue outcomes of alveolar ridge preservation," *The*

International Journal of Oral & Maxillofacial Implants, vol. 33, no. 5, pp. 979–994, 2018.

[6] V. Chappuis, M. G. Araújo, and D. Buser, "Clinical relevance of dimensional bone and soft tissue alterations post-extraction in esthetic sites," *Periodontology 2000*, vol. 73, no. 1, pp. 73–83, 2017.

[7] D. S. Thoma, S. P. Bienz, H. C. Lim, W. Z. Lee, C. H. F. Hämmerle, and R. E. Jung, "Explorative randomized controlled study comparing soft tissue thickness, contour changes, and soft tissue handling of two ridge preservation techniques and spontaneous healing two months after tooth extraction," *Clinical Oral Implants Research*, vol. 31, no. 6, pp. 565–574, 2020.

[8] R. E. Jung, A. Ioannidis, C. H. F. Hämmerle, and D. S. Thoma, "Alveolar ridge preservation in the esthetic zone," *Periodontology 2000*, vol. 77, no. 1, pp. 165–175, 2018.

[9] K. Fischer, S. Mühlemann, R. Jung, A. Friedmann, and S. Fickl, "Dimensional evaluation of different ridge preservation techniques with a bovine xenograft: a randomized controlled clinical trial," *The International Journal of Periodontics & Restorative Dentistry*, vol. 38, no. 4, pp. 549–556, 2018.

[10] D. Halabi, J. Escobar, C. Alvarado, N. Martinez, and C. Muñoz, "Chlorhexidine for prevention of alveolar osteitis: a randomised clinical trial," *Journal of Applied Oral Science*, vol. 26, pp. 1–7, 2018.

[11] E. Varoni, M. Tarce, G. Lodi, and A. Carrassi, "Chlorhexidine (CHX) in dentistry: state of the art," *Minerva Stomatologica*, vol. 61, pp. 399–419, 2012.

[12] G. Botilde, P. E. Colin, O. González-Martín, G. Lecloux, E. Rompen, and F. Lambert, "Hard and soft tissue analysis of alveolar ridge preservation in esthetic zone using deproteinized bovine bone mineral and a saddle connective tissue graft: a long-term prospective case series," *Clinical Implant Dentistry and Related Research*, vol. 22, no. 3, pp. 387–396, 2020.

[13] C. H. F. Hämmerle, M. G. Araújo, M. Simion, and On Behalf of the Osteology Consensus Group 2011, "Evidence-based knowledge on the biology and treatment of extraction sockets," *Clinical Oral Implants Research*, vol. 23, pp. 80–82, 2012.

[14] S. P. Bienz, R. E. Jung, V. M. Sapata, C. H. F. Hämmerle, J. Hüsler, and D. S. Thoma, "Volumetric changes and peri-implant health at implant sites with or without soft tissue grafting in the esthetic zone, a retrospective case–control study with a 5-year follow-up," *Clinical Oral Implants Research*, vol. 28, no. 11, pp. 1459–1465, 2017.

[15] R. E. Jung, I. Sailer, C. H. F. Hämmerle, T. Attin, and P. Schmidlin, "In vitro color changes of soft tissues caused by restorative materials," *The International Journal of Periodontics & Restorative Dentistry*, vol. 27, pp. 251–257, 2007.

[16] R. Faria-Almeida, I. Astramskaite-Januseviciene, A. Puisys, and F. Correia, "Extraction socket preservation with or without membranes, soft tissue influence on post extraction alveolar ridge preservation: a systematic review," *Journal of Oral and Maxillofacial Research*, vol. 10, no. 3, 2019.

[17] D. S. Thoma, M. Zeltner, M. Hilbe, C. H. F. Hämmerle, J. Hüsler, and R. E. Jung, "Randomized controlled clinical study evaluating effectiveness and safety of a volume-stable collagen matrix compared to autogenous connective tissue grafts for soft tissue augmentation at implant sites," *Journal of Clinical Periodontology*, vol. 43, no. 10, pp. 874–885, 2016.

[18] F. Vignoletti, P. Matesanz, D. Rodrigo, E. Figuero, C. Martin, and M. Sanz, "Surgical protocols for ridge preservation after tooth extraction. A systematic review," *Clinical Oral Implants Research*, vol. 23, pp. 22–38, 2012.

[19] L. Fee, "Socket preservation," *British Dental Journal*, vol. 222, no. 8, pp. 579–582, 2017.

[20] R. Cairo, L. Barbato, P. Tonelli, G. Batalocco, G. Pagavino, and M. Nieri, "Xenogeneic collagen matrix versus connective tissue graft for buccal soft tissue augmentation at implant site. A randomized, controlled clinical trial," *Journal of Clinical Periodontology*, vol. 44, no. 7, pp. 769–776, 2017.

[21] I. Sanz-Martín, E. Rojo, E. Maldonado, G. Stroppa, J. Nart, and M. Sanz, "Structural and histological differences between connective tissue grafts harvested from the lateral palatal mucosa or from the tuberosity area," *Clinical Oral Investigations*, vol. 23, no. 2, pp. 957–964, 2019.

24

Autogenous Chin Block Grafts in the Aesthetic Zone: A 20-Year Follow-Up Case Report

Carlo Maiorana, Susanna Ferrario, Pier Paolo Poli, and Mattia Manfredini

Fondazione IRCCS Ca' Granda Ospedale Maggiore Policlinico, Implant Center for Edentulism and Jawbone Atrophies, Maxillofacial Surgery and Odontostomatology Unit, University of Milan, Via della Commenda 10, 20122 Milan, Italy

Correspondence should be addressed to Susanna Ferrario; ferrariosusanna@gmail.com

Academic Editor: Leandro Napier de Souza

The successful use of osseointegrated implants in the treatment of partial or complete edentulism requires a sufficient bone support. Whenever rehabilitation in atrophic edentulous areas is needed, bone augmentation procedures are recommended. The aim is to provide adequate amount of supporting bone to achieve a prosthetically guided implant placement. This in turn leads to functional and aesthetic improvements that can be maintained on the long term. Bone grafting of the atrophic site can be performed either prior to implant placement or at the time of implantation. Irrespective of the timing, bone augmentation by means of autogenous bone grafts is a reliable technique, as confirmed by several studies. On the other hand, long-term evidence on the use of autogenous chin block grafts in preprosthetic implant surgery is still scarce. Thus, the purpose of the present case is to report the 20-year clinical and radiological outcome of autogenous chin block grafts used to augment a bilateral defect due to agenesis of the upper lateral incisors for implant placement purposes.

1. Introduction

The agenesis of the upper lateral incisors is a challenging clinical situation, being an area of high aesthetic value with a limited space available for a correct implant insertion, even after an orthodontic treatment, together with high patient expectations [1].

The agenesis often results in alveolar bone defects, especially at the expense of the buccal plate. The repair of congenital or acquired alveolar defects with autologous bone grafts is one of the most traditional surgical techniques in oral and maxillofacial surgery. Once the ideal amount of bone has been restored, implant treatment assumes an important role in the rehabilitation of these patients [2].

Bone reconstruction techniques have been improved in order to optimize the aesthetic and functional result [3, 4]. Despite this, the functional rehabilitation of atrophic alveolar ridges still remains a challenge in oral implantology. Bone augmentation procedures are often indicated to allow implant placement in an optimal three-dimensional position to achieve long-term function and predictable aesthetic results for prosthetic restorations [3]. The extension of the bone defect determines whether bone augmentation procedures can be performed simultaneously with implant placement or as a separate procedure [5].

Among the various bone augmentation materials available, only autologous bone combines osteoconductive, osteoinductive, and osteogenic features when compared to any other bone substitute [6]. Thanks to its biological properties and also due to the absence of immunological reactions, autologous bone graft is considered the "gold standard" for bone regeneration procedures [7].

However, intraoral harvesting is not free from limitations; these include the extension of the donor site and possible complications that may occur during the bone harvesting procedure [8].

The use of intraoral donor sites such as mandibular symphysis and ramus has several advantages compared to that of extraoral sites such as the iliac crest and the tibial plateau. Some studies have shown that membranous bone grafts, including the mandibular symphysis and ramus, show less resorption and better and faster revascularization than endochondral bone grafts, such as the iliac crest and tibial plateau [9, 10]. Therefore, the embryological origin of the donor site plays a pivotal role in the success of the procedure. An additional important advantage of intraoral donor sites is that bone harvesting can be performed with local anesthetic infiltrations without recurring to general anesthesia. Furthermore, intraoral bone grafts can be easily obtained with lower complications compared to extraoral bone grafts, and also, the postoperative course is easier and faster [11]. Common donor sites in the oral region are mandibular symphysis, retromolar area, and maxillary tuberosity [11, 12].

The mandibular symphysis not only provides a greater graft volume of more than 50% compared to the mandibular ramus but is also characterized by a simpler surgical access. Moreover, it has been proved that the mandibular symphysis graft is composed on average of 65% cortical bone and 36% cancellous bone. Conversely, the mandibular ramus is almost 100% cortical in nature. The corticocancellous nature of the bone harvested from the mandibular symphysis facilitates a faster vascularization once the block is positioned at the recipient site, resulting in more rapid integration. Better postoperative patient morbidity and low rate of wound dehiscence are other reasons why the ramus as a donor site may be preferred [11].

The use of bone substitutes characterized by low turnover rates to cover the graft may reduce the resorption rate of the bone block [13]. Some authors found that deproteinized bovine bone (DBB) particles stabilized by resorbable membranes covering onlay block grafts reduced resorption by almost 50% in comparison to noncovered grafts [1, 14]. Bone substitutes may also contribute to the creation of a smooth connection between the block graft and the recipient bone and can provide a scaffold that promotes bone regeneration [13, 14]. Another advantage of using resorbable rather than nonresorbable membranes is the elimination of a second surgical phase.

Long-term studies evaluating the survival rates of dental implants placed in sites augmented with symphysis onlay grafts are lacking. However, to the best of our knowledge, no studies are currently available reporting on survival analysis performed with more than 10 years of follow-up.

In view of the aforesaid, the aim of the present case report was to evaluate the survival rate of dental implants placed in resorbed alveolar ridges reconstructed with symphysis autogenous onlay bone grafts.

2. Case Presentation

A 19-year-old male affected by agenesis of the upper lateral incisors was referred to the authors' department seeking for an implant-supported fixed rehabilitation.

At the time of presentation, the patient was healthy, nonsmoking, with no local or systemic pathologies nor drug allergies (ASA I according to the American Society of Anesthesiologists physical status classification).

The anatomy of the upper jaw was evaluated by clinical examination and panoramic radiograph. At the clinical examination, it was immediately possible to observe a bilateral bone defect in correspondence with the upper lateral incisor region. The appearance and consistency of the soft tissues were good (Figure 1). The orthopantomograph confirmed the agenesis of the upper lateral incisors with a reduced development of the alveolar process in a mesiodistal direction (Figure 2).

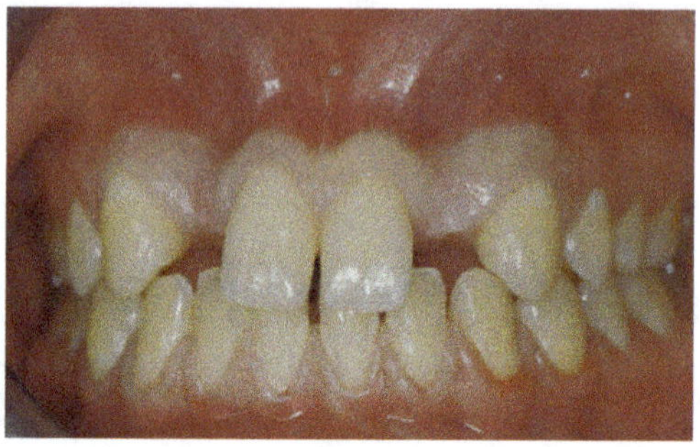

Figure 1: Initial clinical situation.

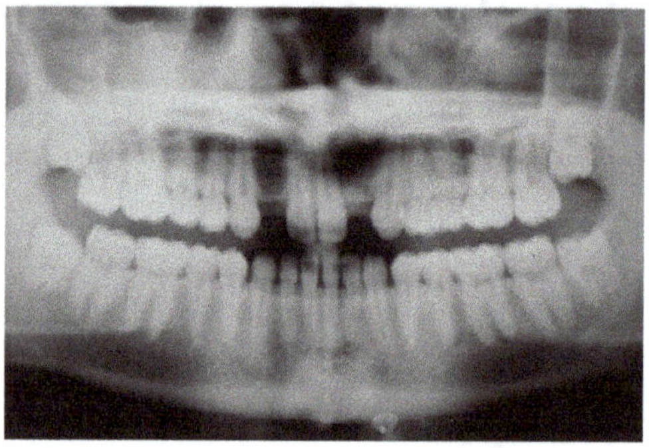

Figure 2: Initial orthopantomography.

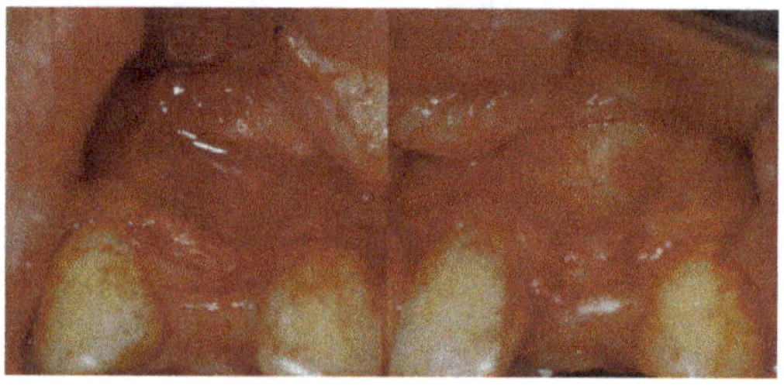

Figure 3: Buccal view of the defects on 12 and 22.

After discussing possible treatment alternatives with the patient, it was decided to proceed with a bone augmentation procedure by means of intraoral autogenous bone harvested from the mandibular symphysis and delayed implant insertion. All surgical and prosthetic procedures were performed by the same team. A signed informed consent was obtained from the patient. All procedures were conducted according to the 1964 Helsinki Declaration and its later amendments.

The first surgical phase was performed on an outpatient basis under local anesthesia after premedication with diazepam 0.2 mg/kg administered orally 30 minutes before surgery. Two monocortical block grafts were collected from the symphysis and fixed at the buccal aspect of the bone defects with osteosynthesis screws (Figures 3–5). At this point, DBB particles (Bio-Oss®, Geistlich Biomaterials,

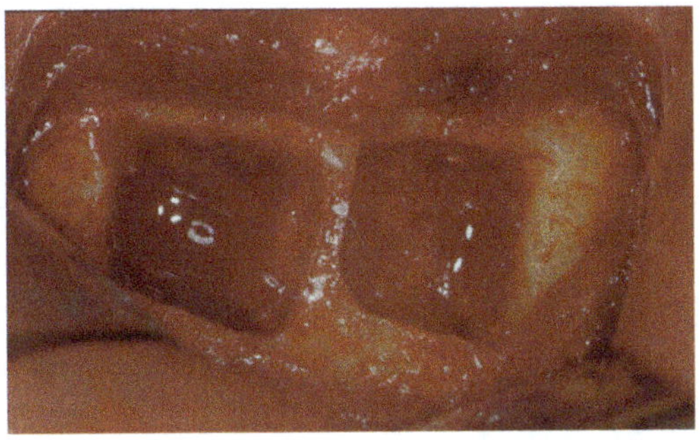

FIGURE 4: Bone blocks' removal from the mandibular symphysis.

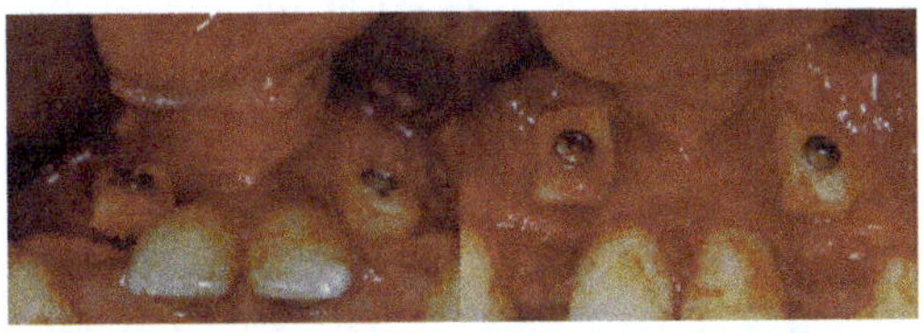

FIGURE 5: Bone block stabilization by screws.

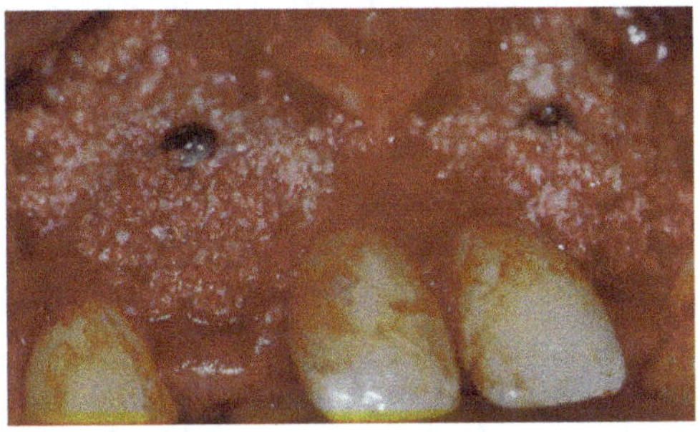

FIGURE 6: Coverage of the surgical site with deproteinized bovine bone (Bio-Oss®, Geistlich Biomaterials, Wolhusen, Switzerland).

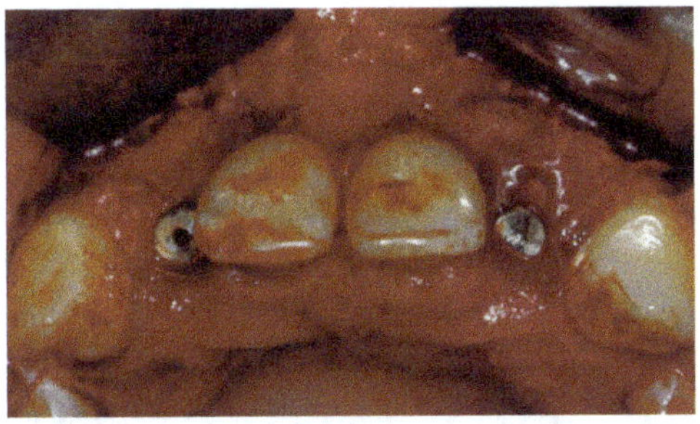

FIGURE 7: Implant placement.

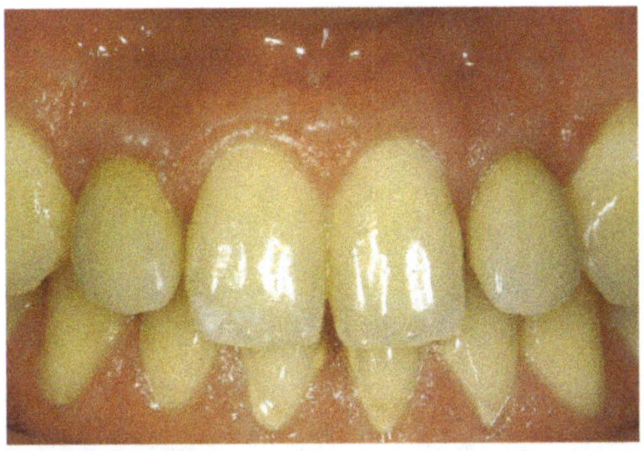

FIGURE 8: Clinical situation at 8 years.

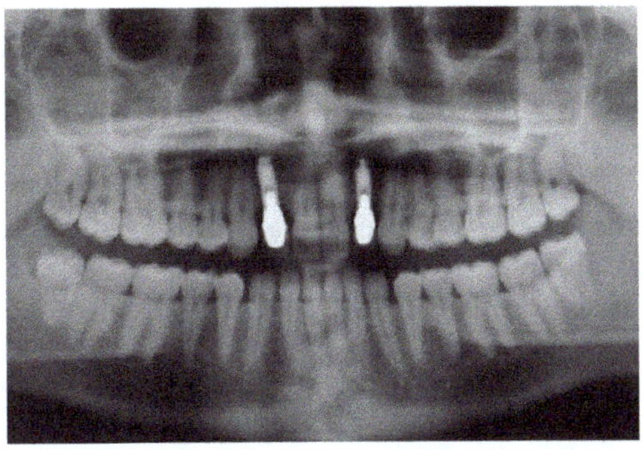

FIGURE 9: Orthopantomography at 8 years.

Wolhusen, Switzerland) and native lyophilized type I resorbable collagen membranes from equine origin (Paroguide®, GABA VEBAS srl, Rome, Italy) were used to cover the block graft at each site (Figure 6). Suture in polyamide was performed with detached stitches to obtain a first-intention seal of the flaps. Silk sutures were instead used at the donor site.

Postoperative medications included amoxicillin 1 g twice daily for 6 days, starting on the day of surgery, naproxen sodium as required every 6 hours, and 0.2% chlorhexidine mouthwashes twice daily for 2 weeks, starting on the day after surgery.

The sutures were removed after 14 days, and an orthopantomograph was performed. After 6 months of uneventful healing, fixation screws were removed, and two 3.25 × 13 mm implants were placed in a prosthetically guided position with the aid of a surgical stent (Figure 7). The insertion torque was >35 Ncm.

After 5 months, implants were uncovered to connect the healing abutments. After proper maturation of the soft tissues, impressions were taken with custom impression trays to start the prosthetic phase. Temporary implant-supported acrylic resin prostheses were connected to the implants for initial load and soft tissue conditioning. After 6 months, definitive implant-supported cemented-retained metal-ceramic prostheses were delivered. A buccal peri-implant gingival plastic surgery was performed with a diamond bur to improve the aesthetic of the soft tissues.

Clinical and radiological evaluations were conducted at 8 years (Figures 8 and 9) and 20 years from the prosthetic loading (Figures 10 and 11). After 20 years, the clinical examination showed healthy and stable soft tissues, with no signs of suppuration and bleeding on probing. Peri-implant probing was performed at six sites per implant, namely, mesiobuccal, buccal, distobuccal, mesiopalatal, palatal, and distopalatal. In all said sites, probing depth values ≤ 4 mm were observed. An adequate amount of attached keratinized tissue was present apically to the gingival margin. The quality and stability of the gingival architecture were supported by the radiographic analysis. The 8-year and 20-year orthopantomographs were scanned to obtain digital images with a resolution of 1200 dpi. The digital images were imported in a specialized

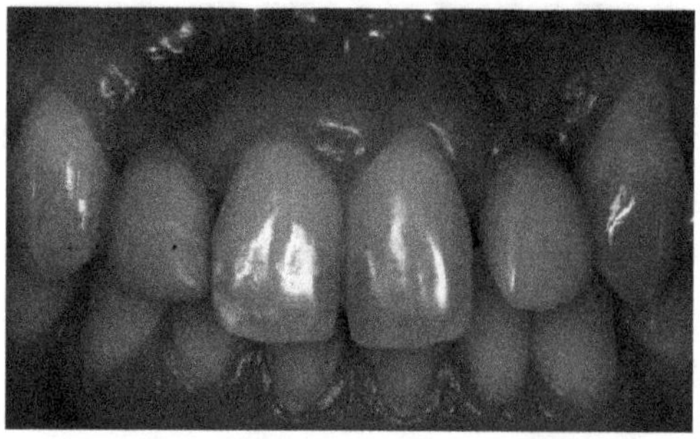

Figure 10: Clinical situation at 20 years.

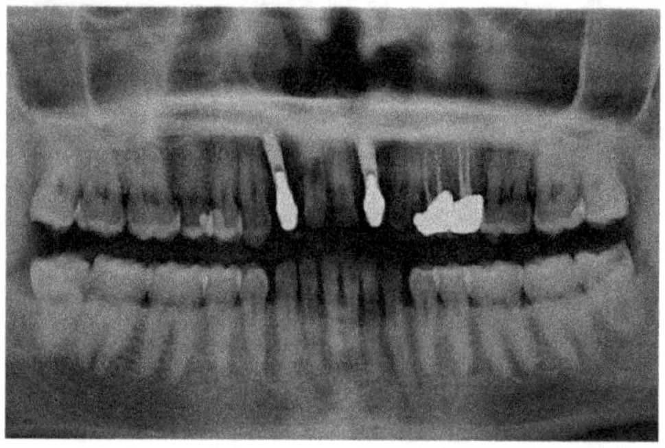

Figure 11: Orthopantomography at 20 years.

computer software (ImageJ 1.49v, Research Services Branch, National Institutes of Health, Bethesda, MD, USA). The calibration of the pixel/millimeter ratio was performed on the basis of a known distance, namely, the length of the implants. The 8-year orthopantomograph revealed no detectable marginal bone resorption, calculated as the distance between the most apical bone-to-implant contact visible in the scanned image and the implant-abutment connection level at the mesial and distal aspects (Figure 9). The same measurements were performed in the 20-year orthopantomography (Figure 11); however, it was not possible to obtain reliable data due to metal artifacts. Nonetheless, the clinical findings suggested the presence of stable marginal bone levels circumferentially around the implants.

3. Discussion

The present case was reported to document clinically and radiographically the long-term survival of dental implants placed in atrophic alveolar ridges augmented with mandibular symphysis autogenous onlay grafts. The rationale was to provide evidence that implant rehabilitations in bone reconstructed with autogenous mandibular grafts might constitute a reliable treatment option on a long-term basis. This strengthens the current evidence, as only few studies reported on the outcome of such implant-supported rehabilitations for periods longer than 10 years.

In a recent retrospective study [15], it has been claimed that intraoral bone grafts harvested from the mandibular symphysis, mandibular ramus, and maxillary tuberosity provide a good treatment modality for ridge augmentation. In addition, the amount of bone available from these sites is sufficient for anatomical defects extended up to the width of three teeth [16]. Harvesting of retromolar and symphysis bone grafts is particularly recommended in those cases involving multiple tooth reconstruction in the mandible. The surgical access to the symphysis has been described as being easier than that of the mandibular ramus [11]. Both techniques can be performed on an outpatient basis, while harvesting of bone from distant sites is associated with inpatient care and increased costs [17]. Both the harvesting and grafting procedures are usually performed in the same surgical field. The use of autologous bone in the present case showed excellent survival and success rates. The success of the bone augmentation was confirmed by the stability of the marginal bone levels assessed at the mesial and distal aspects of the implants over the years. It is worth mentioning that at the 20-year follow-up visit, a horizontal remodeling of the buccal plate was observed. This however did not affect the implant stability. The horizontal bone resorption that was found is attributable to the embryological nature of the bone that was grafted and the duration of the follow-up [18]. From the aesthetic aspect, the gingival parabolas have been maintained over time, and therefore, the aesthetic success has been preserved on the long term [19]. The present study confirmed the long-term effectiveness of alveolar ridge augmentation and implant placement by means of autogenous bone grafts [20]. This procedure resulted in stable bone conditions with low risk of mucosal recession over an observation period of 20 years.

It should be noted, however, that a similar clinical situation, currently, can be solved through the use of narrow implants and careful soft tissue management. As a matter of fact, at present, soft tissue augmentation techniques have demonstrated good aesthetic results so that more invasive bone augmentation procedures may be avoided [21]. Furthermore, at the time of surgery, the patient was only 19 years old and a different approach with an additional waiting period of 3 years might be contemplated to prevent the intrusion of the peri-implant tissues that may occur in case of premature implant insertion [22]. The patient also refused presurgical orthodontic treatment aimed at optimizing the interdental spaces of the anterior sector.

In a recent paper [18], an average follow-up of 23.9 months was calculated for literature articles on follow-up of patients with implant rehabilitation in augmented bone with autogenous bone grafts. It is therefore clear that the resorption evaluated in this 20-year case report is worthy of note. The hypothesis that bone substitutes could effectively replace the use of autologous bone with its osteoinductive, osteoconductive, and osteogenic properties is still under investigation. On the other hand, various studies have proved benefits and appropriateness of autogenous tissue for an ideal reconstruction of atrophied ridges before implant surgery [23].

Regarding surgical complications, the postoperative morbidity is commonly related to the management of the soft tissues. The most frequent postsurgical complications included flap dehiscences with or without exposure of the grafts or membrane [24]. The peri-implant mucosa needs to be supported by an adequate three-dimensional volume of alveolar bone, including an intact buccal plate of sufficient height and thickness [4, 25, 26]. Deficiency of the buccal bone anatomy has a negative impact on the aesthetic outcome and is therefore considered a critical causative factor for implant complications and failures [4, 26, 27]. In the present case, no soft tissue complications occurred at any stage.

Postoperative morbidity after mandibular bone harvesting procedures was reported to be mainly related to temporary or permanent neural disturbances involving the inferior alveolar nerve and its branches [23]. It is clear that although precise anatomical limits have been defined on the localization of the mandibular incisor canal, in the bone removal from the mandibular symphysis, there is no objective limit below which the probability of having neurosensory alterations is eliminated. This is due to physiological changes in the course of the mandibular incisor canal. It is therefore advisable to subjectively evaluate the feasibility of the technique on a case-by-case basis through orthopantomographs and second-level investigations such as computed tomography, dental scan, and stereolithographic prototypes. No drawbacks related to neurosensory complications were noted in the present case.

A limitation of the study is the marginal bone loss measurement on the mesial and distal aspects owing to 2D imaging. The measurement of buccal and lingual bone loss can only be performed using 3D imaging modalities. However, panoramic radiographs are frequently used in clinical settings for the evaluation of bone peak stability [2, 28].

The results of the present study pointed out that, in case of agenesis of the upper lateral incisors, bone grafting from the mandibular symphysis and delayed implant placement may provide satisfactory functional and aesthetic outcomes on the long term. Despite a certain resorption of the graft that may occur, correct management of the peri-implant soft tissues and the prosthesis is pivotal to maintain the success on the long term. To date, a similar clinical situation can be resolved through the use of narrow implants and careful soft tissue management. Furthermore, at the time of surgery, the patient was 19 years old. To prevent intrusion, we would wait additional 3 years before surgery.

References

[1] C. Maiorana, "Histomorphometric evaluation of anorganic bovine bone coverage to reduce autogenous grafts resorption: preliminary results," *The Open Dentistry Journal*, vol. 5, no. 1, pp. 71–78, 2011.

[2] C. Maiorana, P. P. Poli, A. Mascellaro, S. Ferrario, and M. Beretta, "Dental implants placed in resorbed alveolar ridges reconstructed with iliac crest autogenous onlay grafts: a 26-year median follow-up retrospective study," *Journal of Cranio-Maxillofacial Surgery*, vol. 47, no. 5, pp. 805–814, 2019.

[3] C. Maiorana, P. P. Poli, and M. Beretta, "Guided bone regeneration and implant placement in association with a coronally positioned palatal sliding flap: a 17-year follow-up case report," *The Journal of Oral Implantology*, vol. 44, no. 5, pp. 371–376, 2018.

[4] M. Beretta, P. P. Poli, S. Pieriboni et al., "Peri-implant soft tissue conditioning by means of customized healing abutment: a randomized controlled clinical trial," *Materials*, vol. 12, no. 18, p. 3041, 2019.

[5] D. Buser, K. Dula, H. P. Hirt, and R. K. Schenk, "Lateral ridge augmentation using autografts and barrier membranes: a clinical study with 40 partially edentulous patients," *Journal of Oral and Maxillofacial Surgery*, vol. 54, no. 4, pp. 420–432, 1996.

[6] P. Galindo-Moreno, G. Ávila, J. E. Fernández-Barbero, F. Mesa, F. O'Valle-Ravassa, and H. L. Wang, "Clinical and histologic comparison of two different composite grafts for sinus augmentation: a pilot clinical trial," *Clinical Oral Implants Research*, vol. 19, no. 8, pp. 755–759, 2008.

[7] M. Chiapasco, M. Zaniboni, and L. Rimondini, "Autogenous onlay bone grafts vs. alveolar distraction osteogenesis for the correction of vertically deficient edentulous ridges: a 2-4-year prospective study on humans," *Clinical Oral Implants Research*, vol. 18, no. 4, pp. 432–440, 2007.

[8] A. T. Jensen, S. S. Jensen, and N. Worsaae, "Complications related to bone augmentation procedures of localized defects in the alveolar ridge. A retrospective clinical study," *Oral and Maxillofacial Surgery*, vol. 20, no. 2, pp. 115–122, 2016.

[9] J. D. Smith and M. Abramson, "Membranous vs. endochondral bone autografts," *Archives of Otolaryngology*, vol. 99, no. 3, pp. 203–205, 1974.

[10] A. Esen, G. Yıldırım, Ö. İnan, and D. Dolanmaz, "The use of autogeneous mandibular bone block grafts for reconstruction of alveolar defects," *Annals of Maxillofacial Surgery*, vol. 5, no. 1, pp. 71–76, 2015.

[11] C. M. Misch, "Comparison of intraoral donor sites for onlay grafting prior to implant placement," *International Journal of Oral & Maxillofacial Implants*, vol. 12, no. 6, pp. 767–776, 1997.

[12] C. M. Misch, C. E. Misch, R. R. Resnik, and Y. H. Ismail, "Reconstruction of maxillary alveolar defects with mandibular symphysis grafts for dental implants: a preliminary procedural report," *The International Journal of Oral & Maxillofacial Implants*, vol. 7, no. 3, pp. 360–366, 1992.

[13] T. Von Arx and D. Buser, "Horizontal ridge augmentation using autogenous block grafts and the guided bone regeneration technique with collagen membranes: a clinical study with 42 patients," *Clinical Oral Implants Research*, vol. 17, no. 4, pp. 359–366, 2006.

[14] C. Maiorana, M. Beretta, S. Salina, and F. Santoro, "Reduction of autogenous bone graft resorption by means of bio-oss coverage: a prospective study," *International Journal of Periodontics & Restorative Dentistry*, vol. 25, no. 1, pp. 18–25, 2005.

[15] A. Sakkas, F. Wilde, M. Heufelder, K. Winter, and A. Schramm, "Autogenous bone grafts in oral implantology—is it still a "gold standard"? A consecutive review of 279 patients with 456 clinical procedures," *International Journal of Implant Dentistry*, vol. 3, no. 1, p. 23, 2017.

[16] V. Moraschini, L.A. da C. Poubel, V. F. Ferreira, and E. dos S.P. Barboza, "Evaluation of survival and success rates of dental implants reported in longitudinal studies with a follow-up period of at least 10 years: a systematic review," *International Journal of Oral and Maxillofacial Surgery*, vol. 44, no. 3, pp. 377–388, 2015.

[17] G. K. B. Sàndor, I. A. Nish, and R. P. Carmichael, "Comparison of conventional surgery with motorized trephine in bone harvest from the anterior iliac crest," *Oral Surgery, Oral Medicine,*

Oral Pathology, Oral Radiology, and Endodontology, vol. 95, no. 2, pp. 150–155, 2003.

[18] E. Nkenke and F. W. Neukam, "Autogenous bone harvesting and grafting in advanced jaw resorption: morbidity, resorption and implant survival," *European Journal of Oral Implantology*, vol. 7, Supplement 2, pp. S203–S217, 2014.

[19] D. Buser, W. Martin, and U. C. Belser, "Optimizing esthetics for implant restorations in the anterior maxilla: anatomic and surgical considerations," *International Journal of Oral & Maxillofacial Implants*, vol. 19, pp. 43–61, 2004.

[20] V. Chappuis, L. Rahman, R. Buser, S. F. M. Janner, U. C. Belser, and D. Buser, "Effectiveness of contour augmentation with guided bone regeneration: 10-year results," *Journal of Dental Research*, vol. 97, no. 3, pp. 266–274, 2017.

[21] T. Testori, T. Weinstein, F. Scutellà, H. L. Wang, and G. Zucchelli, "Implant placement in the esthetic area: criteria for positioning single and multiple implants," *Periodontol 2000*, vol. 77, no. 1, pp. 176–196, 2018.

[22] L. Bohner, M. Hanisch, J. Kleinheinz, and S. Jung, "Dental implants in growing patients: a systematic review," *The British Journal of Oral & Maxillofacial Surgery*, vol. 57, no. 5, pp. 397–406, 2019.

[23] M. Chiapasco, M. Zaniboni, and M. Boisco, "Augmentation procedures for the rehabilitation of deficient edentulous ridges with oral implants," *Clinical Oral Implants Research*, vol. 17, Supplement 2, pp. 136–159, 2006.

[24] L. Cordaro, F. Torsello, S. Morcavallo, and V. M. di Torresanto, "Effect of bovine bone and collagen membranes on healing of mandibular bone blocks: a prospective randomized controlled study," *Clinical Oral Implants Research*, vol. 22, no. 10, pp. 1145–1150, 2011.

[25] U. Grunder, S. Gracis, and M. Capelli, "Influence of the 3-D bone-to-implant relationship on esthetics," *International Journal of Periodontics & Restorative Dentistry*, vol. 25, no. 2, pp. 113–119, 2005.

[26] D. Farronato, P. M. Pasini, A. A. Orsina, M. Manfredini, L. Azzi, and M. Farronato, "Correlation between buccal bone thickness at implant placement in healed sites and buccal soft tissue maturation pattern: a prospective three-year study," *Materials*, vol. 13, no. 3, p. 511, 2020.

[27] S. Chen, "Clinical and esthetic outcomes of implants placed in postextraction sites," *International Journal of Oral & Maxillofacial Implants*, vol. 24, 2009.

[28] H. Tercanli Alkis and N. Turker, "Retrospective evaluation of marginal bone loss around implants in a mandibular locator-retained denture using panoramic radiographic images and finite element analysis: a pilot study," *Clinical Implant Dentistry and Related Research*, vol. 21, no. 6, pp. 1199–1205, 2019.

25

A Prosthetic and Surgical Approach for Full-Arch Rehabilitation in Atrophic Maxilla Previously Affected by Peri-Implantitis

Angélica Letícia Reis Pavanelli,[1] Erica Dorigatti de Avila,[2] Luiz Antônio Borelli Barros-Filho,[1] Francisco de Assis Mollo Junior,[2] Joni Augusto Cirelli,[1] Luiz Antônio Borelli Barros,[3] and Rafael Scaf de Molon[1]

[1]*Department of Diagnosis and Surgery, São Paulo State University (UNESP), School of Dentistry, Araraquara Sao Paulo, Brazil*
[2]*Department of Dental Materials and Prosthodontics, São Paulo State University (UNESP), School of Dentistry, Araraquara Sao Paulo, Brazil*
[3]*Department of Social Dentistry, São Paulo State University (UNESP), School of Dentistry, Araraquara Sao Paulo, Brazil*

Correspondence should be addressed to Rafael Scaf de Molon; rafael.molon@unesp.br

Academic Editor: Sukumaran Anil

Rehabilitation of atrophic maxilla with dental implants is still a challenge in clinical practice especially in cases of alveolar bone resorption due to peri-implantitis and pneumatization of the maxillary sinuses. Several surgical approaches have been employed to reconstruct the lost tissues allowing the proper tridimensional position of the implants. In this context, the aim of this case report is to describe a surgical and prosthetic approach to fully rehabilitate the atrophic maxilla with dental implants. The patient presented with unsatisfactory functional and esthetical implant-supported prosthesis with some of the implants already lost by peri-implantitis. The remaining three implants were also affected by peri-implantitis. Reversal prosthetic planning was performed, and a provisional prosthesis was fabricated and anchored in two short implants. Sinus floor augmentation procedure and onlay bone graft were then accomplished. After a healing period of 8 months, digital-guided surgery approach was performed to place the implants. Finally, a definitive prosthesis was installed. One-year follow-up has revealed stabilization of the bone tissue level, successful osseointegration, and a pleasant esthetic and functional result. A proper diagnosis and careful planning play an important role to enhance precision and to achieve patient esthetic and functional outcomes.

1. Introduction

Dental implants have been extensively used to rehabilitate partial or total edentulous patients in the recent decades [1, 2]. To obtain appropriate implant retention, it is essential to have sufficient amount of bone volume in the receptor area, and in many cases, this condition is not suitable, for instance, in cases of long-term tooth loss leading to alveolar bone atrophy, bone defects due to different types of trauma, and pneumatization of the maxillary sinuses [3]. All of those issues impair the installation of dental implants in a proper tridimensional position [2, 4].

When teeth are lost due to periodontal disease, dental cavities, or trauma and the oral rehabilitation is not performed in a reasonable amount of time, the alveolar process tends to resorb. In this regard, the reduction in bone density, resorption of the alveolar ridge, and pneumatization of the maxillary sinuses are characteristics that usually affect patients that have lost their teeth for a long time [5, 6]. In this context, several approaches have been used to rehabilitate atrophic areas in the maxilla with dental implants. Among the various techniques used for rehabilitation of atrophic jaw, some of them can be highlighted: guided bone regeneration with rhBMP-2 [7–9]; osteogenesis by alveolar distraction [10, 11]; autogenous, homogenous,

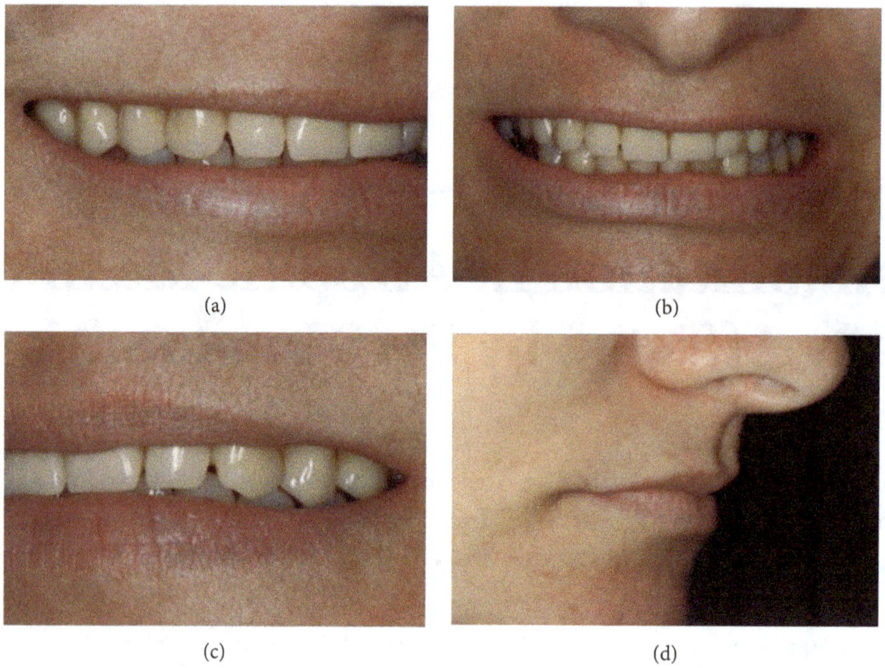

FIGURE 1: Clinical images of the patient's smile.

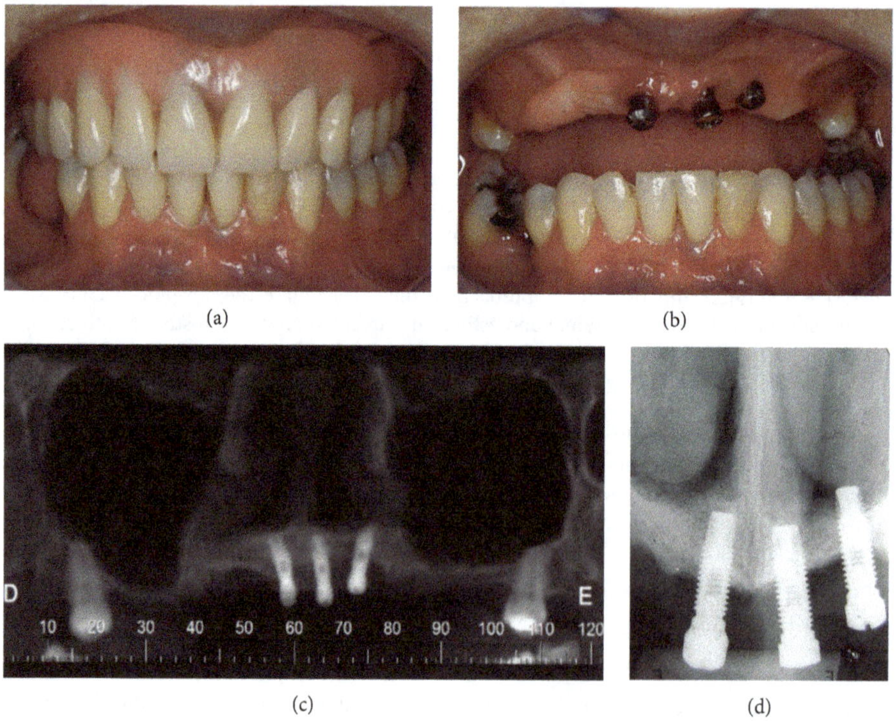

FIGURE 2: Intraoral images of the prosthesis in placement (a). After prosthesis removal, it is possible to observe gingival inflammation and swelling of the implants (b). Panoramic and periapical radiographies show evident bone resorption around the implant threads and severe pneumatization of the maxillary sinuses (c, d).

and xenogenous bone graft [7–9, 12–14]; bone reconstruction with vascularized free flap [15]; and the use of short dental implants (dental implants with less than 8 mm in length) [2, 16–18]. The use of autogenous bone graft is still the gold standard to rehabilitate atrophic jaws due to its osteogenic, osteoinductive, and osteoconductive properties [19]. However, in cases of severe atrophy of the maxilla, the amount of bone graft necessary to fully reconstruct the area is quite high, which requires an extra oral donor area such as the iliac crest region [20] or calvarial bone graft [21, 22]. Autogenous bone graft

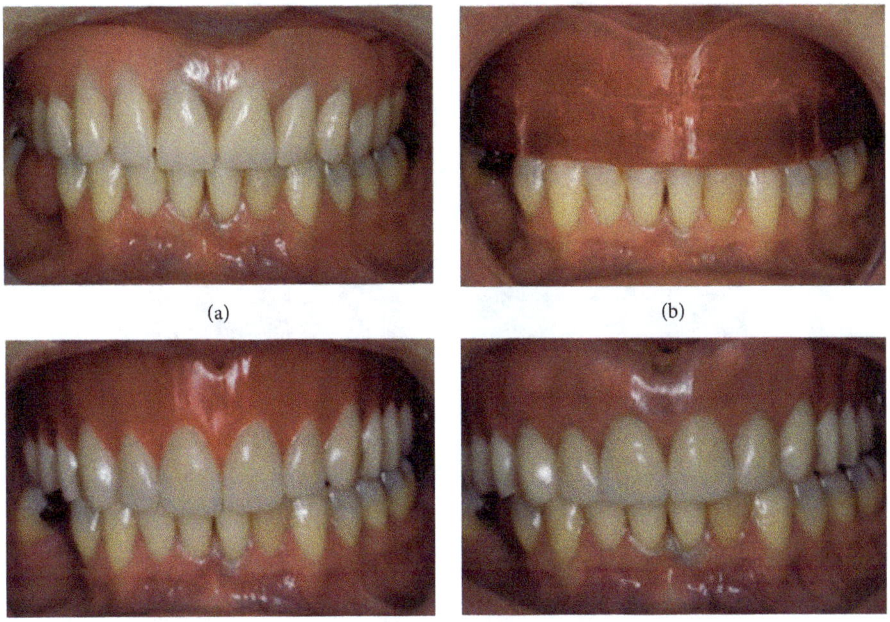

(a) (b) (c) (d)

FIGURE 3: Prosthetic procedures were carried out to install a provisional prosthesis attached to two short implants by means of o-ring connection (a–d).

has some drawbacks, for instance, limited amount of bone graft that can be harvested (intraoral approach), increased surgical time and rehabilitation, high costs, intensive postsurgical care, and excessive morbidity to the patient especially when extraoral graft is harvested.

Trying to overcome the disadvantages of autogenous bone graft, guided bone regeneration with bone substitute materials and growth factors (recombinant human bone morphogenetic protein-2 (rhBMP-2), plasma-rich platelets (PRP), and leukocyte- and platelet-rich fibrin (L-PRF)) have been proposed and tested [23, 24]. Although positive results have been demonstrated with guided bone regeneration and rhBMP-2 [25, 26], the elevated costs of rhBMP-2 (infuse bone graft), healing time, surgical morbidity, and risk of membrane and biomaterial exposure decrease patient acceptance. On the other hand, L-PRF seems to allow early placement of dental implant in maxillary sinuses [27] and increased bone formation when combined with demineralized bovine bone mineral (DBBM) [28]. In order to minimize patient discomfort, morbidity, costs, and healing time, bone substitute materials such as demineralized bovine bone mineral (DBBM) have been extensively used to fill maxillary sinuses in atrophic upper jaw with high success rate and low morbidity to the patient [29, 30]. This approach permits implant placement with a sufficient length allowing proper osseointegration and anchorage of the implant. This approach is aimed at reducing comorbidities and allowing faster implant rehabilitation with minimal complications to the patient.

Finally, implant design, implant abutment connections (implant platform), and physical-chemical surface characteristics play pivotal role in the osseointegration process enhancement (implant microtopography) and in primary implant stability (macrotopography) especially in patients requiring immediate implant loading and in patients with poor bone quality and quantity [31–33]. Thus, this case report is aimed at presenting a complex case of oral rehabilitation with dental implants in a patient with severe atrophy of the posterior maxilla, associated with the presence of some implants with peri-implantitis. The clinical management of this case is fully presented, and the chosen approaches are therefore discussed.

2. Case Report

A 45-year-old Caucasian female patient sought for dental treatment in the Department of Periodontology with the main complaints of dissatisfaction with the use of a total upper denture (Figures 1(a)–1(d)). Patient medical records were not significant, and she denied use of alcohol or smoking. Her clinical history was marked by premature tooth loss in her adult age and by the use of removable prosthesis thereafter. She underwent implant rehabilitation in the maxilla eight years ago, and some implants were lost due to peri-implantitis in the posterior area of the maxilla. Clinical and radiographic examination revealed poor oral hygiene and the presence of three dental implants in the anterior area with gingival bleeding, swelling, and localized calculus in the implant surface (Figures 2(a) and 2(b)). Panoramic radiography showed extensive pneumatization of the maxillary sinuses, a radiolucent area around the remaining implant threads, and alveolar bone loss around the implant threads near the apical third of the fixation (Figures 2(c) and 2(d)).

Based on her medical history and clinical and radiographic analyses, the treatment plan was proposed in different stages. The first treatment phase encompassed new provisional prosthesis, surgical removal of the implants affected by peri-implantitis followed by the installation of

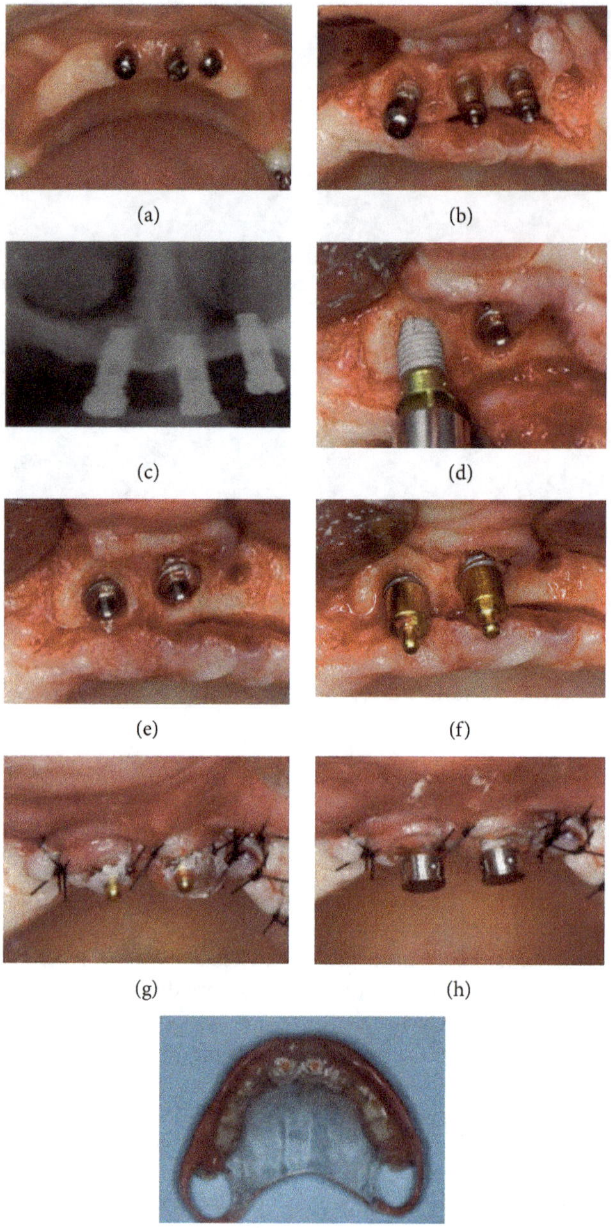

(a) (b) (c) (d) (e) (f) (g) (h) (i)

FIGURE 4: The first step in the surgical procedures was to expose the area where the implants were installed, and then, the implants were removed (a–c). After implant removal, two short implants were immediately installed. An appropriate abutment was installed in each of the implants to allow provisional prosthesis installation with appropriate retention (d–i).

two short implants with immediate loading, and provisional prosthesis installation. In the second phase, the surgical approaches included maxillary sinus floor augmentation bilaterally with concomitant graft with DBBM plus PRF membranes, autogenous block bone graft, implant placement, and definitive prosthetic rehabilitation. The planned surgical reconstruction in different phases of the treatment was intended to allow the patient to use provisional prosthesis during her treatment without functional and esthetic complaints. Written informed consent was obtained prior to initial treatment.

The first step of treatment involved the confection of new provisional prosthesis previous to implant removal. In this moment, all the expectations of the patient regarding her tooth characteristics (color, size, position, etc.) and all the necessary changes in her prosthesis were taken into account to achieve all the patient's functional and esthetic requirements. The prosthetic procedures are represented by Figures 3(a)–3(d). Subsequently, two remote vertical releasing incisions were performed in the alveolar crest followed by a crestal incision on the area where the implants were installed (Figures 4(a) and 4(b)). Periapical radiography was taken to evaluate the implants (Figure 4(c)). A full-thickness flap was elevated on the buccal and palatal aspects. The removal of the implants was performed with the aid of a trephine drill trying to preserve the remaining alveolar bone

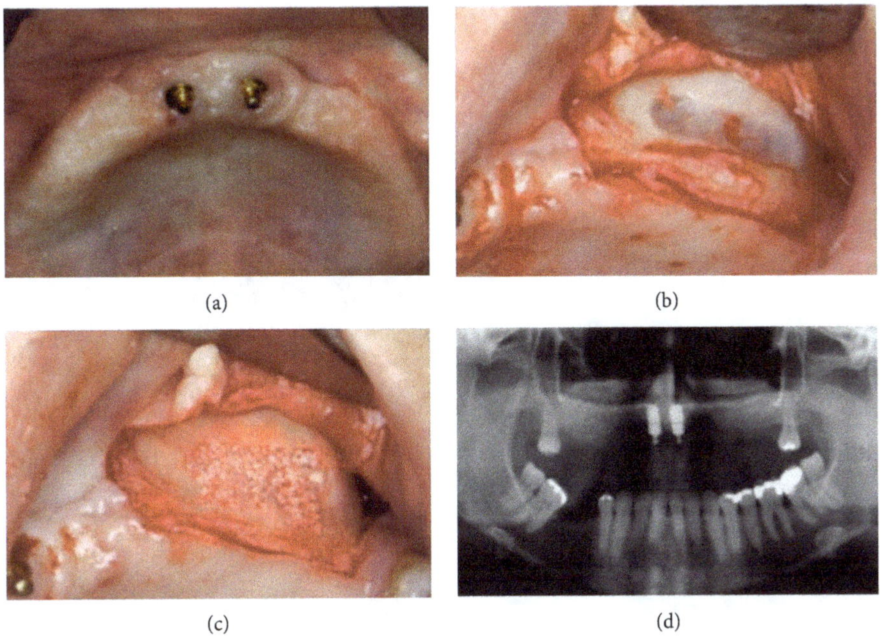

FIGURE 5: The second surgical procedure was carried out to augment the maxillary sinuses. DBBM plus L-PRF was used to fill the sinuses aiming at increasing bone height to allow proper implant length installation (a–c). Panoramic radiography shows the maxillary sinuses immediately after bone graft (d).

as much as possible. Then, two short implants were installed in the remaining alveolar bone crest (Figures 4(d)–4(f)) (Conexao® Sistema de Protese, external hexagons, 5.0 × 5.5 and 4.3 × 5.5 mm). The implant insertion torque for both implants was higher as 45 Ncm, which permitted the immediate function of the implants. The prosthetic abutment connection was installed, and the soft tissue was closed by means of simple suture (Figures 4(g) and 4(h)). The o-ring connection was able to assist the retention of the provisional total prosthesis (Figure 4(i)).

The next step in the process of rehabilitation was to perform the maxillary sinus floor augmentation. This procedure was completed four months after short implant placement. The surgical procedure consisted by a midcrestal and vertical releasing incisions alongside the remaining alveolar bone to reveal the lateral sinus wall [28]. A lateral window approach was performed to access the sinus wall using diamond round bur. The surgical access respected the position of implant placement planning and the maxillary sinus anatomy [27, 28]. After careful sinus membrane elevation, the maxillary sinuses were filled with a mixture of L-PRF and large particles [29, 30] (1-2 mm) of DBBM (Bio-Oss, Geistlich Pharma AG, Wolhusen, Switzerland). Membranes of L-PRF were also used to cover the lateral window of the sinus cavity. The soft tissue was then sutured with absorbable sutures (Vicryl, Ethicon, Somerville, NJ, USA). After the surgical procedure, a panoramic radiography was taken to evaluate the maxillary sinus bone gain (Figure 5(d)).

After four months of the maxillary sinus augmentation procedure, it was planned to increase the bone thickness in the maxillary anterior area with autogenous block bone graft. The autogenous bone graft was harvested from the mandibular ramus. For this, an access preparation was carried out with a crestal and vertical releasing incision in the retromolar region. Then, a mucoperiosteal flap was obtained by exposing the buccal wall and the oblique line. The osteotomy was performed with rotating instruments and the cortical block was obtained with a hammer and chisel, as described [34]. The mucoperiosteal flap was repositioned, and the defect was sutured with Vicryl 4-0 thread (Figures 6(a)–6(d)). Thereafter, the autogenous bone was split in two parts and then were placed in position in the receptor area and fixed with cortical screws (Figures 6(e) and 6(f)). Panoramic radiography was taken immediately after graft placement (Figure 6(g)). The patient was instructed to apply chlorhexidine (0.12%) twice a day. Ibuprofen 600 mg three times a day for 3 days was prescribed for pain relief and amoxicillin 875 mg plus 125 mg of potassium clavulanate three times a day for 7 days. The area healed uneventfully, and sutures were removed at two weeks. The patient reported minimal swelling and discomfort postoperatively.

The implants were placed with the aid of guided surgical approach after a 4-month onlay graft healing. Initially, the provisional prosthesis was filled with proper acrylic material (due to the internal prosthesis wear performed after graft placement) and was adjusted to allow precise adaptation to the augmented area, with ideal occlusion, fitting, and esthetics. The prosthesis was then duplicated to be used as multifunctional guide. Four vestibular gutta-percha fillings assisted as radiographic markers. A silicone interocclusal record was made to maintain the denture in a stable interarch position, during the cone beam computed tomography (CBCT) scan. A cone beam technique (I-CAT Cone Beam; Hatfield, PA, USA) was used to scan the patient. A second scan was made of the prosthesis extraorally. Virtual planning was performed with seven implants in the posterior area of the maxilla (three in the right side), as described [35]. Three guided anchor pins were planned to fix the surgical guide. A 3D planning was made with the aid of computerized images.

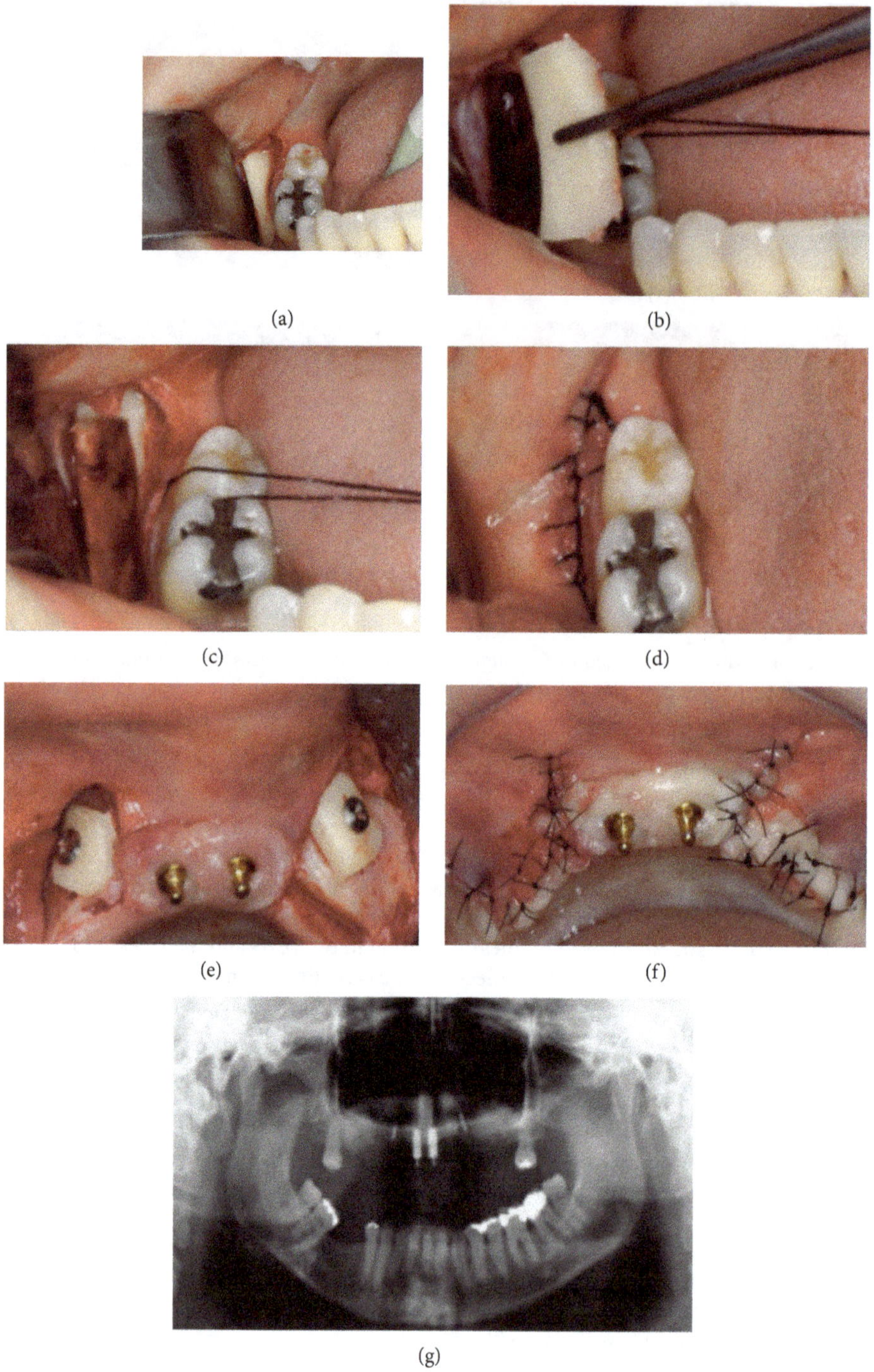

FIGURE 6: The third surgical approach was to install an onlay autogenous block bone graft harvested from the mandibular ramus. The graft was split and was installed in the receptor area in the posterior maxilla to augment the alveolar crest width and consequently to allow implant installation in an ideal tridimensional position (a–f). Panoramic radiography was taken immediately after graft placement (g).

The diameter, length, and positioning of the implants were defined, and the files were sent to Bioparts (Brasilia, DF, Brazil) to manufacture the surgical templates (Figures 7(a)–7(c)). The surgical template was stabilized with three screws, before the instrumentation for implant installation. The Cone Morse Due implants (Implacil De Bortoli, Sao Paulo, SP, Brazil) with 3.5 mm in diameter and varied lengths were used to rehabilitate the patient. After implant installation, the cover screws were installed to all implants (due to low insertion torque) and a healing period of 3 months was set to tissue healing (Figures 7(d)–7(h)).

After the healing period of 3 months, the implants were exposed and the cover screws were removed (Figures 8(a)–8(d)). A miniconical abutment was chosen for all implants, and the mini pillars were then installed (Figures 8(e)–8(h)). Finally, definitive prosthesis was carried out following all the necessary steps of prosthesis fabrication (Figures 9(a)–9(j)). The definitive prosthesis was installed in the patient

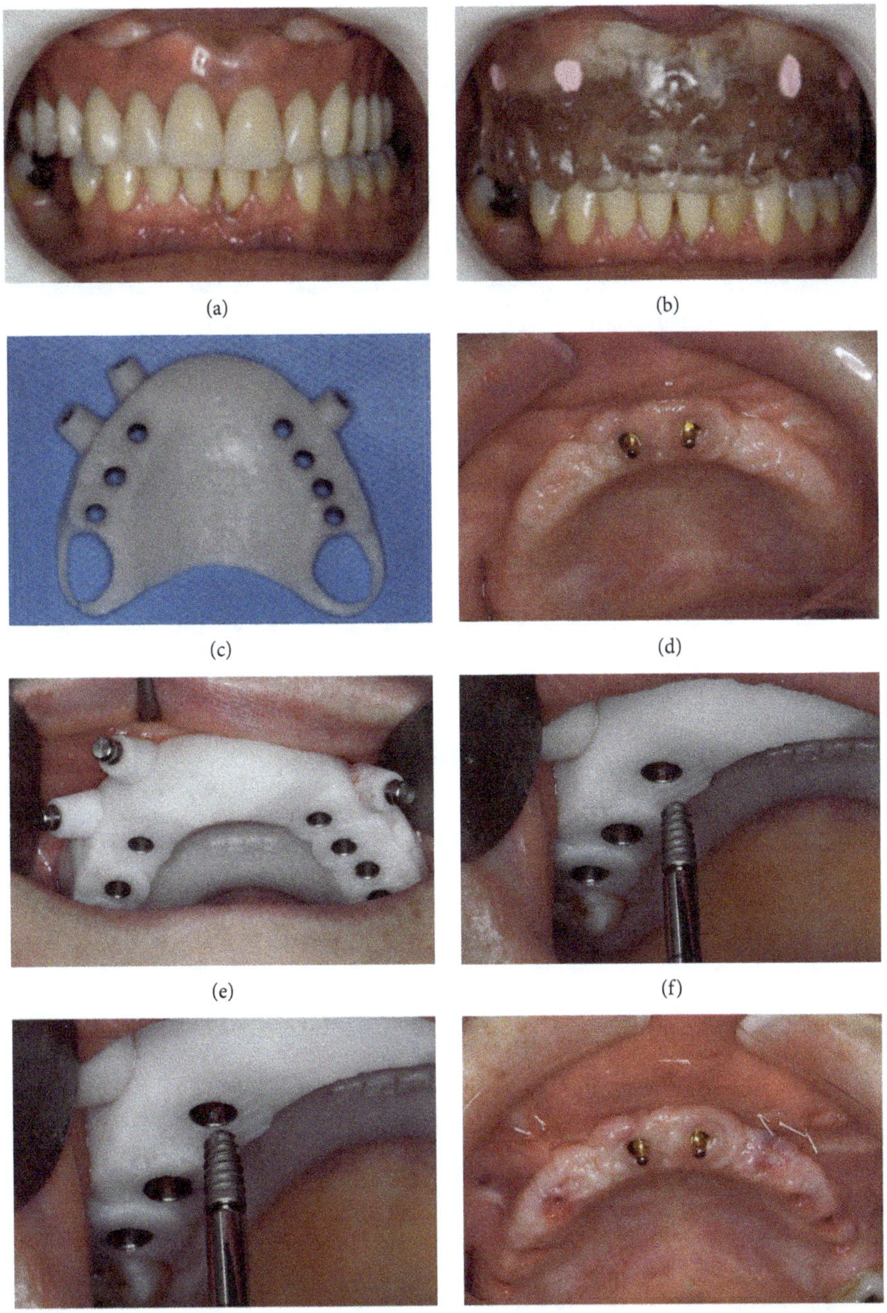

(a) (b) (c) (d) (e) (f) (g) (h)

Figure 7: After a healing period of 8 months from the maxillary sinus augmentation procedure, the implants were installed by means of guided surgery. Seven implants were planned and installed in the posterior area of the maxilla (a–h).

(Figures 10(a)–10(d)). After one year of follow-up, the patient was satisfied with the final result in relation to the esthetics and function (Figures 11(a)–11(c)). Panoramic radiography was taken after one year to show the implants without any signs of infection and proper osseointegration (Figure 11(d)).

3. Discussion

Rehabilitation of maxillary deficiencies with dental implants can be a challenge for most of the clinicians and surgeons, and in many instances, a multidisciplinary approach with the involvement of several disciplines is mandatory to achieve satisfactory functional and esthetic outcomes. The increased expectation for a pleasant esthetic result from the patient is something that increases the challenge for a successful oral rehabilitation. In this context, the advancements in tissue engineering, bone regeneration, bone substitute biomaterials, implant surface, and design have promoted the development of new materials and techniques for the successful treatment of complex cases. Moreover, the introduction of new technologies, such as cone beam computed

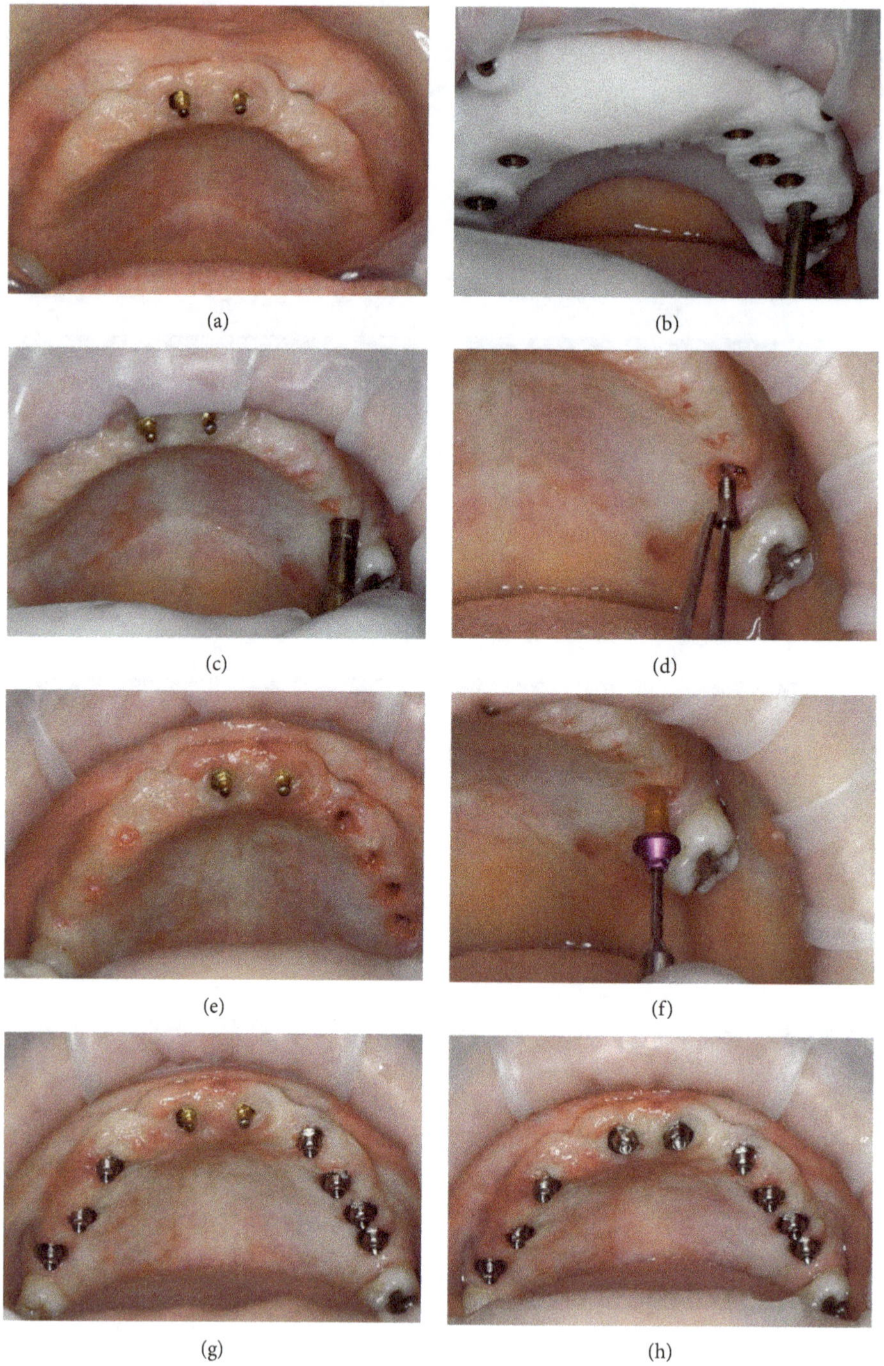

Figure 8: The implants were allowed to heal for 4 months, and then, the procedures to expose the implants were initiated (a, b). The cover screws of all implants were removed with the aid of the surgical template (c–f). Appropriate abutments were chosen and installed (g, h).

tomography, guided implant surgery, and new software, allow the achievement of more predictable and safe surgical procedures. Although interdisciplinary treatments usually result in better clinical outcomes, the increased treatment duration, costs, and miscommunication between clinicians should be taken into account when planning a complex oral rehabilitation.

In the case presented, it was chosen to perform the treatment in several steps. The initial treatment plan, i.e., the confection of provisional prosthesis supported by two short implants, was selected to allow the proper rehabilitation of the patient without affecting the masticatory functions, esthetics, and social behavioral. As the previous prosthesis was not adequate in terms of esthetics and functions due to the loss of the implants by peri-implantitis [36], the prosthesis was disregarded and a new one was confectioned. The placement of two short implants in the anterior region was capable to support the prosthesis with the o-ring connection. This surgical and prosthetic treatment also allowed us to evaluate the patient smile, lip support, phonetics, tooth size, and satisfaction with the new implant-supported prosthesis. This approach called reverse planning is indicated in pretty

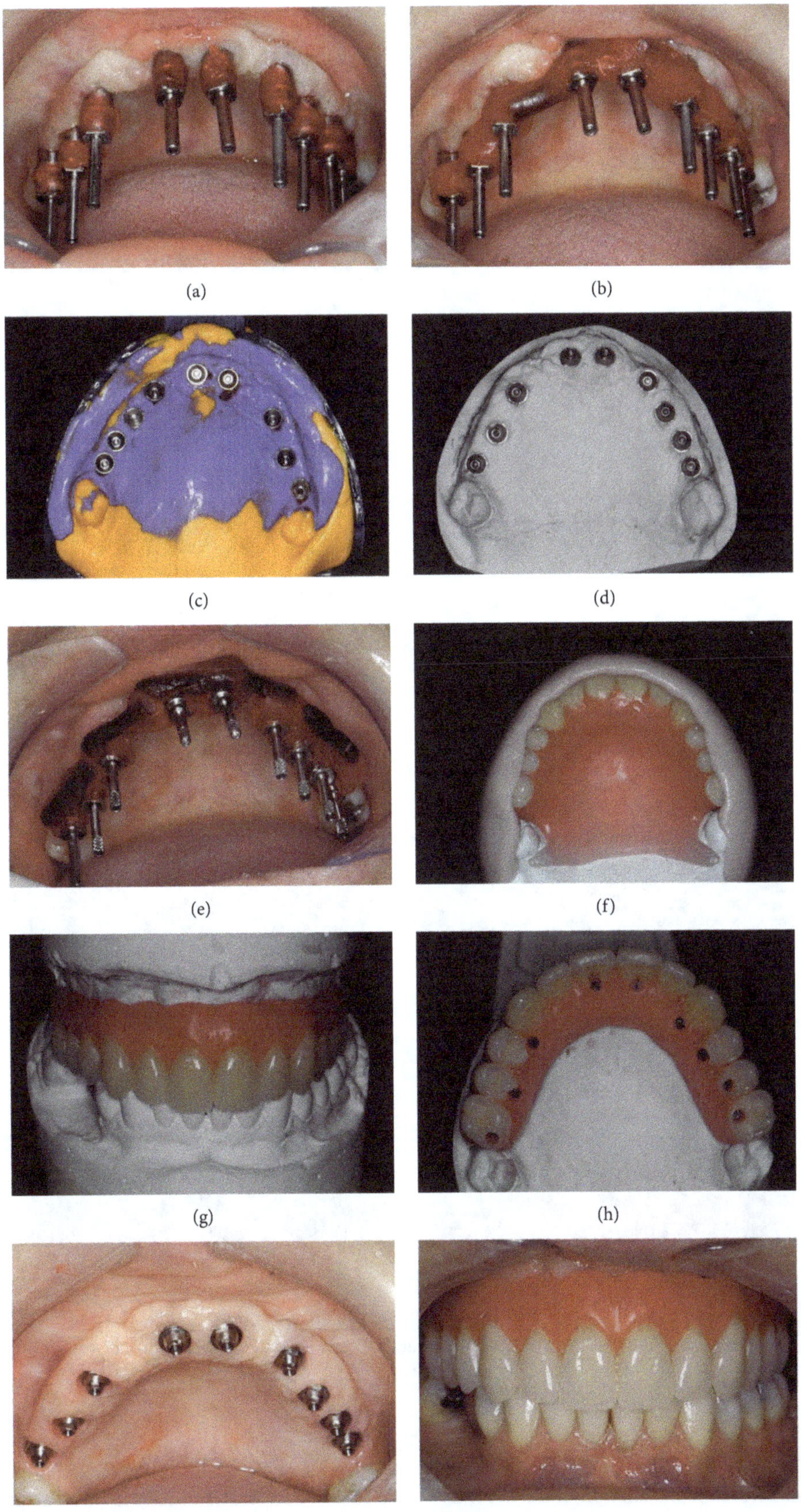

(a) (b) (c) (d) (e) (f) (g) (h) (i) (j)

FIGURE 9: Prosthetic procedures to manufacture the definitive prosthesis were performed. All the necessary steps to create the definitive prosthesis were carried out (a–j).

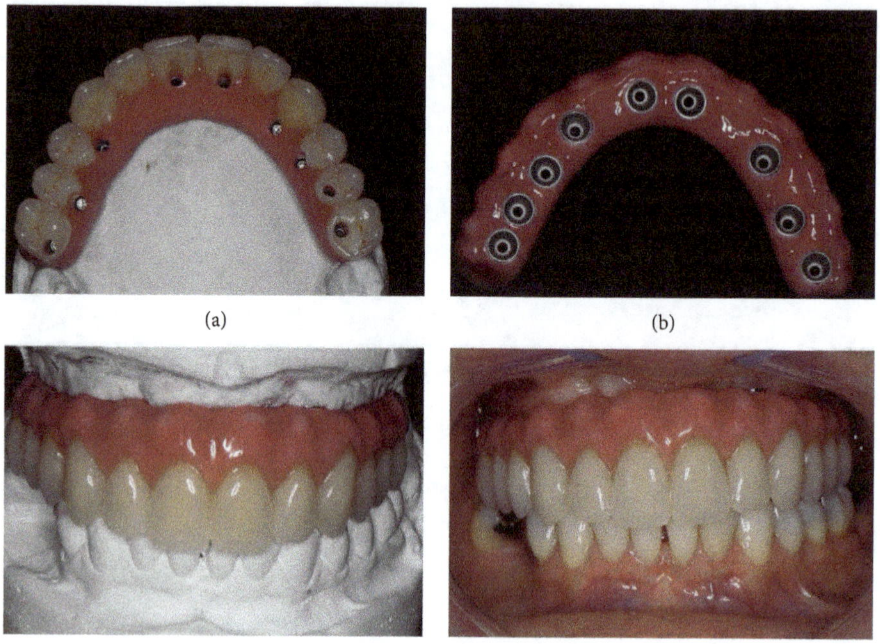

(a) (b) (c) (d)

Figure 10: The definitive prosthesis was installed.

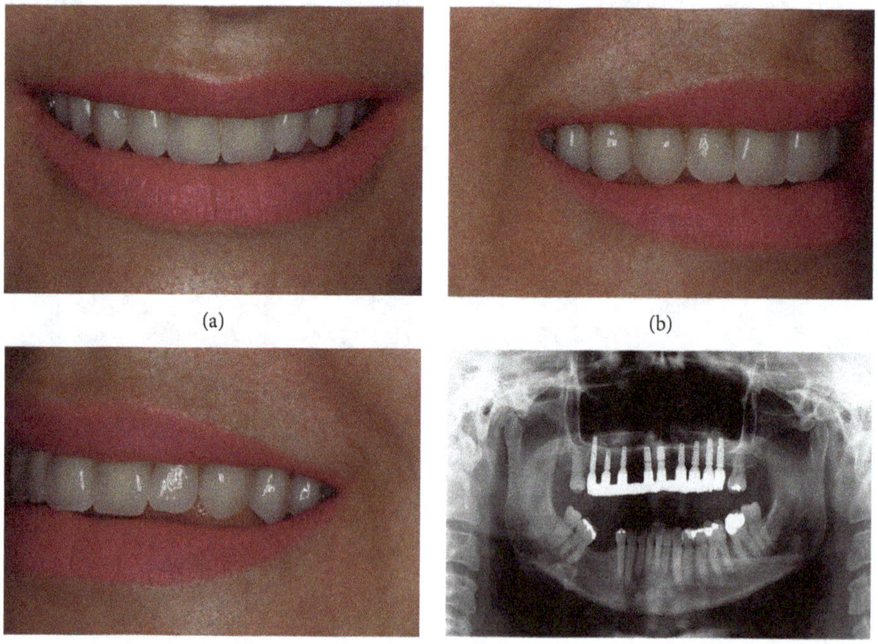

(a) (b) (c) (d)

Figure 11: (a–c) One-year follow-up shows the successful functional and esthetic outcomes and proper osseointegration of the implants without any signs of infection.

much all cases because the patient can adapt and accept the new clinical condition before the installation of the definitive prosthesis.

The placement of conventional length implants (>10 mm) in the posterior maxilla in the presence of insufficient bone height usually requires sinus floor augmentation procedures. Several studies in the literature have demonstrated successful results with dental implants in maxillary sinus grafted with autogenous, bone substitute materials, and combinations thereof. Thus, after a healing period of 4 months, it was decided to perform the sinus floor augmentation procedure using a combination of DBBM and

L-PRF. This approach was chosen because previous studies have demonstrated beneficial effects when the maxillary sinus is graft with combination of DBBM and growth factor, allowing early implant placement and more new natural bone formation [27, 28, 37, 38]. The rationale behind the use of growth factor in maxillary sinus is to provide a stable scaffold when mixing with the DBBM and also to increase the process of angiogenesis and osteogenesis. The healing period after maxillary sinus augmentation was set as 8 months to allow proper maturation of the bone.

During the follow-up visits, it was decided to graft the anterior alveolar crest with an onlay autogenous bone graft to increase the width of the alveolar bone. This surgical procedure is aimed at correcting horizontal deficiencies in the maxillary area allowing the installation of implants in an ideal tridimensional position. According to Buser et al. [39], an improper implant positioning might lead to esthetic and functional complications and should be avoided to achieve satisfactory outcomes. Therefore, the autogenous bone was harvested from the mandibular ramus, placed in position with titanium screws, and the area was let to heal for 4 months. The rationale to perform the surgical procedures for bone augmentation (in maxillary sinus and alveolar crest) in two different time points is to decrease patient comorbidities and discomfort. Moreover, as the healing period for maxillary sinus augmentation with DBBM takes longer than autogenous bone graft, the treatment duration was not affected.

After the healing period, the placement of implants was planned by means of computed guided surgery. After CBCT scan of the patient and denture, the virtual planning was performed and the files were sent to Bioparts (Brasilia, DF, Brazil) to manufacture the surgical templates. The conical implants were installed with the flapless approach, which facilitates would healing and decreased postoperative pain [35]. Virtual planning and flapless approach are very reliable and accurate treatment modalities and present some advantages over the conventional implant surgery, such as correct implant positioning, high level of accuracy, faster implant placement, faster wound healing, better treatment planning, and less amount of anesthetics necessary. As the implants were installed over the bone graft and the primary stability of the implants were lower than 40 Ncm, it was decided to not load the implants immediately after surgery. Three months were waited before the definitive prosthesis was confectioned. Finally, the prosthetic procedures were comprehensively performed and the definitive prosthesis was installed.

Despite the fact that the present treatment approaches have led to a satisfactory functional and esthetic result, it also presents some disadvantages that need to be taken into account. The virtual planning of the implants is time-consuming and comes with a higher cost due to multiple CBCT scans and template fabrication. This method necessitates good communication with the dental technician. Moreover, implant graft (maxillary sinus and onlay autogenous bone) increases the treatment duration and costs and might lead to postoperative discomfort.

4. Conclusions

In summary, this case report illustrates an efficient surgical-prosthetic approach for the management of a complex case of peri-implantitis, which required surgical reconstruction of the maxillary bone, dental implants, and prosthetic rehabilitation. A proper diagnosis and careful planning play an important role to enhance precision and to achieve patient esthetic and functional outcomes. Moreover, bone regenerative procedures by means of onlay autogenous bone graft and maxillary sinus augmentation allowed implant placement in an ideal tridimensional position, which favored the manufacturing of a proper prosthesis regarding function, esthetics, and biological properties, known as periodontal prosthesis.

References

[1] V. Moraschini, L. A. Poubel, V. F. Ferreira, and E. S. Barboza, "Evaluation of survival and success rates of dental implants reported in longitudinal studies with a follow-up period of at least 10 years: a systematic review," *International Journal of Oral and Maxillofacial Surgery*, vol. 44, no. 3, pp. 377–388, 2015.

[2] T. T. H. Nguyen, M. Y. Eo, T. S. Kuk, H. Myoung, and S. M. Kim, "Rehabilitation of atrophic jaw using iliac onlay bone graft combined with dental implants," *International Journal of Implant Dentistry*, vol. 5, no. 1, p. 11, 2019.

[3] M. Cordaro, S. Donno, F. Ausenda, and L. Cordaro, "Influence of bone anatomy on implant placement procedures in edentulous arches of elderly individuals: a cross-sectional study on computed tomography images," *The International Journal of Oral & Maxillofacial Implants*, vol. 35, no. 5, pp. 995–1004, 2020.

[4] E. D. de Avila, R. S. de Molon, M. A. Cardoso et al., "Aesthetic implant rehabilitation in periodontally compromised patients: a surgical and prosthetic rationale," *Journal of the International Academy of Periodontology*, vol. 18, pp. 120–128, 2016.

[5] F. Pieri, E. Caselli, C. Forlivesi, and G. Corinaldesi, "Rehabilitation of the atrophic posterior maxilla using splinted short implants or sinus augmentation with standard-length implants: a retrospective cohort study," *The International Journal of Oral & Maxillofacial Implants*, vol. 31, no. 5, pp. 1179–1188, 2016.

[6] A. Sharan and D. Madjar, "Maxillary sinus pneumatization following extractions: a radiographic study," *The International Journal of Oral & Maxillofacial Implants*, vol. 23, no. 1, pp. 48–56, 2008.

[7] R. S. de Molon, E. D. de Avila, J. A. Cirelli, A. Cardoso Mde, L. Capelozza-Filho, and L. A. Borelli Barros, "Optimizing maxillary aesthetics of a severe compromised tooth through orthodontic movement and dental implants," *Case Reports in Dentistry*, vol. 2014, Article ID 103808, 10 pages, 2014.

[8] R. S. de Molon, E. D. de Avila, J. A. Cirelli et al., "A combined approach for the treatment of resorbed fresh sockets allowing immediate implant restoration: a 2-year follow-up," *The Journal of Oral Implantology*, vol. 41, no. 6, pp. 712–718, 2015.

[9] R. S. de Molon, E. D. de Avila, L. A. de Barros-Filho et al., "Reconstruction of the alveolar buccal bone plate in compro-

mised fresh socket after immediate implant placement followed by immediate provisionalization," *Journal of Esthetic and Restorative Dentistry*, vol. 27, no. 3, pp. 122–135, 2015.

[10] S. Yalcin, M. Ordulu, Y. Emes, H. Gur, I. Aktas, and C. Caniklioglu, "Alveolar distraction osteogenesis before placement of dental implants," *Implant Dentistry*, vol. 15, no. 1, pp. 48–52, 2006.

[11] T. Kanno, M. Mitsugi, Y. Furuki, M. Hosoe, H. Akamatsu, and T. Takenobu, "Overcorrection in vertical alveolar distraction osteogenesis for dental implants," *International Journal of Oral and Maxillofacial Surgery*, vol. 36, no. 5, pp. 398–402, 2007.

[12] B. F. Mello, F. M. de Carvalho, L. F. de Souza da Silva, C. G. Dos Santos, and J. A. Shibli, "Horizontal Ridge Augmentation Using a Xenograft Bone Substitute for Implant- Supported Fixed Rehabilitation: A Case Report with Four Years of Follow-Up," *Case Reports in Dentistry*, vol. 2020, Article ID 6723936, 2020.

[13] R. Spin-Neto, A. Stavropoulos, F. L. Coletti, L. A. Pereira, E. Marcantonio Jr., and A. Wenzel, "Remodeling of cortical and corticocancellous fresh-frozen allogeneic block bone grafts–a radiographic and histomorphometric comparison to autologous bone grafts," *Clinical Oral Implants Research*, vol. 26, no. 7, pp. 747–752, 2015.

[14] R. Spin-Neto, A. Stavropoulos, F. L. Coletti, R. S. Faeda, L. A. Pereira, and E. Marcantonio Jr., "Graft incorporation and implant osseointegration following the use of autologous and fresh-frozen allogeneic block bone grafts for lateral ridge augmentation," *Clinical Oral Implants Research*, vol. 25, no. 2, pp. 226–233, 2014.

[15] M. Chiapasco, M. Zaniboni, and M. Boisco, "Augmentation procedures for the rehabilitation of deficient edentulous ridges with oral implants," *Clinical Oral Implants Research*, vol. 17, Suppl 2, pp. 136–159, 2006.

[16] A. A. Al-Hashedi, T. B. Taiyeb Ali, and N. Yunus, "Short dental implants: an emerging concept in implant treatment," *Quintessence International*, vol. 45, no. 6, pp. 499–514, 2014.

[17] D. Nisand and F. Renouard, "Short implant in limited bone volume," *Periodontol 2000*, vol. 66, no. 1, pp. 72–96, 2014.

[18] R. S. de Molon, F. S. Lages, C. P. Rivera, A. P. de Souza Faloni, R. Margonar, and T. P. Queiroz, "Evaluation of short and regular implants after prosthesis placement in the mandible: a nonrandomized controlled clinical trial," *The Journal of Contemporary Dental Practice*, vol. 18, no. 12, pp. 1122–1129, 2017.

[19] A. Mordenfeld, T. Albrektsson, and M. Hallman, "A 10-year clinical and radiographic study of implants placed after maxillary sinus floor augmentation with an 80:20 mixture of deproteinized bovine bone and autogenous bone," *Clinical Implant Dentistry and Related Research*, vol. 16, no. 3, pp. 435–446, 2014.

[20] A. Sethi, T. Kaus, J. I. Cawood, H. Plaha, M. Boscoe, and P. Sochor, "Onlay bone grafts from iliac crest: a retrospective analysis," *International Journal of Oral and Maxillofacial Surgery*, vol. 49, no. 2, pp. 264–271, 2020.

[21] A. Yousif, G. M. Raghoebar, T. F. Putters, A. Vissink, and J. Schortinghuis, "Calvarial bone grafts to augment the alveolar process in partially dentate patients: a prospective case series," *International Journal of Implant Dentistry*, vol. 6, no. 1, p. 57, 2020.

[22] D. E. Wortmann, J. Klein-Nulend, L. J. van Ruijven, A. Vissink, G. M. Raghoebar, and J. Schortinghuis, "Histomorphometric and micro-CT analyses of calvarial bone grafts used to reconstruct the extremely atrophied maxilla," *Clinical Implant Dentistry and Related Research*, vol. 22, no. 5, pp. 593–601, 2020.

[23] R. M. Freitas, R. Spin-Neto, E. Marcantonio Junior, L. A. Pereira, U. M. Wikesjo, and C. Susin, "Alveolar ridge and maxillary sinus augmentation using rhBMP-2: a systematic review," *Clinical Implant Dentistry and Related Research*, vol. 17, no. 1, pp. e192–e201, 2015.

[24] R. M. de Freitas, C. Susin, R. Spin-Neto et al., "Horizontal ridge augmentation of the atrophic anterior maxilla using rhBMP-2/ACS or autogenous bone grafts: a proof-of-concept randomized clinical trial," *Journal of Clinical Periodontology*, vol. 40, no. 10, pp. 968–975, 2013.

[25] L. M. S. Zanettini, F. Vieira, G. G. Fritscher, R. M. Pagnoncelli, and C. Heitz, "Use of recombinant human bone morphogenetic protein-2 associated with lyophilized bovine bone in reconstruction of atrophic maxilla," *The Journal of Craniofacial Surgery*, vol. 29, no. 7, pp. 1934–1938, 2018.

[26] R. M. de Freitas, C. Susin, W. M. Tamashiro et al., "Histological analysis and gene expression profile following augmentation of the anterior maxilla using rhBMP-2/ACS versus autogenous bone graft," *Journal of Clinical Periodontology*, vol. 43, no. 12, pp. 1200–1207, 2016.

[27] E. C. Pichotano, R. S. de Molon, L. G. Freitas de Paula, R. V. de Souza, E. Marcantonio Jr., and D. L. Zandim-Barcelos, "Early placement of dental implants in maxillary sinus grafted with leukocyte and platelet-rich fibrin and deproteinized bovine bone mineral," *The Journal of Oral Implantology*, vol. 44, no. 3, pp. 199–206, 2018.

[28] E. C. Pichotano, R. S. de Molon, R. V. de Souza, R. S. Austin, E. Marcantonio, and D. L. Zandim-Barcelos, "Evaluation of L-PRF combined with deproteinized bovine bone mineral for early implant placement after maxillary sinus augmentation: a randomized clinical trial," *Clinical Implant Dentistry and Related Research*, vol. 21, no. 2, pp. 253–262, 2019.

[29] R. S. de Molon, F. S. Magalhaes-Tunes, C. V. Semedo et al., "A randomized clinical trial evaluating maxillary sinus augmentation with different particle sizes of demineralized bovine bone mineral: histological and immunohistochemical analysis," *International Journal of Oral and Maxillofacial Surgery*, vol. 48, no. 6, pp. 810–823, 2019.

[30] T. L. Dos Anjos, R. S. de Molon, P. R. Paim, E. Marcantonio, E. Marcantonio Jr., and R. S. Faeda, "Implant stability after sinus floor augmentation with deproteinized bovine bone mineral particles of different sizes: a prospective, randomized and controlled split-mouth clinical trial," *International Journal of Oral and Maxillofacial Surgery*, vol. 45, no. 12, pp. 1556–1563, 2016.

[31] M. A. Eskan, G. Uzel, and S. Yilmaz, "A fixed reconstruction of fully edentulous patients with immediate function using an apically tapered implant design: a retrospective clinical study," *International Journal of Implant Dentistry*, vol. 6, no. 1, p. 77, 2020.

[32] E. D. de Avila, R. S. de Molon, B. P. Lima et al., "Impact of physical chemical characteristics of abutment implant surfaces on bacteria adhesion," *The Journal of Oral Implantology*, vol. 42, no. 2, pp. 153–158, 2016.

[33] E. D. de Avila, R. S. de Molon, C. E. Vergani, F. de Assis Mollo Jr., and V. Salih, "The relationship between biofilm and

physical-chemical properties of implant abutment materials for successful dental implants," *Materials (Basel)*, vol. 7, no. 5, pp. 3651–3662, 2014.

[34] R. S. de Molon, W. N. de Paula, R. Spin-Neto et al., "Correlation of fractal dimension with histomorphometry in maxillary sinus lifting using autogenous bone graft," *Brazilian Dental Journal*, vol. 26, no. 1, pp. 11–18, 2015.

[35] R. A. Landazuri-Del Barrio, J. Cosyn, W. N. De Paula, H. De Bruyn, and E. Marcantonio Jr., "A prospective study on implants installed with flapless-guided surgery using the all-on-four concept in the mandible," *Clinical Oral Implants Research*, vol. 24, no. 4, pp. 428–433, 2013.

[36] G. A. de Barros Lucena, R. S. de Molon, A. J. Moretti, J. A. Shibli, and D. M. Rego, "Evaluation of microbial contamination in the inner surface of titanium implants before healing abutment connection: a prospective clinical trial," *The International Journal of Oral & Maxillofacial Implants*, vol. 33, no. 4, pp. 853–862, 2018.

[37] B. Molemans, S. Cortellini, R. Jacobs, N. Pinto, W. Teughels, and M. Quirynen, "Simultaneous sinus floor elevation and implant placement using leukocyte- and platelet-rich fibrin as a sole graft material," *The International Journal of Oral & Maxillofacial Implants*, vol. 34, no. 5, pp. 1195–1201, 2019.

[38] M. Kumar, S. Chopra, D. Das, M. Gupta, J. Memoalia, and G. Verma, "Direct maxillary sinus floor augmentation for simultaneous dental implant placement," *Ann Maxillofac Surg*, vol. 8, no. 2, pp. 188–192, 2018.

[39] D. Buser, W. Martin, and U. C. Belser, "Optimizing esthetics for implant restorations in the anterior maxilla: anatomic and surgical considerations," *The International Journal of Oral & Maxillofacial Implants*, vol. 19, pp. 43–61, 2004.

26

Autotransplantation of Two Immature Third Molars with the use of L-PRF

Manon Rey Lescure,[1] Nicola Alberto Valente,[2] Sibylle Chatelain,[3] Chiara Cinquini,[4] and Antonio Barone[4]

[1]Unit of Oral Surgery and Implant Dentistry, Department of Oral and Maxillofacial Surgery, University Hospital of Geneva, 1205 Geneva, Switzerland
[2]Department of Stomatology, Faculty of Dentistry, University of Seville, 41009 Seville, Spain
[3]Department of Oral and Maxillofacial Surgery, Lausanne University Hospital (CHUV), 1011 Lausanne, Switzerland
[4]Department of Surgical, Medical, Molecular and of Critical Area Pathologies, Complex Operative Unit of Stomatology and Oral Surgery, University-Hospital of Pisa, University of Pisa, 56126 Pisa, Italy

Correspondence should be addressed to Antonio Barone; barosurg@gmail.com

Academic Editor: Leandro Napier de Souza

Tooth autotransplantation is a procedure which provides the extraction of an erupted or impacted tooth and its repositioning to another site in the oral cavity. This Case Report describes a successful case of two autotransplantations of open-apex mandibular third molars in place of the hopeless first mandibular molars with the use of L-PRF in a growing patient. A 15-year-old male patient was referred to the Dental Clinic for the extractions of the two hopeless mandibular first molars. Autotransplantation was considered the best treatment option for both sites 36 and 46, because the presence of two impacted mandibular third molars (38 and 48) with an incomplete root formation. Teeth 36 and 46 were extracted and replaced with teeth 38 and 48. The patient had an uneventful healing. At follow-up visits, the two autotransplanted teeth showed physiologic mobility, absence of inflammation and discomfort, and absence of infection; probing depth values were within normal range, and the vitality tests were positive. After 2 years, the teeth in position 36 and 46 showed absence of infection and mobility, and positive pulp vitality tests and the radiographic examinations exhibited closure of the root apices as well as absence of any periapical radiolucency or root resorption. Tooth autotransplantation is a good treatment option in case of tooth loss offering an alternative to traditional or implant-supported prosthesis especially for growing patients.

1. Introduction

Tooth autotransplantation is a procedure that involves extraction of an erupted or impacted tooth and its repositioning to another site within the same individual's oral cavity [1]. This treatment has shown several advantages and should always be taken in consideration together with other restorative treatment options such as removable or fixed restorative treatment, orthodontic treatment, and osseointegrated implants [2]. In contrast to a dental implant—which cannot be placed in those patients who have not completed the craniofacial skeletal growth—tooth transplantation is remarkably helpful in growing patients because it allows the tooth to maintain its function and proprioception and to follow the patient's facial growth pattern [3]. After a complete healing of the tooth transplantation, the preservation of its periodontal ligament allows orthodontic movement, if required. In addition, the pulp vitality of the transplanted tooth can be easily preserved in cases of open apex tooth; therefore, the donor tooth could undergo a complete root formation and growth [4]. In a long-term study, the authors revealed that the apical root foramen should be greater than 1 mm to have a predictable pulp revascularization [5]. On the contrary, teeth with closed apices had less frequent pulp

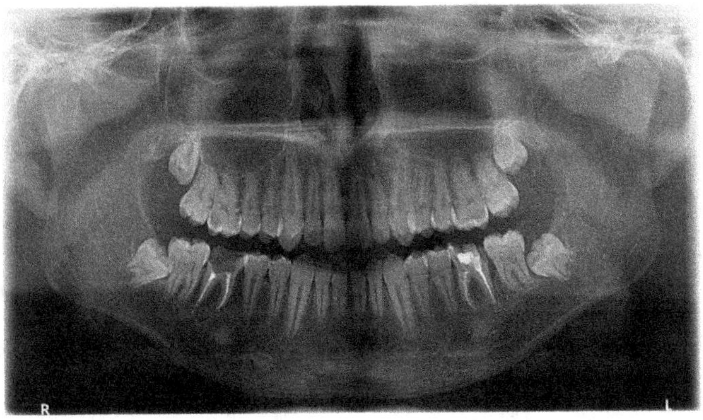

FIGURE 1: Initial panoramic radiograph.

healing and revascularization, thus, requiring endodontic treatment beforehand or at 2 weeks after tooth transplantation [6]. As in almost all surgical procedures, some complications have been reported in tooth transplantations, such as pulp necrosis, infections, root resorption, and ankylosis [7]. The scientific literature has reported various success and survival rates with a wide range of percentages that go from 60% to 95% [1, 3, 8]. Although at present no evidence-based parameters exist to evaluate the clinical success for autotransplantation, the following outcomes could be considered successful: complete healing for gingival and bone tissues, a restored tooth vitality, a tooth mobility within a physiological range, and an absence of root resorption. Recently, in a systematic review, some authors observed an average survival rate of 89.1% for transplanted teeth, showing that this procedure could be considered a reliable treatment option even when compared to single implants that had a survival rate of 96% [9].

Leukocyte-Platelet-Rich Fibrin (L-PRF) is an autologous blood-derived product containing a fibrin clot with serum and platelets, which enhances healing processes [10]. L-PRF is characterized by the absence of any additives in the blood sample and plays a role in improving wound healing processes by promoting cellular proliferation and angiogenesis [11]. Although many studies have focused on the use of L-PRF in oral surgical procedures such as impacted tooth extractions and bone grafting, there is still a lack of knowledge on its application in tooth autotransplantations.

This case report describes a successful case of autotransplantation of open-apex mandibular third molars in place of the first mandibular molars with the use of L-PRF and preservation of their vitality over 2 years of follow-up.

2. Case Report

A 15-year-old male patient in good general health was referred to the Dental Clinic at the University of Geneva (Switzerland) for the extractions of the two mandibular first molars (46 and 36) that were hopeless because of extensive caries. The two teeth had been endodontically treated, and both had shown perforation of the pulp chamber's floor due to decay, and, additionally, tooth 36 had shown a distal vertical bone defect. The patient's medical history was noncontributory, and an extensive clinical examination revealed poor oral hygiene and a few other carious lesions. The patient showed a full mouth plaque score > 30% and a full mouth bleeding score > 35%. To keep etiologic factors under control, the patient underwent scaling and received oral hygiene instructions. After evaluating multiple rehabilitative solutions, including orthodontic treatment and temporary partial removable prosthesis, autotransplantation was considered the best treatment option for both site 46 and 36. Teeth 38 and 48 were considered as donor teeth because they had open apices, not-completed root development and were impacted (Figure 1).

The patient's parents provided verbal and written informed consent after explanation and discussion of the treatment plan and before starting any procedures. The perioral skin and intraoral mucosa disinfection were performed with 0.1% chlorhexidine swab, and local anesthesia was administered using 4% articain solution for block and periapical anesthesia.

The first mandibular molars were extracted trying to reduce the trauma as much as possible. The roots were separated using high-speed fissure burs and were carefully luxated (Figures 2 and 3). The extraction sockets were thoroughly cleaned and irrigated with NaCl solution to remove all residual granulation tissues.

Platelet-Rich-Fibrin (L-PRF, IntraSpin®, Boca Raton, FL, USA) was prepared according to the manufacturer's guidelines. Four 9 ml tubes were filled with peripheral blood by venipuncture. The tubes were centrifuged at 2700 rpm using the IntraSpin® centrifuge for 12 minutes, the fibrin clots were transferred to the Xpression™ box (IntraSpin®, Boca Raton, FL, USA), and after 5 minutes, the L-PRF membranes were ready for use.

At the donor tooth sites, a full thickness envelope flap was raised, and bone removal was performed on the distal and buccal sites down to the cervical line of the tooth in order to completely expose the crown and make the tooth extraction as atraumatic as possible. The donor teeth were gently removed taking care to avoid any pressure and mechanical damage to the periodontal ligament. Once extracted, the donor teeth were stored in the L-PRF exudate, taken from the Xpression™ box, and the receiving sites were prepared by removing the interradicular bone. A minimal shaving of

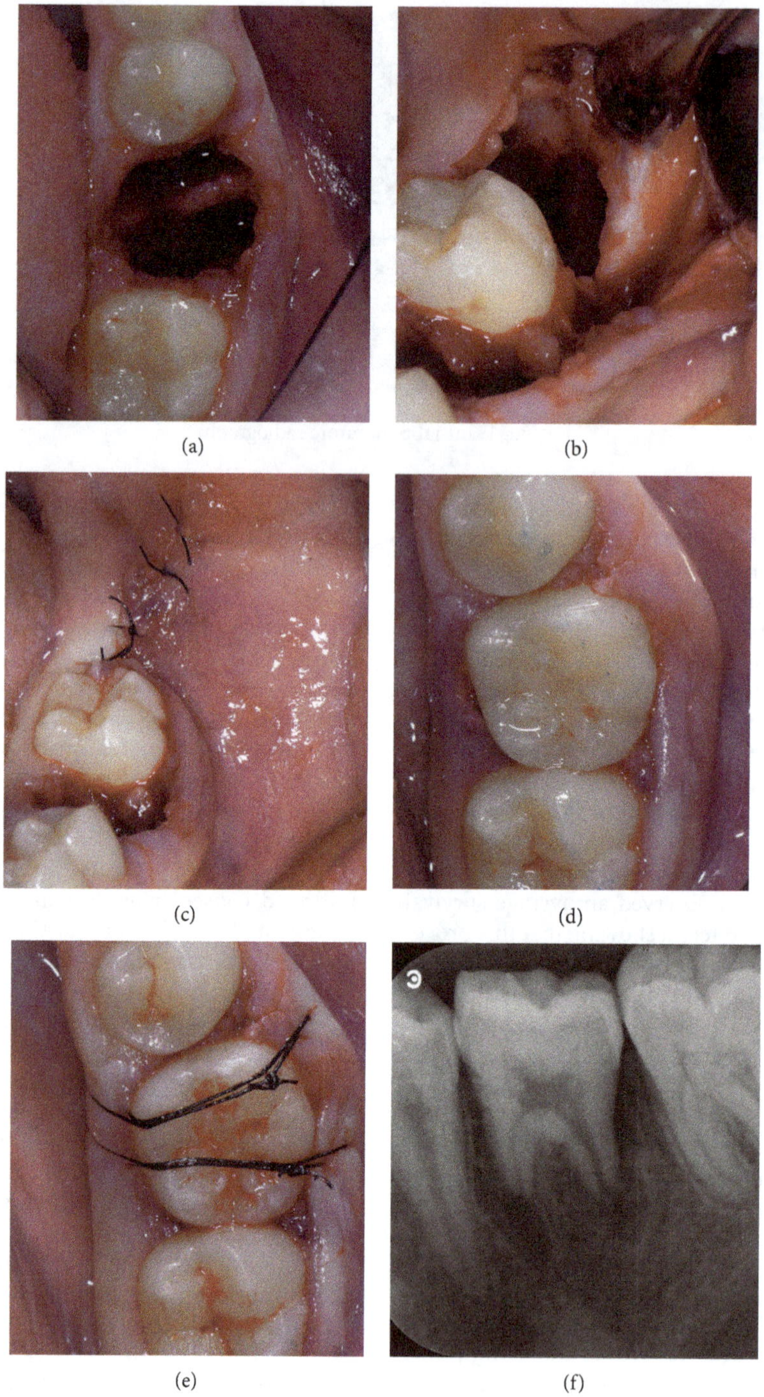

FIGURE 2: Tooth 36: (a) alveolar extraction socket; (b) alveolar extraction socket of left third molar; (c) sutures of third molar extraction site; (d) transplanted tooth in position 36; (e) cross-sutures for stabilization; (f) periapical radiograph immediately after transplantation.

third molar crowns was necessary to adjust the mesiodistal width to the space available, and all efforts were taken to minimize tooth extraoral permanence to less than 7 minutes. The L-PRF membranes were placed in the receiving sites, and, subsequently, the mandibular third molars were placed in the first molar extraction sites. A good fit of the donor tooth into the receiving sites was achieved.

Sutures were placed across the occlusal surfaces to better stabilize the transplanted teeth and to reposition the flaps. The two transplanted teeth showed a good stability in their position, thus, not requiring any additional stabilization.

During the postoperative period, the patient was prescribed 2 grams of amoxicillin daily for 5 days, 1000 mg of paracetamol every 8 hours according to pain, and 0.12% chlorhexidine mouth-rinse for the following 4 weeks. The patient was also instructed to avoid brushing and interdental cleaning in the surgical areas for 4 weeks and to follow a soft diet for 2 weeks.

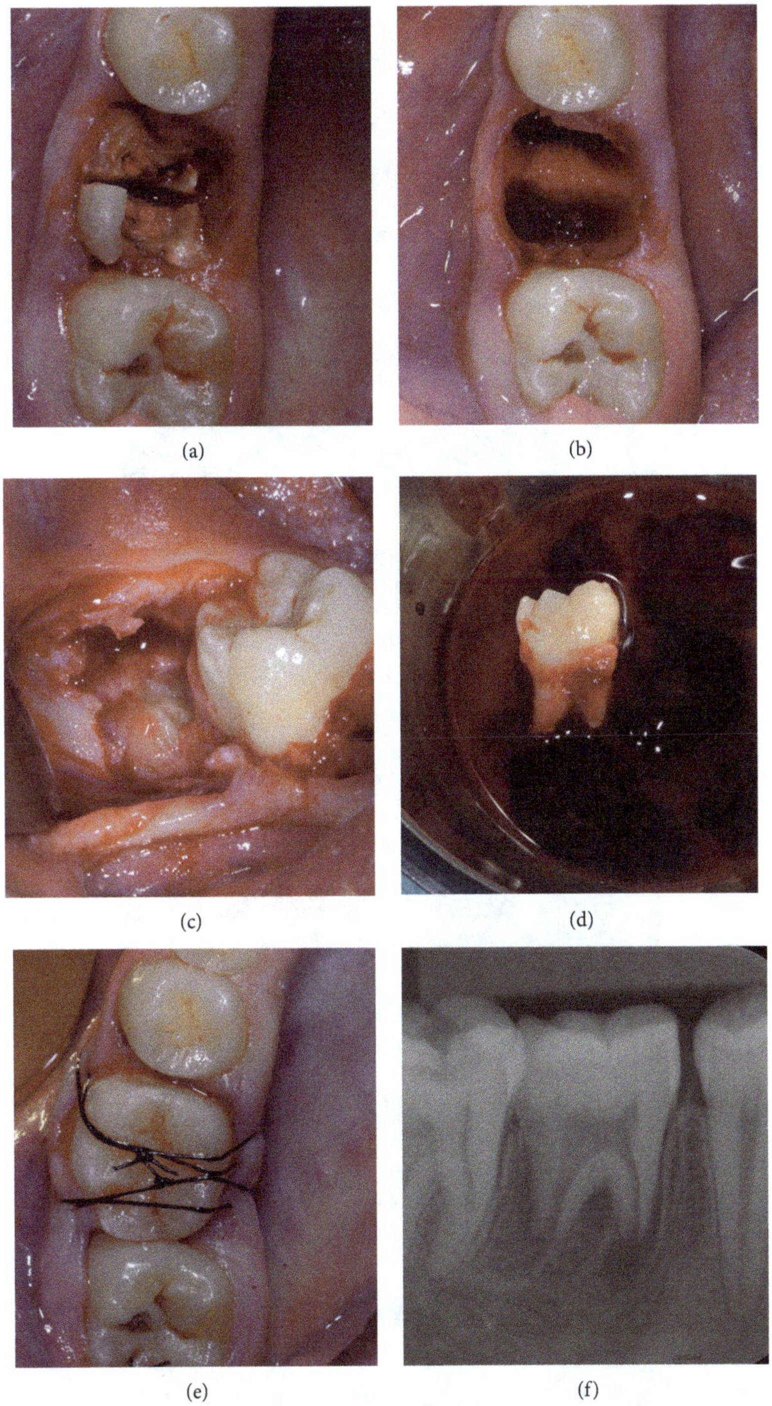

Figure 3: Tooth 46: (a) root's separation; (b) alveolar fresh extraction socket; (c) impacted right third molar; (d) third molar donor tooth extracted and stored in the L-PRF exudate; (e) transplanted tooth in position 46 and cross-sutures for stabilization; (f) periapical radiograph immediately after transplantation.

Patient healing was uneventful, and the sutures were removed after 1 week. The decision to avoid endodontic treatment was based on the presence of open apices and undeveloped roots. A large consensus, based on reports and reviews, underlines that in presence of developing roots with open apices, the best practice is to allow for a natural pulp healing with a strict clinical monitoring. At 2-month follow-up, the clinical examination revealed that both autotransplanted teeth had physiologic mobility, absence of inflammation, and discomfort. At 6-month follow-up, the patient showed absence of inflammation or infection, probing depth values within normal range, and the vitality tests were positive for both autotransplanted teeth. After 1- (Figures 4 and 5) and 2-year (Figures 6–8) follow-up, the teeth in position 36 and 46 showed absence of infection and mobility, and positive pulp vitality tests and the radiographic

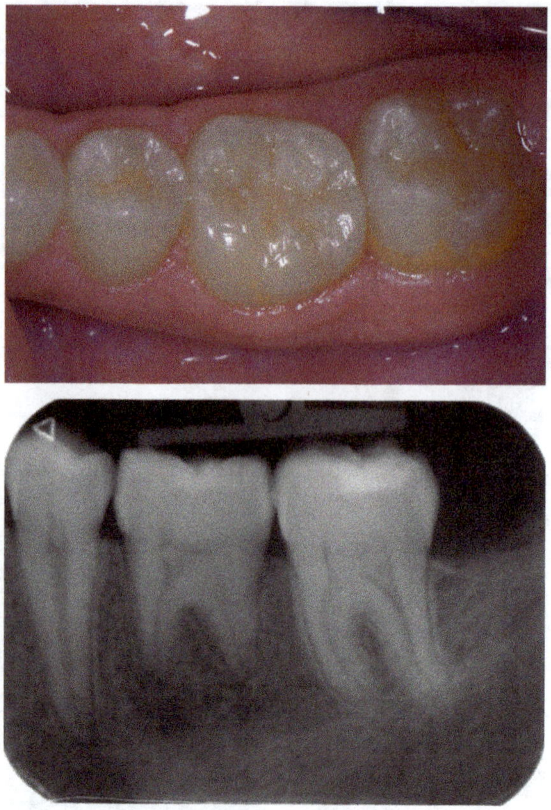

FIGURE 4: Tooth 36 at 1 year of follow-up.

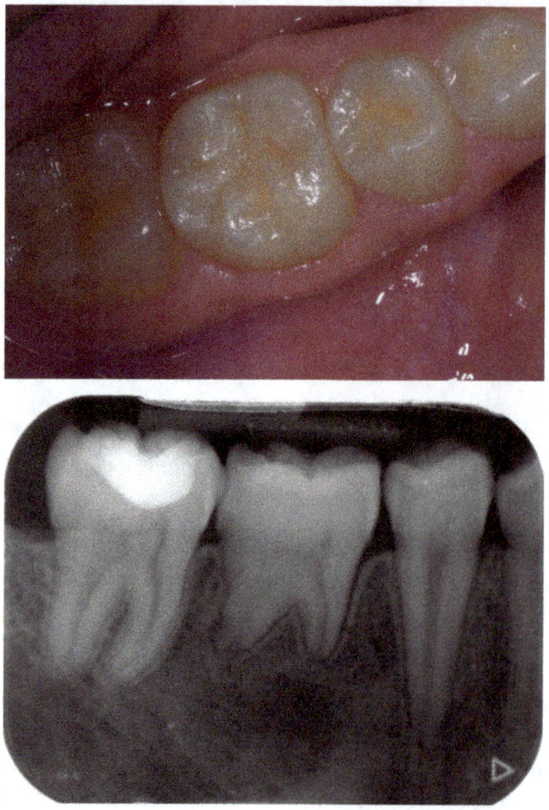

FIGURE 5: Tooth 46 at 1 year of follow-up.

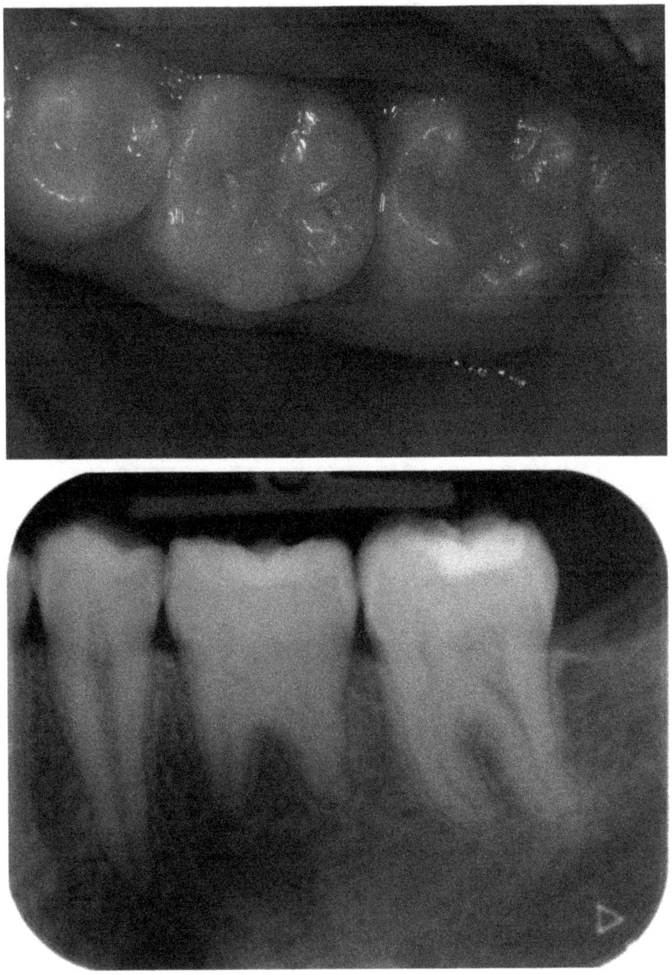

FIGURE 6: Tooth 36 at 2 years of follow-up.

examinations exhibited closure of the root apices and absence of any periapical radiolucency or root resorption. The patient reported satisfactory masticatory function and absence of pain, discomfort, or other adverse events.

3. Discussion

This report shows a successful case of two open apex third-molar autotransplantations that maintained their pulp vitality and function after 2 years of follow-up.

Tooth autotransplantation makes it possible to replace teeth with an unfavorable prognosis due to extensive carious lesions, tooth anomalies, and fractures, which can be caused by traumatic injuries. In the past years, some cases of oral piercing-associated tooth fractures were described, especially in young patients [12].

Dental implants are generally considered an ideal treatment option in case of missing teeth for patients with permanent dentition but a few clinical issues should be considered when this treatment is evaluated in young patients. First, dental implants are not free from biological and mechanical complications, and the longer the implants will be used, the higher the risk of complications could be. Second, the impact of facial growth and development on dental implants is well known as well as the risks of implant infraocclusion and displacement especially for implants in the esthetic area. Therefore, the autotransplantation should be considered a viable option because it can be performed in young growing patients, when implants are fully contraindicated, as it allows the maintenance of periodontal ligaments, and, consequently, the transplanted tooth can follow the facial growth pattern and can be moved orthodontically. An important consideration is the cost-effectiveness of autotransplantation: the treatment cost for an autotransplantation is definitely lower than for an implant rehabilitation. This is fully in agreement with a retrospective study where the authors have reported that the choice for the autotransplantation approach was based on the economic cost evaluation in 35% of patients [13].

Some recent reviews and meta-analyses have found that the overall survival and success rates for the autotrasplantation approach were high and ranged between 75% and 95%. Although the percentages of success are very high, a careful analysis of the scientific data could reveal a remarkable variety of the success/survival rates. Indeed, the discordance in the clinical outcomes presumably indicates a wide variety between the different scientific reports. Despite the amount of studies present in the scientific literature, the quality of

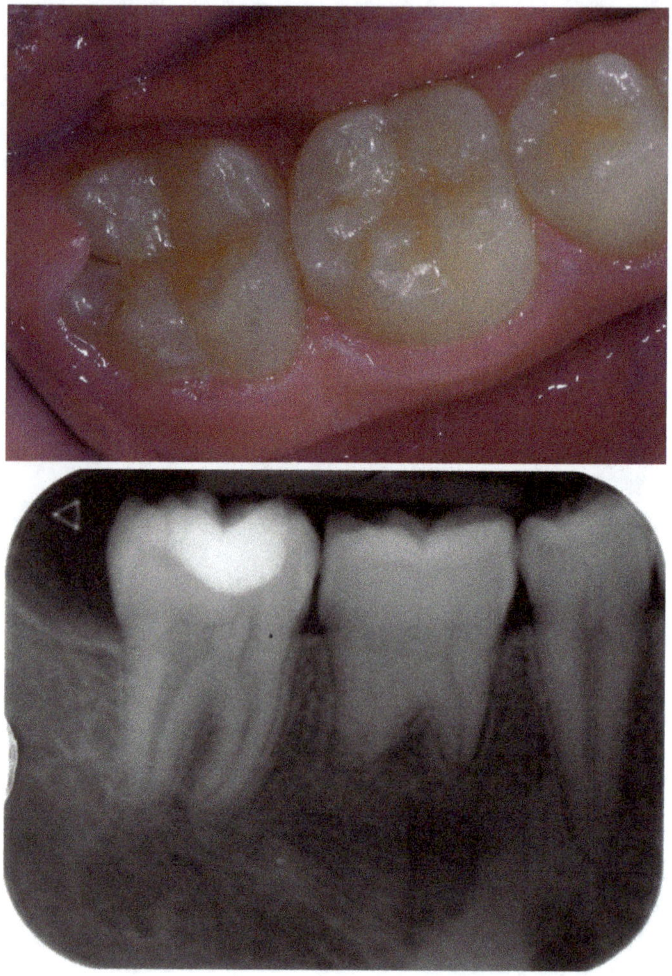

FIGURE 7: Tooth 46 at 2 years of follow-up.

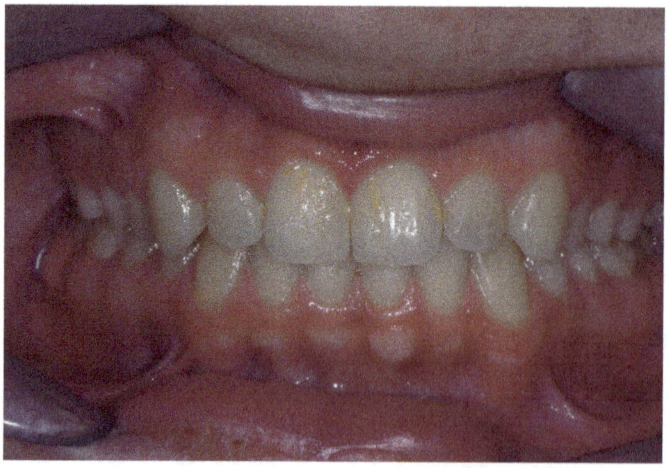

FIGURE 8: Clinical view at 2 years of follow-up.

evidence is still low because of methodological limitations and technical discrepancies among the different studies. Moreover, it has been clearly shown that multirooted teeth like molars have a significantly less favorable prognosis than single rooted teeth [14].

Several criteria have been observed as key factors for obtaining a successful autotrasplantation. The recipient sites have to be free from infections and need to have enough bone to allow an adequate stabilization for the transplanted tooth. In terms of donor sites, the teeth with uncomplete root development are the ideal candidates for transplantation because they have potential for root formation and maintained pulp vitality. Some other prognostic factors that could impact the success rates of autotransplantation are the atraumatic tooth extraction, the limitations of injuries of the root and of the periodontal ligament, minimal handling of the root, and reduced extraoral storage time. All the above reported factors are associated with minimizing the risk for periodontal ligament damage, which would predispose to the most frequent complications reported with autotransplants such as internal/external root resorption and ankylosis.

L-PRF has been claimed to promote wound healing processes and angiogenesis [10]. In the present case, the use of L-PRF at donor sites may have improved the natural process of revascularization of the transplanted teeth. Moreover, the storage of the extracted teeth in the L-PRF exudate may have contributed to the maintenance of viability of the cells of both pulp and periodontal ligament, improving the clinical outcomes.

However, the overall cumulative occurrence of complications appears to be extremely nonconsistent among different studies; ankylosis, for instance, was reported to be 40% in some studies [14] and 0% in some others [13]. Recently, a study showed that a radiographic-guided approach with the use of a replica would significantly improve the predictability of the treatment when compared to a conventional approach [15]. The hypothesis was that the use of a surgical tooth-replica to shape the receiving site could significantly decrease the risk of damaging the periodontal ligament of donor tooth and, therefore, could increase the success/survival rates of autotransplanted teeth.

The autotransplantation is a good treatment option in case of tooth loss especially for young and/or growing patients, in which dental implants are contraindicated. Moreover, the use of L-PRF in our clinical case seems to have played a beneficial role in the surgical procedure outcomes.

The absence of a good level of scientific evidence should encourage randomized controlled studies to better evaluate the usefulness of this procedure.

Authors' Contributions

All the authors approved the final version of the manuscript and agreed to be accountable for all aspects of the work.

References

[1] C. Atala-Acevedo, J. Abarca, M. J. Martínez-Zapata, J. Díaz, S. Olate, and C. Zaror, "Success rate of autotransplantation of teeth with an open apex: systematic review and meta-analysis," *Journal of Oral and Maxillofacial Surgery : Official Journal of the American Association of Oral and Maxillofacial Surgeons*, vol. 75, no. 1, pp. 35–50, 2017.

[2] S. Yang, B.-Y. Jung, and N.-S. Pang, "Outcomes of autotransplanted teeth and prognostic factors: a 10-year retrospective study," *Clinical Oral Investigations*, vol. 23, no. 1, pp. 87–98, 2019.

[3] K. Martin, S. Nathwani, and R. Bunyan, "Autotransplantation of teeth: an evidence-based approach," *British Dental Journal*, vol. 224, no. 11, pp. 861–864, 2018.

[4] K. Almpani, S. N. Papageorgiou, and M. A. Papadopoulos, "Autotransplantation of teeth in humans: a systematic review and meta-analysis," *Clinical Oral Investigations*, vol. 19, no. 6, pp. 1157–1179, 2015.

[5] J. O. Andreasen, H. U. Paulsen, Z. Yu, T. Bayer, and O. Schwartz, "A long-term study of 370 autotransplanted premolars. Part II. Tooth survival and pulp healing subsequent to transplantation," *European Journal of Orthodontics*, vol. 12, no. 1, pp. 14–24, 1990.

[6] W.-C. Chung, Y.-K. Tu, Y.-H. Lin, and H.-K. Lu, "Outcomes of autotransplanted teeth with complete root formation: a systematic review and meta-analysis," *Journal of Clinical Periodontology*, vol. 41, no. 4, pp. 412–423, 2014.

[7] J. O. Andreasen, H. U. Paulsen, Z. Yu, and O. Schwartz, "A long-term study of 370 autotransplanted premolars. Part III. Periodontal healing subsequent to transplantation," *European Journal of Orthodontics*, vol. 12, no. 1, pp. 25–37, 1990.

[8] S. A. Nagori, O. Bhutia, A. Roychoudhury, and R. M. Pandey, "Immediate autotransplantation of third molars: an experience of 57 cases," *Oral Surgery, Oral Medicine, Oral Pathology and Oral Radiology*, vol. 118, no. 4, pp. 400–407, 2014.

[9] A. Mainkar, "A systematic review of the survival of teeth intentionally replanted with a modern technique and cost-effectiveness compared with single-tooth implants," *Journal of Endodontics*, vol. 43, no. 12, pp. 1963–1968, 2017.

[10] J. Choukroun, A. Diss, A. Simonpieri et al., "Platelet-rich fibrin (PRF): a second-generation platelet concentrate. Part IV: clinical effects on tissue healing," *Oral Surgery, Oral Medicine, Oral Pathology, Oral Radiology, and Endodontics*, vol. 101, no. 3, pp. e56–e60, 2006.

[11] R. J. Miron, M. Fujioka-Kobayashi, M. Bishara, Y. Zhang, M. Hernandez, and J. Choukroun, "Platelet-rich fibrin and soft tissue wound healing: a systematic review," *Tissue Engineering. Part B, Reviews*, vol. 23, no. 1, pp. 83–99, 2017.

[12] M. R. Giuca, M. Pasini, S. Nastasio, S. D'Ercole, and D. Tripodi, "Dental and periodontal complications of labial and tongue piercing," *Journal of Biological Regulators and Homeostatic Agents*, vol. 26, no. 3, pp. 553–560, 2012.

[13] L. Boschini, M. Melillo, and F. Berton, "Long term survival of mature autotransplanted teeth: A retrospective single center analysis," *Journal of Dentistry*, vol. 98, article 103371, 2020.

[14] J. Juslin, P. Jääsaari, T. Teerijoki-Oksa, A. Suominen, and H. Thorén, "Survival of Autotransplanted Teeth With Open Apices: A Retrospective Cohort Study," *Journal of Oral and Maxillofacial Surgery : Official Journal of the American Association of Oral and Maxillofacial Surgeons*, vol. 78, no. 6, pp. 902.e1–902.e9, 2020.

[15] M. EzEldeen, J. Wyatt, A. Al-Rimawi et al., "Use of CBCT guidance for tooth autotransplantation in children," *Journal of Dental Research*, vol. 98, no. 4, pp. 406–413, 2019.

27

One-Piece Titanium Implants: Retrospective Case Series

Gunar Wagner[1] **and Dieter Hartung**[2]

[1]*Department of Restorative Dentistry and Periodontology, University Medical Center Leipzig, 04103 Leipzig, Germany*
[2]*Dental Practice, 37213 Witzenhausen, Germany*

Correspondence should be addressed to Gunar Wagner; gwa@rheinbogenklinik.de

Academic Editor: Sukumaran Anil

Purpose. One-piece titanium implants are not routinely used for reconstruction after tooth loss. Several limitations seemed to be apparent although the concept provides a straightforward approach for different clinical situations. A clinical documentation of five prosthetic restorations with one-piece titanium implants serving as a relevant treatment option in dental surgery is pursued. We demonstrate the feasibility and benefits of one-piece titanium implants for fixed dental prosthesis. Detailed descriptions of the technical features and the surgical approach by means of clinical cases are given. The prosthetic workflow when working with one-piece titanium implants is depicted in detail as well as examples for implant-supported tooth replacement in the posterior region and the esthetic zone. Conditions of applications regarding different timing of implant placement using the system and its limitations are discussed. *Results.* Clinical cases with a follow-up period of up to 10 years are presented to prove the long-term success of one-piece titanium implants in terms of bone and soft-tissue stability respecting the biological criteria for periodontal health. *Conclusions.* One-piece titanium implants represent a reliable treatment method for single-tooth replacements. Clinical success with long-time bone stability around the implantation site can be achieved. Taken into account the requirements for periodontal tissue stability, uneventful healing without extensive tissue loss is demonstrated by means of clinical cases presenting patients with periodontitis.

1. Introduction

Although dental implant therapy can be considered a standard procedure, various biological and technical aspects must be considered to avoid incidence and progression of peri-implant mucositis and peri-implantitis [1]. Clinical success of dental titanium implants to preserve marginal bone and soft-tissue levels is still one of the most commonly studied subjects in modern dentistry leading to the emergence of various technical and surgical developments [2–4]. The majority of dental implants used in the clinical field remain two-piece implants. The implant-abutment interface of two-piece implants is usually positioned at the epicrestal or subcrestal level. Frequently bone loss of 1.5-2 mm vertically and 1.5 mm horizontally can be observed around dental implants. This is widely accepted if later bone loss within one year after loading does not exceed 0.2 mm annually [5–7]. Nonetheless, peri-implantitis progresses in a nonlinear accelerating pattern and the majority of cases occur within 3 years of function [8]. Several factors are being discussed to be of significant importance to maintain peri-implant health. Hard- and soft-tissue deficiencies can lead to complications and impaired implant survival [9]. The clinical circumstances in patients with periodontitis are challenging and should be taken into account during implant therapy. A common threat for recession formation around dental implants is posed by repeated changes of the implant-abutment interface [10, 11]. To stabilize the soft-tissue thickness around dental implants, platform-switching concepts or the one abutment-one time protocol was developed to eliminate the potential for disturbances to the peri-implant mucosal barrier [3, 12]. One-piece titanium implants were originally introduced to the market with a sturdy design for minimally invasive and conventional prosthetic methods enabling restoration of single-tooth defects. Due to high primary stability, it was proposed that early loading using immediate implant placement could therefore be performed [13, 14]. The absence of a microgap and abutment complications remains favourable in the oral cavity [15]. The macroconfiguration design of one-piece titanium implants facilitates high insertion torque in situations with varying bone density. This could be of importance considering the vulnerable implant-abutment connection in two-piece implants leading to technical failures. This concept was not further extended due to lower success rates and evident bone loss after one year within a specific titanium implant system [16, 17]. Within the limitations of the current case series, different clinical situations are used to illustrate recent developments and benefits introducing the one-piece titanium implant system FairOne™ (FairImplant GmbH, Bönningstedt, Germany) to achieve periodontal stability and long-term success.

2. One-Piece Implant System

The one-piece titanium implant FairOne™ (FairImplant GmbH, Bönningstedt, Germany) was introduced to the market in 2006. The macro geometry and the surface design are constructed with an emphasis on periodontal soft-tissue integration and peri-implant stability to achieve best clinical results. The conical-shaped implant made of titanium medical grade four is composed of self-tapping threads and congruent drills. Three prosthetic flanks at the coronal part ensure precise immediate impression or performance of digital scanning processes. Taken into account the complex interplay between scalloped bone topography and different gingival profiles, this one-piece implant is designed with a continuous rough surface promoting long-term clinical stability [18, 19]. Lack of an implant-abutment connection with formation of a microgap is beneficial for one-piece implants since this could promote adherence of inflammatory cells accompanied with a significant peri-implant bone loss [20]. The moderately rough surface at the prosthetic head promotes an adequate transition from soft- to hard-tissue connection which is aimed at combining undisturbed osseointegration and periodontal healing [21]. Osteoconduction on both etched and commercially pure titanium surfaces could be significantly increased with modified nanoscale deposits of calcium phosphate crystals on the implant surface [22, 23]. Therefore, implant threads are additionally coated with a resorbable calcium phosphate layer for improved osseointegration (BONIT®, DOT GmbH, Rostock, Germany). The conical shape of the implant body was designed to achieve high primary stability [24]. The FairOne™ is designed with a round apex to work as a bone condenser and to protect surrounding anatomical structures. Maxillary sinus lift procedures could be facilitated by preservation of the fragile mucosa (Figure 1).

A drilling-protocol with depth and diameter conformed instruments was specially developed for this system. During osteotomy, a shaping-drill with conical design corresponding to the tapered design of the implant is able to avoid unnecessary damage of osseous structures during implant bed preparation. Additionally, given the design of the drill, it is easy to harvest autologous bone chips with high quality at the site of osteotomy. When necessary, a thread cutter allows for low insertion-torque during preparation but in the large majority

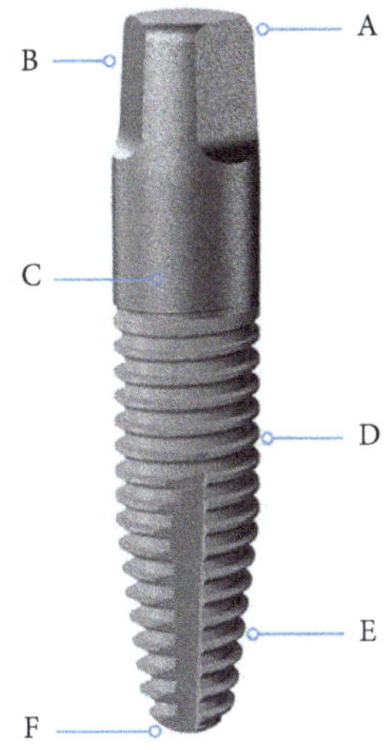

FIGURE 1: Features of the one-piece conical titanium implant FairOne™: (a) preparable head: 3°, (b) three prosthetic flanks for immediate impressions or digital scanning processes, height: 3.5 mm; (c) transition zone with continuous rough surface (1.5-2.5 μm), height: 4 mm; (d) surface with resorbable CaP-coating (BONIT®), roughness: 4 μm, conical shape for high primary stability; (e) self-tapping threads and congruent drills for iBIC; (f) round apex designed to protect anatomical structures.

of cases, the self-tapping threads on the implant surface allow for ideal primary stability (Figure 2).

When placing implants, a continuous stability during the healing phase is one of the key factors for success. Usually after three to four weeks, primary stability is minimized due to increased osteoclastic activity around implants. New bone formation leading to secondary stability has not yet occurred, and the overall stability receives a significant drop [25]. The bone metabolic activity could also be significantly influenced depending on the magnitude and period of loading [26]. The one-piece implant and the concerted drilling protocol are aimed at achieving an optimized initial bone-implant contact (iBIC) to facilitate immediate implant placement.

3. Clinical Case 1: Surgical Procedure Placing One-Piece Implants

In the following case, a 60-year-old, healthy male patient received restorative therapy with a one-piece implant after tooth loss. The patient has undergone periodontal treatment in the past. Keratinized gingiva around dental implants is important for long-term success of the rehabilitation. If the tissue thickness is 2.0 mm or less, crestal bone loss up to 1.45 mm may occur [27]. The amount of KG at the desired site for implantation was sufficient, and surgery could be performed without soft-tissue grafting. Bone sounding was performed to assess the defect morphology presurgically and provide sufficient information for the design of the flap (Figure 3(a)). The surgical procedures were performed using a microsurgical approach. Surgical access was obtained by

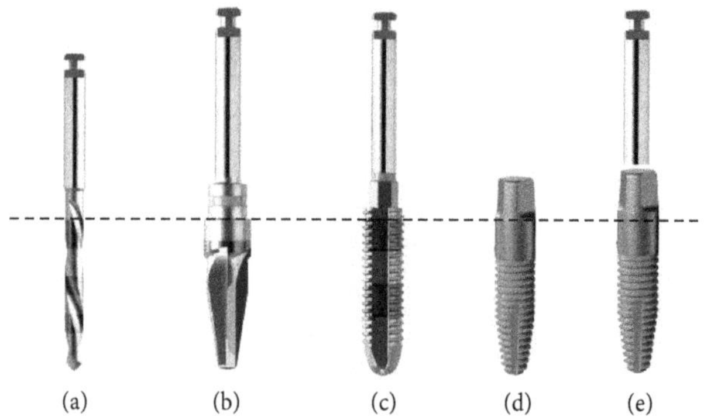

FIGURE 2: (a) Predrilling instrument ø 2.0 mm; (b) shaping-drill with conical design for bone harvesting during preparation, variable diameter and length; (c) thread cutter (optional); (d) one-piece implant (FairOne™) with self-tapping thread; (e) overlapping view of shaping-drill with corresponding tapered design of the FairOne™ (B+D).

preparation of a trapezoidal full-thickness flap. Particular attention was paid in the preservation of the adjacent soft tissue. The oral portion of the interdental periodontal complex was left undetached. The flap was gently elevated to the buccal site before implantation (Figure 3(b)). After implant-bed preparation using the drilling-protocol, a one-piece implant (FairOne™; diameter: 5.0 mm and length: 10 mm) was placed (Figures 3(c) and 3(d)). The insertion torque of 50 Ncm was applied. Special attention should be paid since the buccal area of the bone crest is usually positioned more apically than the mesial and distal flanks of the implant site. The flap was apically repositioned and sutured in a tension-free condition (Seralon®, D1S 15, 5-0, Serag-Wiessner, Naila, Germany) providing a sufficient buccal preservation of at least 4 mm of KG at the healing site (Figures 3(e) and 3(f)). After one week of nonsubmerged healing, the surgical site showed proper conditions showing no signs of recession formation (Figure 3(g)). Sutures were removed postsurgically, and the patient was asked to abstain from mechanical oral hygiene in the area for two weeks. A chlorhexidine mouth rinse CHX 0.2%, (Dynexidin® forte, Kreussler & Co. GmbH, Wiesbaden, Germany) was used for chemical biofilm control. After 12 weeks of implantation, the surgical site showed perfect conditions for single-tooth replacement with a thick KG around the implant (Figure 3(h)). The prosthetic treatment could be finalized using a metal-supported ceramic. The crown was designed with a mesial cantilever achieving a pontic design in order to allow for a proper interdental cleaning (Figure 3(i)). The postinterventional maintenance protocol included professional biofilm debridement at 1-month intervals up to 3 months postoperatively, followed by a recall visit at 6 months postoperatively. Motivation for personal plaque control was reinforced at each recall visit. The radiographic evaluation showed no signs of bone resorption and a biological stable situation even after nine years of implant treatment (Figures 3(j)–3(l)). The patient had not experienced complications during the procedure and recovered without complaints.

4. Clinical Case 2: Demonstrating the Prosthetic Workflow Using FairOne™

For single crown restorations, the following case is aimed at illustrating the prosthetic procedure. A 23-year-old, healthy female patient diagnosed with periodontitis suffered from apical periodontitis after root canal treatment on tooth 36. Due to a hopeless prognosis, a decision was made to extract the tooth and to use delayed implantation with a one-piece implant. The clinical situation after atraumatic extraction showed no signs of inflammation and sufficient quantity of soft tissue (Figure 4(a)). Assessment of the correct position and dimensions for the planned reconstruction was realized using a radiograph with calibration ball. After implantation with a one-piece implant (FairOne™; diameter: 5.0 mm and length: 10 mm), it was ensured that no interference in the static or dynamic occlusion is occurring during healing. Minimal adjustments can be performed by means of the preparable head. In order to achieve accurate transmission for the prosthetic restoration, the geometric design should be preserved. This provides the possibility for direct impressions or digital scanning with high-detail reproduction and precision. In the posterior region, no provisional restoration was necessary during the healing phase, since there is no additional surgery for uncovering of the implant and no abutment dis-/reconnection shaping of the emergence profile occurred early during the initial healing phase on the continuous rough surface (Figure 4(b)). Additionally, the baseline of the bone crest in the mesial and distal direction is documented (Figure 4(g)). The impression could be performed using a double-mix technique with a polyether (Impregum™, 3M, Landsberg am Lech, Germany) (Figure 4(c)). Within the laboratory process, a master cast in conjunction with an implant analog and gingival mask was used adjusting the prosthetic restoration and ensuring that the emergence profile of the crown is optimally contoured (Figure 4(d)). In cases were the clinical situation causes interference with the crown design, a transfer coping joined with pattern resin is fabricated. This could enable the surgeon to realize defined adjustments for the prosthetic head prior to the crown fitting and cementation process (Figure 4(e)). CAD/CAM processing is possible with the use of a digital implant model analog (CAM-Analog, FairImplant GmbH, Bönningstedt, Germany). The final restoration was placed using a metal-supported ceramic crown (Figure 4(f)). Provisional cementation for up to four weeks securing the final fitting of the contact situation in the approximal area and adjustment of the occlusal situation as well as the color of the crown was conducted with eugenol-free temporary cement (TempBondNE™, Kerr GmbH, Bioggio, Switzerland). The permanent cementation was usually conducted using a dual-curing dimethacrylate composite with a custom analog for precementation to significantly reduce excess cement (PANAVIA F™, Kuraray Noritake, Tokyo, Japan). Implant placement should ideally by controlled by periapical radiographs that were taken by the use of a long-cone paralleling technique. After 10 weeks of implant treatment, a slight loss in bone height adjacent to the implant in the mesial and distal direction could be observed but no excess of cement is

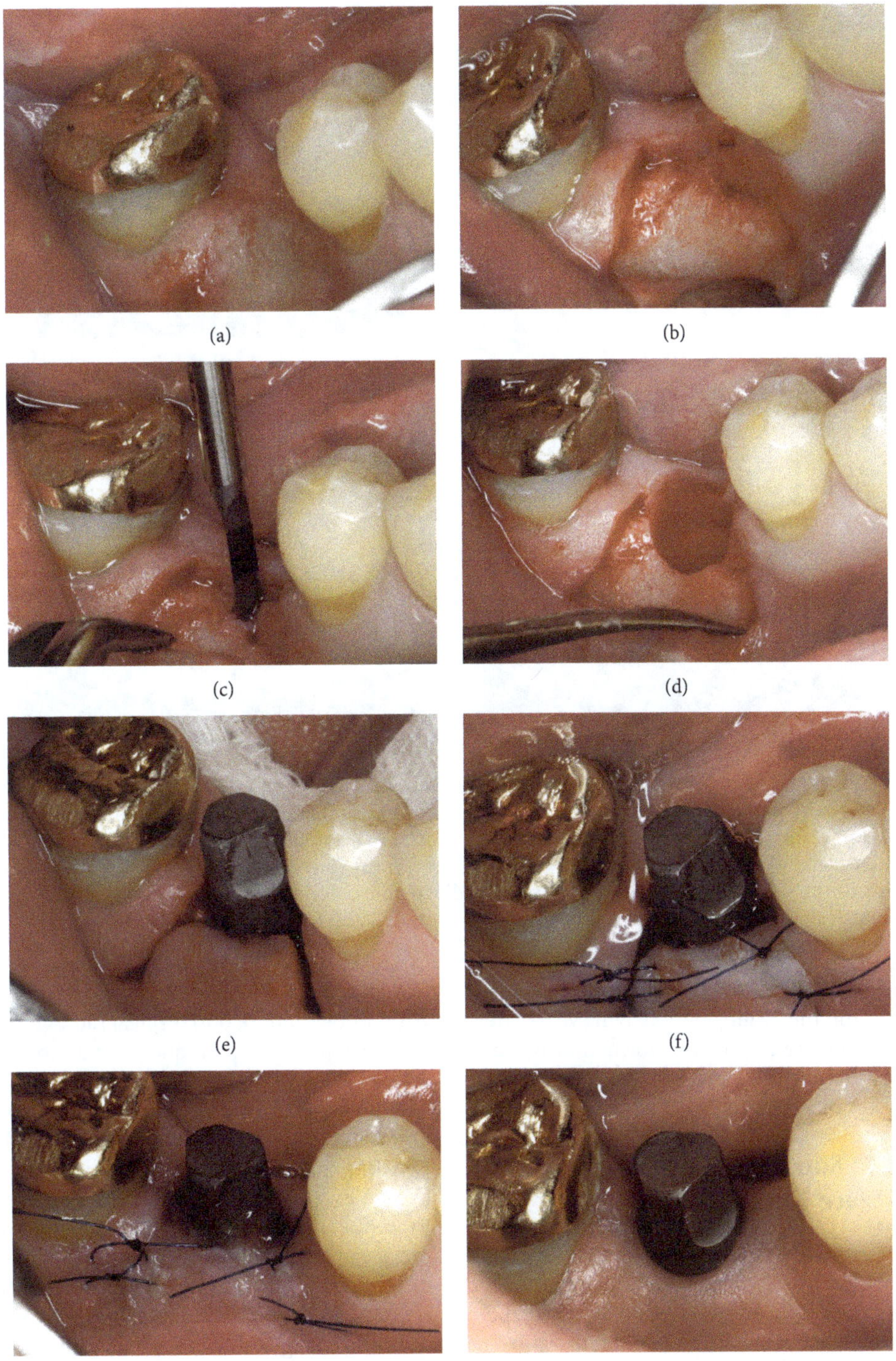

(a) (b) (c) (d) (e) (f) (g) (h)

Figure 3: Continued.

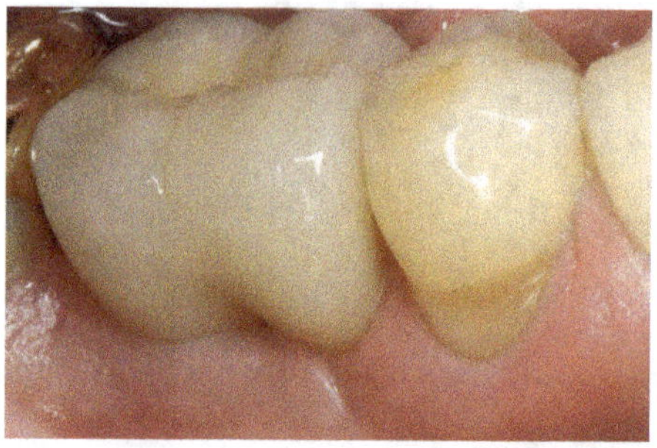

(i)

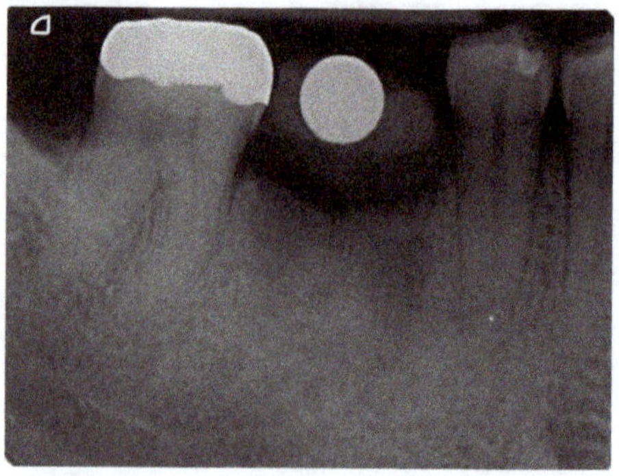

(j)

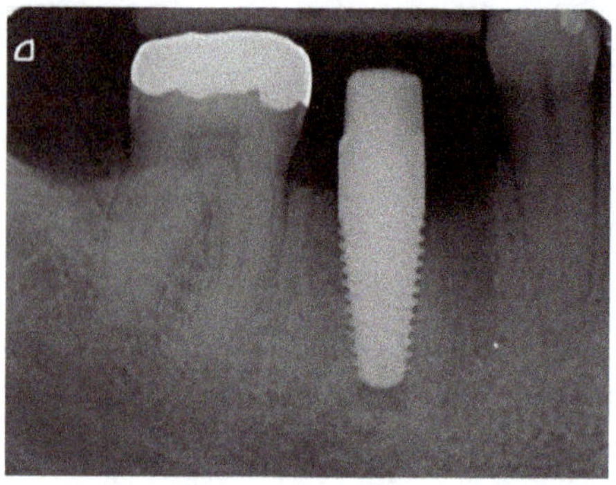

(k)

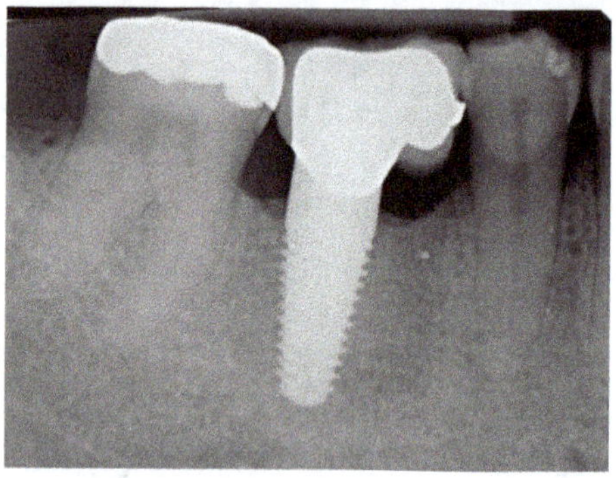

(l)

Figure 3: Implantation of one-piece implant (clinical procedure): (a) clinical situation presurgically; (b) elevation of full-thickness flap with preservation of peripheral periodontium at adjacent teeth; (c) implant bed preparation, predrilling instrument; (d) processed implantation site using drilling protocol; (e) placement of one-piece implant with spatial orientation aligned to the natural dentition; (f) apical repositioned and sutured flap; (g) clinical situation one week after surgery; (h) clinical situation 12 weeks after surgery; (i) single crown prosthetic restoration with mesial pontic design; (j) presurgical radiographic control, calibration ball for planning of implantation; (k) postsurgical radiograph taken directly after implant placement; (l) radiographic control nine years after treatment.

evident (Figure 4(h)). The patient reported no complications during the procedure and the healing period. Nine years after implant placement, remineralisation and formation of new bone at the peri-implant interface can be observed presenting stable biological conditions (Figure 4(i)).

5. Clinical Case 3: Soft-Tissue Augmentation around One-Piece Implants

Single-tooth replacements of interdental spaces or edentulous areas can be achieved with one-piece implants. In the following case, a 50-year-old, healthy male patient who experienced periodontal treatment in the past, demonstrating a thin alveolar crest, was treated with one-piece titanium implants at the left side of the mandible. The keratinized tissue around the targeted implant site was reduced (Figure 5(a)). After augmentation of a free gingival graft (FGG) harvested from the palate, the buccal aspect of the recipient site could be notably expanded to assure thick gingival conditions with keratinized tissue (Figures 5(b) and 5(c)). After uneventful healing of the graft, implant placement with adequate alignment of two implants could be performed (FairOne™; diameter: 4.2 mm and length: 10 mm). An insertion torque of 30 Ncm was applied. A tension-free suturing was conducted (Seralon®, D1S 15, 5-0, Serag-Wiessner, Naila, Germany) providing a sufficient buccal preservation of at least 4 mm of KG at the healing site (Figure 5(d)). After implantation, postsurgical radiographs were taken with a proper parallel technique to monitor the bone crest and correct positioning of the implants (Figure 5(g)). After a healing period of thirteen weeks, successful periodontal integration could be documented (Figure 5(e)). Splinting of the two implants was performed using a flowable composite (Tetric Evo Ceram®, Ivoclar Vivadent, Schaan, Lichtenstein) to support osseointegration. Implants were restored with metal-supported ceramic crowns to allow for full recovery of the masticatory function within the jaw segment (Figure 5(f)). No patient reported complaints could be noticed during the whole procedure. To control for excess cement and proper positioning of the crown, a radiographic control was performed (Figure 5(h)). Nine years after implant placement, a stable osseous situation could be documented and the clinical situation does not indicate the presence of peri-implantitis (Figure 5(i)).

6. Clinical Case 4: Delayed Implantation in the Esthetic Area

The following case illustrates the performance of one-piece titanium implants for complete functional and esthetic rehabilitation in the esthetic zone. A 49-year-old male patient suffering from glaucoma and hypertension was

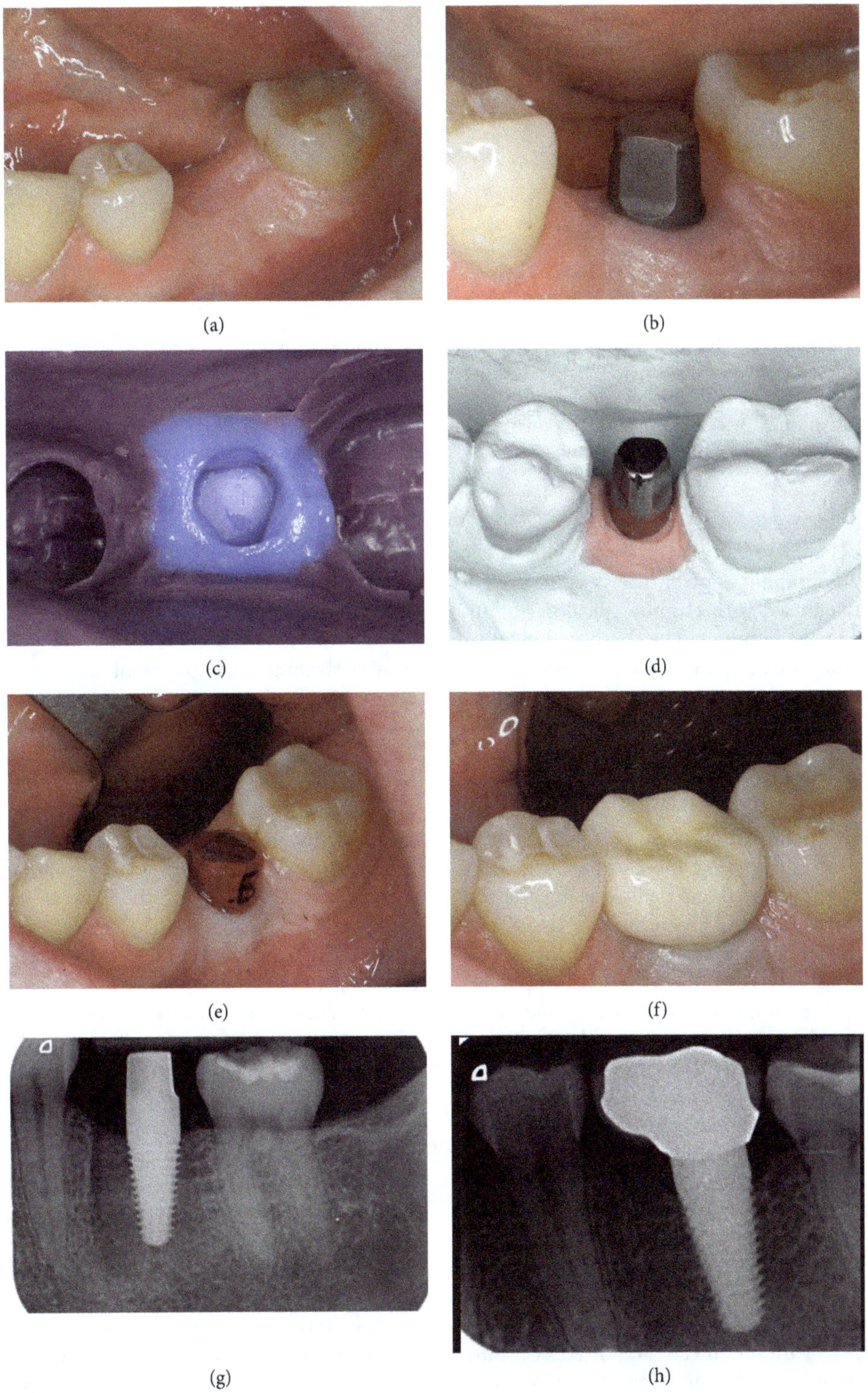

(a) (b) (c) (d) (e) (f) (g) (h)

FIGURE 4: Continued.

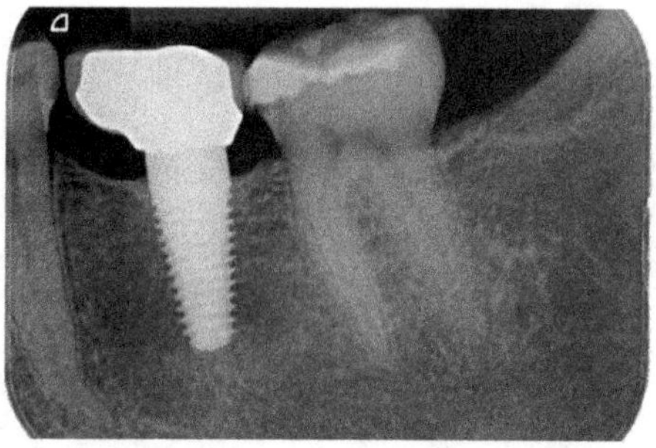

(i)

Figure 4: Prosthetic workflow for the one-piece implant FairOne™: (a) clinical situation presurgically presenting sufficient keratinized gingiva around implant site; (b) clinical situation after healing period of 12 weeks; (c) impression with double-mix technique; (d) laboratory processing, master cast with implant analog, and gingival mask; (e) clinical preparation using a transfer coping for occlusal adaption; (f) clinical situation with cemented implant crown (mesial pontic design); (g) postoperative radiographic control after delayed implantation; (h) radiographic evaluation four months after prosthetic restoration; (i) radiographic control nine years after implant treatment.

seeking help at the dental practice with complaints in the upper jaw. After radiographic control, the maxillary right lateral incisor was diagnosed with chronic apical periodontitis following root canal treatment. The tooth had a hopeless prognosis but the surrounding bone was assessed to be appropriate for implantation (Figure 6(d)). Subsequent to minimal invasive extraction, socket preservation with soft-tissue augmentation by means of a free gingival graft was conducted (Figure 6(a)). Healing occurred uneventful, and soft-tissue dimensions could be preserved (Figure 6(b)). The implantation was performed three months after extraction. To support the alveolar ridge during implantation, a connective tissue pedicle using the roll technique was performed [28]. The connective tissue was prepared from the palatinal area and rotated to the buccal site of the implantation site (Figure 6(c)). After implantation of the one-piece implant (FairOne™; diameter: 5.0 mm and length: 10 mm) (Figure 6(e)), the flap was repositioned and tension-free suturing was secured (Figure 6(f)). A temporary provisional composite crown for esthetic demands was delivered directly after implantation (Figure 6(g)). After implantation, postsurgical radiographs were taken with a proper parallel technique to monitor the bone crest and correct positioning of the implants (Figure 6(h)). One week after uneventful healing, sutures could be removed with interdental papilla remained well preserved (Figure 6(i)). The patient reported only slight pain directly postoperative. The composite crown was replaced with a metal-supported ceramic crown, and after four months of healing, stable soft-tissue conditions without recession formation could be documented (Figure 6(j)). The clinical and radiological situation remained stable even 10 years after intervention with a good prognosis (Figures 6(k) and 6(l)).

7. Clinical Case 5: Immediate Implantation in the Esthetic Area

Immediate placement using one-piece titanium implants could be part of routine clinical practice. After fracture of the maxillary left central incisor, a 54-year-old, healthy patient who received periodontal treatment in the past was administered to implant therapy using FairOne™. The clinical situation does not support any symptoms of severe infection or traumatic damages of the surrounding soft tissue (Figure 7(a)). Preoperative radiographs provide information about the osseous environment prior to implant therapy. These served as a baseline image to monitor the height of the bone to implant contact for further diagnosis and prevention of peri-implantitis (Figures 7(g) and 7(h)). The patient decided for immediate implant therapy after discussing treatment options. During atraumatic minimal invasive extraction, debonding of the neighboring implant crown took place presenting healthy soft-tissue conditions (Figure 7(b)). After complete extraction, a precise cleaning and rinsing of the extraction socket was conducted (Figure 7(c)). Immediate placement using a one-piece titanium implant (FairOne™; diameter: 4.2 mm and length: 13 mm) was performed, and complete wound closure could be carried out establishing primary stability (Figure 7(d)). A temporary provisional composite crown for esthetic demands was delivered, and rebonding of the adjacent implant crown was conducted. Appropriate design of the provisional restoration was considered to preserve soft-tissue stability around the implants during healing period (Figure 7(e)). Following healing, a temporary metal-supported ceramic crown could be provided five months after implant therapy (Figure 7(f)). The patient was satisfied and had no complaints during the whole procedure. The radiographic control showed stable osseous conditions for the one-piece implant of the maxillary first central incisor (Figure 7(i)). Eight years after the first implantation, a second one-piece implant had to be inserted for the left lateral incisor. A postsurgical radiograph taken directly after immediate implantation of the left central incisor did not show further bone loss evident in the area of interest. The preceding interventions using FairOne™ at adjacent teeth are clinically and radiologically inconspicuous (Figure 7(j)). The radiographic control of nine months after immediate implantation revealed bone stability for all one-piece titanium implants (Figure 7(k)).

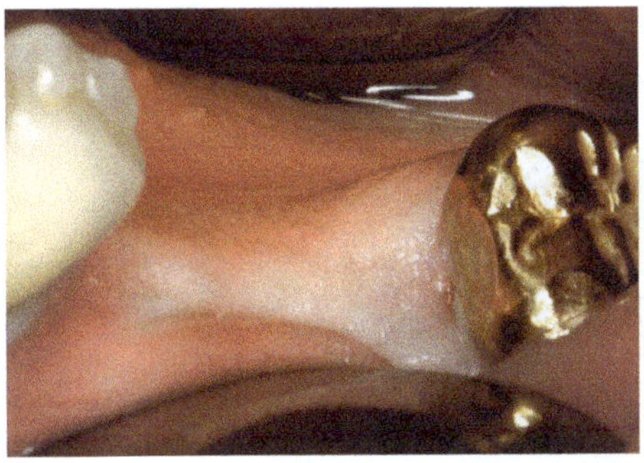

(a)

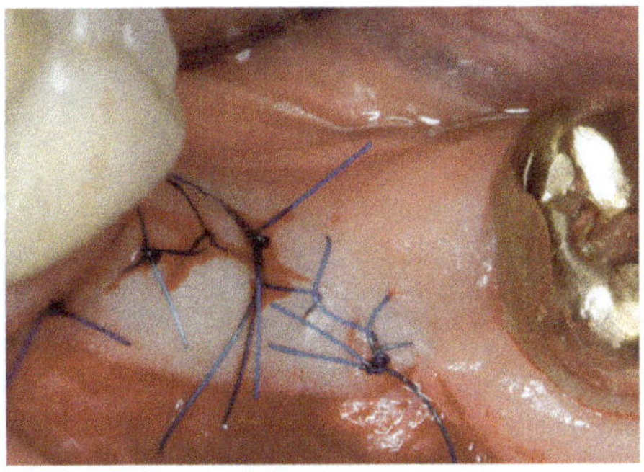

(b)

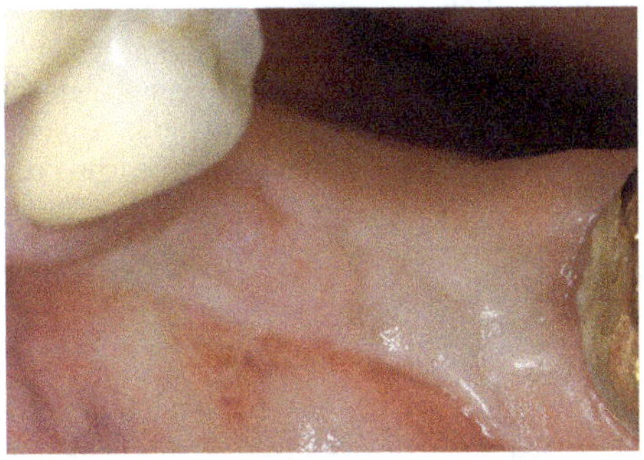

(c)

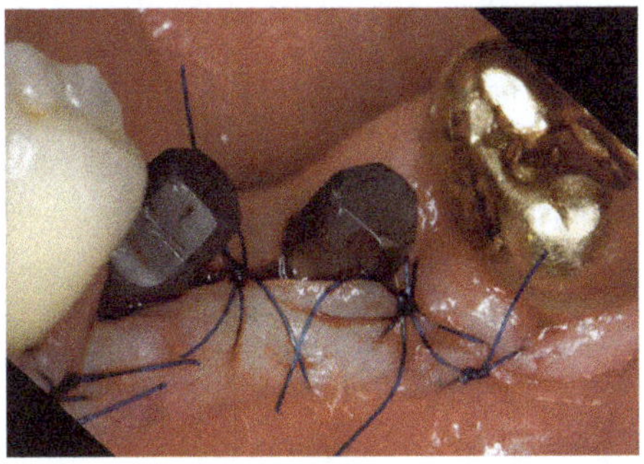

(d)

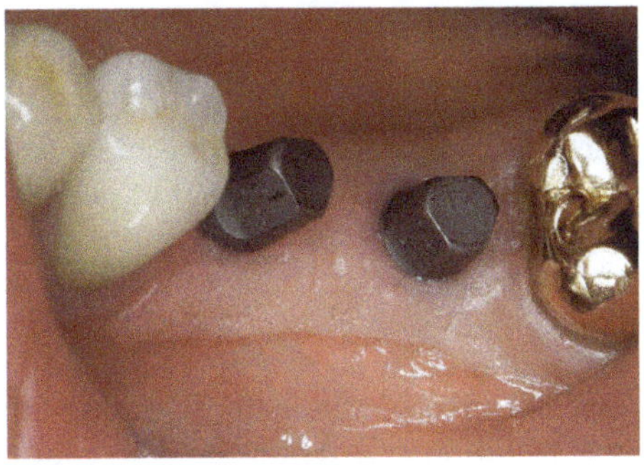

(e)

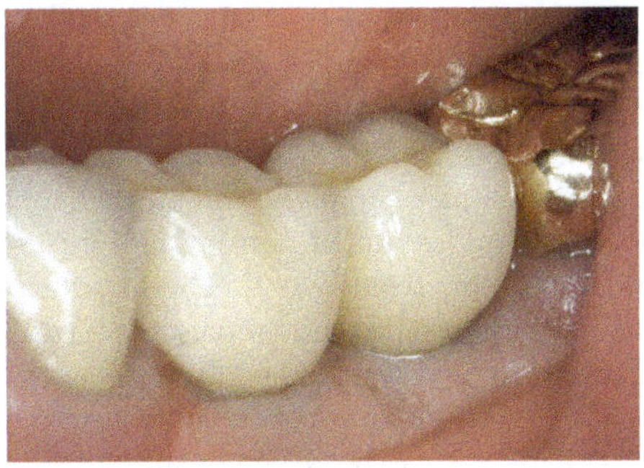

(f)

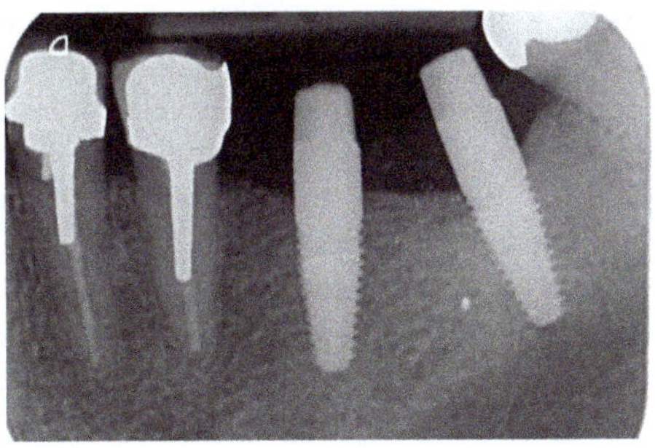

(g)

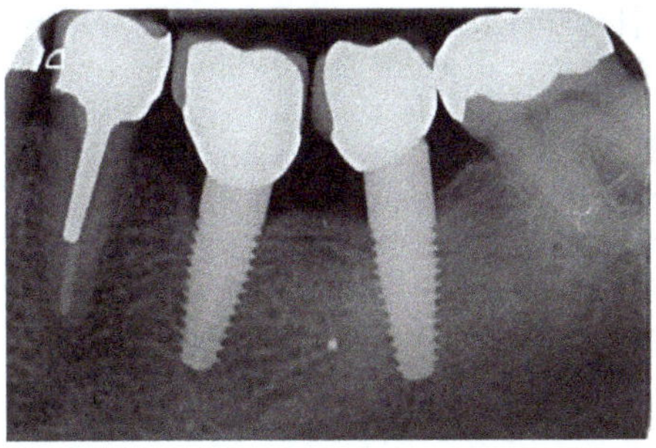

(h)

FIGURE 5: Continued.

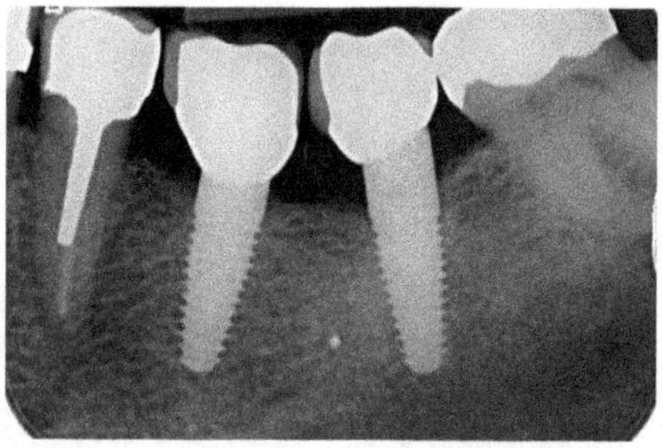

(i)

Figure 5: Soft-tissue augmentation in the region of the planned implantation: (a) clinical situation presurgically presenting small alveolar crest and reduced width of keratinized gingiva around implant site; (b) augmentation of free gingival graft at the buccal aspect; (c) clinical situation six weeks after healing; (d) postoperative clinical situation after implantation of two one-piece implants, flap closure; (e) clinical situation after 12 weeks of transgingival healing; (f) prosthetic restoration six months after implantation, cemented single crowns; (g) radiographic control after implantation; (h) postsurgical radiograph taken directly after cementation of single crowns; (i) radiographic control nine years after implant treatment.

8. Discussion

Critical evaluations revealed lower success rates and more bone resorption for one-piece implants with direct loading [16]. It must be considered that the clinical success for restorations using one piece-implants is determined by the implant design, insertion depth, and loading protocols. Marginal bone loss around two-piece implants of more than 0.44 mm/year could be an indication of peri-implant bone loss progression and should be avoided [29]. The fact that transgingival healing of one-piece implants represents a risk factor for microbial infection by direct contact via pathogens from the oral cavity at the mucogingival border is a common argument. In contrast, no differences between nonsubmerged and submerged healing in terms of significant soft-tissue loss could be revealed [15]. Furthermore, experimental studies concluded that the biological width (BW) dimensions for one-piece implants are favourable compared to two-piece implants and were more similar to the natural dentition [30]. Taken into account the criteria for periodontal stability, we could demonstrate successful healing of one-piece implants in the posterior region without loss of the BW resulting in long-term success. Disadvantages discussed leading to impairments of peri-implant health are the inevitable cementation process of one-piece implants without the possibility of screw-retained restorations. In this context, one has to take into account that two-piece implants with prefabricated abutments and a plain platform connection in the crestal area could not compensate the natural course of the peri-implant soft-tissue outline or the scalloped alveolar leading to situations where the cementation gap is positioned much deeper subgingivally than necessary. Consequently, the crown margin does not remain accessible for cleansing and oral hygiene resulting in increased probability for cementation-associated peri-implantitis [31]. Although recent evidence found no significant influence on the positioning of the implant regarding the alveolar crest [32], bacterial colonization of the implant-abutment junction could be facilitated with a subcrestal positioning of the implant [33]. Correct positioning of the crown margin at the level of the mucosal margin could easily be achieved with one-piece implants. Through the continuous rough surface of the FairOne™, possible resorption processes occurring in the early phase of healing could be prevented, as the alignment of the implant-abutment interface with the bone crest is not required. It is important to note that excessive cleansing after cementation of the implant-crown and postsurgical radiographic documentation is recommended not only to control for excess cement but also to document the baseline conditions of the surrounding bone [34]. Systematic analysis revealed that soft-tissue thickness around implants is a decisive factor for early remodeling. In contrast to natural teeth, implants have to be supported with approximately 4 mm of vertical soft tissue as the minimum required height for biological stability [24]. Lack of attached gingiva around dental implants could otherwise lead to increased inflammation and the occurrence of mucositis [35]. Hence, there is a higher risk of gingival recession around implants, and marginal bone loss is more likely to occur [36, 37]. This could additionally lead to patient discomfort especially during brushing and hygiene [38]. In order to prevent soft-tissue dehiscence's caused by the lack of limited peri-implant soft-tissue thickness and the absence of adequate keratinized mucosa, a consequent periodontal management using mucogingival surgery to boost the biotype should be a prerequisite for dental implants [39, 40]. A stable soft-tissue seal as protection barrier from a contaminated intraoral environment is an important factor stabilizing the BW around dental implants [41]. Soft-tissue augmentation remains recommended if necessary when using one-piece implant as demonstrated. Additionally, a significant influence of the presence/absence of a microgap between the implant and the abutment is a decisive factor [42]. X-ray microtomographic imaging on different types of implant-abutment joints reveals bacterial penetration that could be responsible for peri-implant pathologies [43, 44]. Considering these findings, one-piece implants

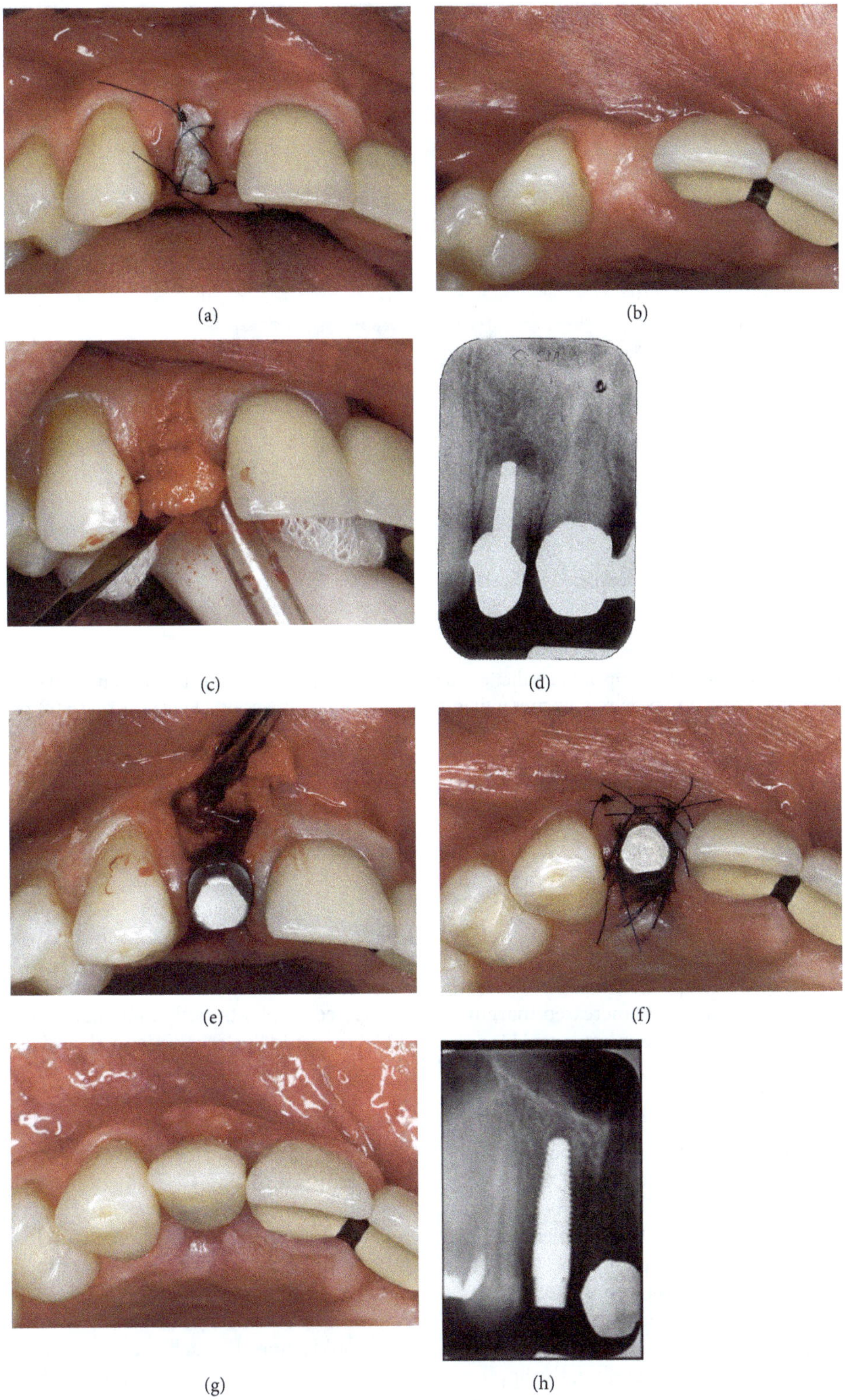

Figure 6: Continued.

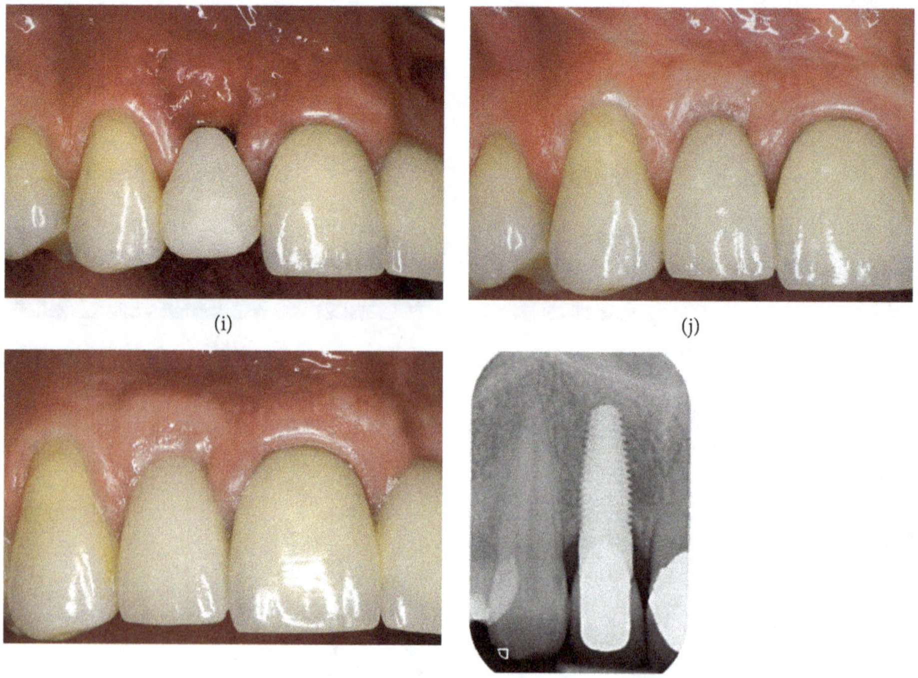

(i) (j) (k) (l)

FIGURE 6: Delayed implantation of one-piece implant in esthetic zone: (a) clinical situation after extraction and socket preservation with soft-tissue augmentation; (b) clinical situation presurgically presenting small horizontal dimension of alveolar ridge; (c) reflection of connective tissue pedicle using roll technique with implant placement; (d) initial radiographic situation with hopeless tooth; (e) clinical situation after implant placement; (f) suturing and fixation of connective tissue at the buccal site; (g) healing after one week and suture removal, immediate provisional restoration (occlusal view); (h) radiographic control after implantation; (i) healing period one week after implantation with provisional restoration (buccal view); (j) prosthetic restoration with single crown four months after healing; (k) clinical situation 10 years after intervention; (l) radiographic control 10 years after implant treatment.

without the formation of a microgap could possibly reduce the bacterial load at critical sites. Repeated abutment disconnections and reconnections considerably increased marginal bone loss and buccal recession in two-piece implants [11, 45]. Data from meta-analyses proofed that less bone resorption and soft-tissue shifts occur by preventing repeated abutment changes for platform switched implants [46]. Further investigations demonstrated a superior method to compensate such peri-implant tissue changes by using one-time abutments [47]. These findings support the idea of undisturbed healing and periodontal integration provided by one-piece dental implants. When placing immediate implants, the goal is to achieve the most beneficial initial bone-implant contact (iBIC) enabling a transition from primary mechanical stability, provided by the design of the implant body, to biologic stability due to new bone formation. Therefore, the application of an ideal insertion torque is of particular interest when placing implants. High insertion torque (≥40 Ncm) was discussed to cause strong compression and distortion in the peri-implant bone leading to necrosis of the osteocytes due to disturbed microcirculation. In contrast, clinical and radiographical studies proofed that high insertion torque does not impair crestal bone levels [48]. Although small cracks at the implant sites could be revealed histologically, no bone resorption was detected supporting the possibility of increased remodeling processes that occur to repair microcracked bone [49]. In this context, the application of one-piece implants with high insertion torque of at least 32 Ncm could be recommended and is supported by the design of the FairOne™. This is of particular interest when performing immediate implant placement securing primary stability even in challenging situations. However, a recent systematic review demonstrates that loading protocols are not likely to influence the clinical outcomes, including implant survival and peri-implant stability regarding implant therapy for single tooth [50]. One-piece implants could meet the requirements for esthetic success providing a scalloped gingival line similar to natural teeth. Nevertheless, in situations where primary stability could not be achieved, one-piece implants have limitations. In such cases, a submerged healing using a two-piece implant would be the treatment of choice. Spatial positioning with profound backward planning is decisive for the prosthetic treatment as the implant system is limited for modifications compared to an individual abutment system using two-piece implants. Systematic analysis for one-piece implants revealed long-term survival rates similar to two-piece designs. Nonetheless, technical and biological complications are still being observed frequently for both systems [51, 52]. The design and the

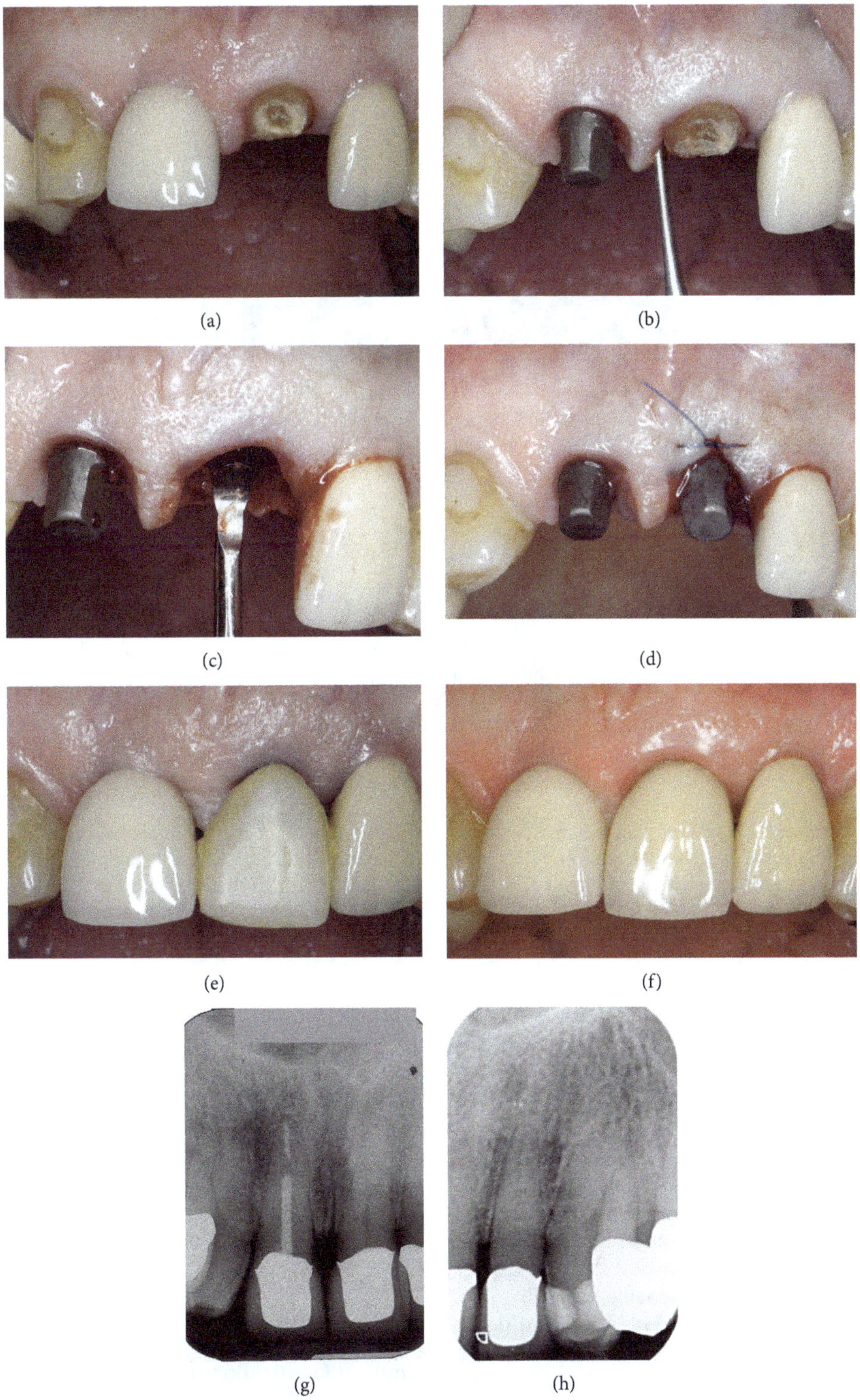

Figure 7: Continued.

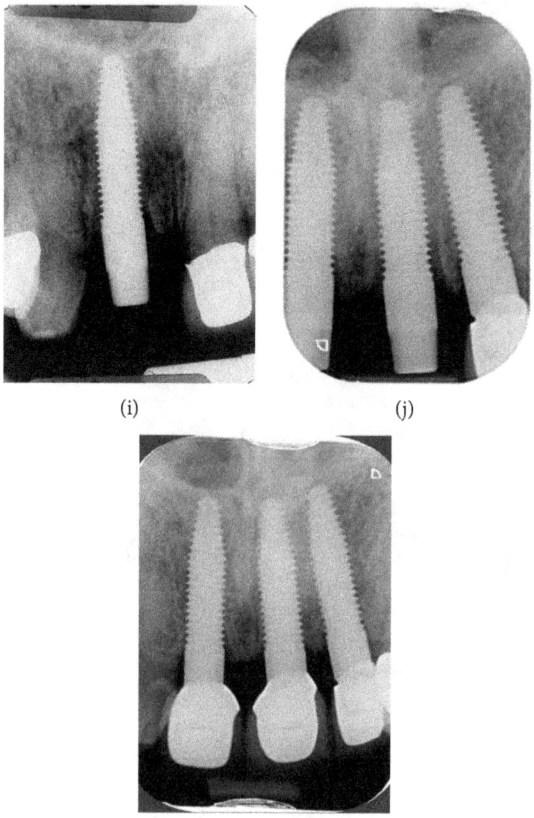

(i) (j) (k)

Figure 7: Immediate restoration of one-piece implant in esthetic zone: (a) clinical situation after fracture of left central incisor, (b) atraumatic extraction of remaining tooth, (c) complete extraction and cleaning of alveolar ridge, (d) clinical situation after immediate implant placement, (e) provisional restoration, reattachment of implant crown for right central incisor, (f) prosthetic restoration with single crown five months after healing, (g) initial radiographic situation with hopeless right central incisor, (h) radiographic situation before implantation of left lateral incisor, (i) radiographic control after implantation of first right incisor, (j) radiographic control after immediate implantation of left central incisor, and (k) radiographic situation nine months after immediate implant placement for left central incisor.

surgical guidelines of the FairOne™ seek to overcome those challenges.

9. Conclusions

One-piece implants proved to be a useful tool for implant-supported tooth replacement in the posterior region as well as in the esthetic zone with benefits regarding the implant design and the surgical workflow. We could demonstrate long-term results of up to 10 years proving that preservation of the biological width including the level of the bone crest to achieve periodontal stability can be realized. Patients who received periodontal treatment in the past are usually compromised due to extensive attachment loss or higher susceptibility for peri-implantitis. Surgical treatment using one-piece titanium implants did not reveal increased tissue loss or frequency of peri-implant diseases in patients with periodontitis. Further clinical studies should evaluate the present findings in comparison with two-piece implant systems using profound clinical data and adequate observation periods.

Consent

Every patient gave the informed consent form prior to intervention.

Acknowledgments

Assistance and valuable support provided by Dirk Ziebolz in reviewing this manuscript was greatly appreciated. Support for Article Processing Charges was kindly provided by Fair-Implant GmbH, Bönningstedt, Germany.

References

[1] S. Jepsen, T. Berglundh, R. Genco et al., "Primary prevention of peri-implantitis: managing peri-implant mucositis," *Journal of Clinical Periodontology*, vol. 42, pp. S152–S157, 2015.

[2] M. Handelsman, "Surgical guidelines for dental implant placement," *British Dental Journal*, vol. 201, no. 3, pp. 139–152, 2006.

[3] E. Salamanca, J. C. Lin, C. Y. Tsai et al., "Dental Implant Surrounding Marginal Bone Level Evaluation: Platform Switching versus Platform Matching—One-Year Retrospective Study," *BioMed Research International*, vol. 2017, Article ID 7191534, 8 pages, 2017.

[4] R. Smeets, B. Stadlinger, F. Schwarz et al., "Impact of dental implant surface modifications on osseointegration," *BioMed Research International*, vol. 2016, Article ID 6285620, 16 pages, 2016.

[5] T. Albrektsson, G. Zarb, P. Worthington, and A. R. Eriksson, "The long-term efficacy of currently used dental implants: a review and proposed criteria of success," *The International Journal of Oral & Maxillofacial Implants*, vol. 1, no. 1, pp. 11–25, 1986.

[6] G. Cardaropoli, U. Lekholm, and J. L. Wennström, "Tissue alterations at implant-supported single-tooth replacements: a 1-year prospective clinical study," *Clinical Oral Implants Research*, vol. 17, no. 2, pp. 165–171, 2006.

[7] M. C. Manz, "Factors associated with radiographic vertical bone loss around implants placed in a clinical study," *Annals of Periodontology*, vol. 5, no. 1, pp. 137–151, 2000.

[8] J. Derks, D. Schaller, J. Hakansson, J. L. Wennstrom, C. Tomasi, and T. Berglundh, "Peri-implantitis - onset and pattern of progression," *Journal of Clinical Periodontology*, vol. 43, no. 4, pp. 383–388, 2016.

[9] C. H. F. Hammerle and D. Tarnow, "The etiology of hard- and soft-tissue deficiencies at dental implants: a narrative review," *Journal of Clinical Periodontology*, vol. 45, pp. S267–S277, 2018.

[10] I. Abrahamsson, T. Berglundh, and J. Lindhe, "The mucosal barrier following abutment dis/reconnection. An experimental study in dogs," *Journal of Clinical Periodontology*, vol. 24, no. 8, pp. 568–572, 1997.

[11] X. Rodriguez, X. Vela, V. Mendez, M. Segala, J. L. Calvo-Guirado, and D. P. Tarnow, "The effect of abutment dis/reconnections on peri-implant bone resorption: a radiologic study of platform-switched and non-platform-switched implants placed in animals," *Clinical Oral Implants Research*, vol. 24, no. 3, pp. 305–311, 2013.

[12] V. Perrotti, D. Zhang, A. Liang, J. Wong, and A. Quaranta, "The effect of one-abutment at one-time on marginal bone loss around implants placed in healed bone: a systematic review of human studies," *Implant Dentistry*, vol. 28, no. 6, pp. 603–612, 2019.

[13] J. Hahn, "One-piece root-form implants: a return to simplicity," *The Journal of Oral Implantology*, vol. 31, no. 2, pp. 77–84, 2005.

[14] S. M. Parel and S. R. Schow, "Early clinical experience with a new one-piece implant system in single tooth sites," *Journal of Oral and Maxillofacial Surgery*, vol. 63, no. 9, pp. 2–10, 2005.

[15] Y. Sasada and D. L. Cochran, "Implant-abutment connections: a review of biologic consequences and peri-implantitis implications," *The International Journal of Oral & Maxillofacial Implants*, vol. 32, no. 6, pp. 1296–1307, 2017.

[16] P. O. Ostman, M. Hellman, T. Albrektsson, and L. Sennerby, "Direct loading of Nobel Direct and Nobel Perfect one-piece implants: a 1-year prospective clinical and radiographic study," *Clinical Oral Implants Research*, vol. 18, no. 4, pp. 409 418, 2007.

[17] L. Sennerby, A. Rocci, W. Becker, L. Jonsson, L. A. Johansson, and T. Albrektsson, "Short-term clinical results of Nobel Direct implants: a retrospective multicentre analysis," *Clinical Oral Implants Research*, vol. 19, no. 3, pp. 219–226, 2008.

[18] R. Jimbo and T. Albrektsson, "Long-term clinical success of minimally and moderately rough oral implants: a review of 71 studies with 5 years or more of follow-up," *Implant Dentistry*, vol. 24, no. 1, pp. 62–69, 2015.

[19] A. Wennerberg, T. Albrektsson, and B. Chrcanovic, "Long-term clinical outcome of implants with different surface modifications," *European Journal of Oral Implantology*, vol. 11, pp. S123–S136, 2018.

[20] N. Broggini, L. M. McManus, J. S. Hermann et al., "Persistent acute inflammation at the implant-abutment interface," *Journal of Dental Research*, vol. 82, no. 3, pp. 232–237, 2003.

[21] T. Albrektsson and A. Wennerberg, "Oral implant surfaces: part 1–review focusing on topographic and chemical properties of different surfaces and in vivo responses to them," *The International Journal of Prosthodontics*, vol. 17, no. 5, pp. 536–543, 2004.

[22] T. A. Dantas, C. S. Abreu, M. M. Costa et al., "Bioactive materials driven primary stability on titanium biocomposites," *Materials Science & Engineering. C, Materials for Biological Applications*, vol. 77, pp. 1104–1110, 2017.

[23] V. C. Mendes, R. Moineddin, and J. E. Davies, "Discrete calcium phosphate nanocrystalline deposition enhances osteoconduction on titanium-based implant surfaces," *Journal of Biomedical Materials Research. Part A*, vol. 90, no. 2, pp. 577–585, 2009.

[24] L. Gaviria, J. P. Salcido, T. Guda, and J. L. Ong, "Current trends in dental implants," *Journal of the Korean Association of Oral and Maxillofacial Surgeons*, vol. 40, no. 2, pp. 50–60, 2014.

[25] S. Raghavendra, M. C. Wood, and T. D. Taylor, "Early wound healing around endosseous implants: a review of the literature," *The International Journal of Oral & Maxillofacial Implants*, vol. 20, no. 3, pp. 425–431, 2005.

[26] H. Sasaki, S. Koyama, M. Yokoyama, K. Yamaguchi, M. Itoh, and K. Sasaki, "Bone metabolic activity around dental implants under loading observed using bone scintigraphy," *The International Journal of Oral & Maxillofacial Implants*, vol. 23, no. 5, pp. 827–834, 2008.

[27] T. Linkevicius, P. Apse, S. Grybauskas, and A. Puisys, "The influence of soft tissue thickness on crestal bone changes around implants: a 1-year prospective controlled clinical trial," *The International Journal of Oral & Maxillofacial Implants*, vol. 24, no. 4, pp. 712–719, 2009.

[28] S. H. Park and H. L. Wang, "Pouch roll technique for implant soft tissue augmentation: a variation of the modified roll technique," *The International Journal of Periodontics & Restorative Dentistry*, vol. 32, no. 3, pp. e116–e121, 2012.

[29] P. Galindo-Moreno, A. León-Cano, I. Ortega-Oller, A. Monje, F. O'Valle, and A. Catena, "Marginal bone loss as success criterion in implant dentistry: beyond 2 mm," *Clinical Oral Implants Research*, vol. 26, no. 4, pp. e28–e34, 2015.

[30] J. S. Hermann, D. Buser, R. K. Schenk, J. D. Schoolfield, and D. L. Cochran, "Biologic width around one- and two-piece titanium implants," *Clinical Oral Implants Research*, vol. 12, no. 6, pp. 559–571, 2001.

[31] T. Linkevicius, E. Vindasiute, A. Puisys, and V. Peciuliene, "The influence of margin location on the amount of undetected cement excess after delivery of cement-retained implant restorations," *Clinical Oral Implants Research*, vol. 22, no. 12, pp. 1379–1384, 2011.

[32] N. Palacios-Garzón, E. Velasco-Ortega, and J. López-López, "Bone loss in implants placed at subcrestal and crestal level: a systematic review and meta-analysis," *Materials*, vol. 12, no. 1, p. 154, 2019.

[33] C. do Nascimento, P. K. Miani, V. Pedrazzi, K. Muller, and R. F. de Albuquerque Jr., "Bacterial leakage along the implant-abutment interface: culture and DNA checkerboard hybridization analyses," *Clinical Oral Implants Research*, vol. 23, pp. 1168–1172, 2012.

[34] N. Staubli, C. Walter, J. C. Schmidt, R. Weiger, and N. U. Zitzmann, "Excess cement and the risk of peri-implant disease - a systematic review," *Clinical Oral Implants Research*, vol. 28, no. 10, pp. 1278–1290, 2017.

[35] D. M. Chung, T. J. Oh, J. L. Shotwell, C. E. Misch, and H. L. Wang, "Significance of keratinized mucosa in maintenance of dental implants with different surfaces," *Journal of Periodontology*, vol. 77, no. 8, pp. 1410–1420, 2006.

[36] A. Bouri Jr., N. Bissada, M. S. Al-Zahrani, F. Faddoul, and I. Nouneh, "Width of keratinized gingiva and the health status of the supporting tissues around dental implants," *The International Journal of Oral & Maxillofacial Implants*, vol. 23, no. 2, pp. 323–326, 2008.

[37] F. Suarez-Lopez Del Amo, G. H. Lin, A. Monje, P. Galindo-Moreno, and H. L. Wang, "Influence of soft tissue thickness on peri-implant marginal bone loss: a systematic review and meta-analysis," *Journal of Periodontology*, vol. 87, no. 6, pp. 690–699, 2016.

[38] A. B. Souza, M. Tormena, F. Matarazzo, and M. G. Araujo, "The influence of peri-implant keratinized mucosa on brushing discomfort and peri-implant tissue health," *Clinical Oral Implants Research*, vol. 27, no. 6, pp. 650–655, 2016.

[39] I. Abrahamsson, T. Berglundh, I. S. Moon, and J. Lindhe, "Peri-implant tissues at submerged and non-submerged titanium implants," *Journal of Clinical Periodontology*, vol. 26, no. 9, pp. 600–607, 1999.

[40] T. Linkevicius, A. Puisys, M. Steigmann, E. Vindasiute, and L. Linkeviciene, "Influence of vertical soft tissue thickness on crestal bone changes around implants with platform switching: a comparative clinical study," *Clinical Implant Dentistry and Related Research*, vol. 17, no. 6, pp. 1228–1236, 2015.

[41] J. S. Hermann, D. Buser, R. K. Schenk, F. L. Higginbottom, and D. L. Cochran, "Biologic width around titanium implants. A physiologically formed and stable dimension over time," *Clinical Oral Implants Research*, vol. 11, no. 1, pp. 1–11, 2000.

[42] D. Lauritano, G. Moreo, A. Lucchese, C. Viganoni, L. Limongelli, and F. Carinci, "The impact of implant-abutment connection on clinical outcomes and microbial colonization: a narrative review," *Materials (Basel)*, vol. 13, no. 5, p. 1131, 2020.

[43] G. N. King, J. S. Hermann, J. D. Schoolfield, D. Buser, and D. L. Cochran, "Influence of the size of the microgap on crestal bone levels in non-submerged dental implants: a radiographic study in the canine mandible," *Journal of Periodontology*, vol. 73, no. 10, pp. 1111–1117, 2002.

[44] A. Scarano, L. Valbonetti, M. Degidi et al., "Implant-abutment contact surfaces and microgap measurements of different implant connections under 3-dimensional X-ray microtomography," *Implant Dentistry*, vol. 25, no. 5, pp. 656–662, 2016.

[45] M. Tallarico, M. Caneva, S. M. Meloni, E. Xhanari, U. Covani, and L. Canullo, "Definitive abutments placed at implant insertion and never removed: is it an effective approach? A systematic review and meta-analysis of randomized controlled trials," *Journal of Oral and Maxillofacial Surgery*, vol. 76, no. 2, pp. 316–324, 2018.

[46] Q. Q. Wang, R. Dai, C. Y. Cao, H. Fang, M. Han, and Q. L. Li, "One-time versus repeated abutment connection for platform-switched implant: a systematic review and meta-analysis," *PLoS One*, vol. 12, no. 10, 2017.

[47] S. Roffel, G. Wu, I. Nedeljkovic, M. Meyer, T. Razafiarison, and S. Gibbs, "Evaluation of a novel oral mucosa in vitro implantation model for analysis of molecular interactions with dental abutment surfaces," *Clinical Implant Dentistry and Related Research*, vol. 21, no. S1, pp. 25–33, 2019.

[48] J. M. Ottoni, Z. F. Oliveira, R. Mansini, and A. M. Cabral, "Correlation between placement torque and survival of single-tooth implants," *The International Journal of Oral & Maxillofacial Implants*, vol. 20, no. 5, pp. 769–776, 2005.

[49] R. Delgado-Ruiz, J. Gold, T. Somohano Marquez, and G. Romanos, "Under-drilling versus hybrid osseodensification technique: differences in implant primary stability and bone density of the implant bed walls," *Materials*, vol. 13, no. 2, p. 390, 2020.

[50] Q. Cheng, Y. Y. Su, X. Wang, and S. Chen, "Clinical outcomes following immediate loading of single-tooth implants in the esthetic zone: a systematic review and meta-analysis," *The International Journal of Oral & Maxillofacial Implants*, vol. 35, no. 1, pp. 167–177, 2020.

[51] J. M. Barrachina-Díez, E. Tashkandi, S. Stampf, and W. Att, "Long-term outcome of one-piece implants. Part II: prosthetic outcomes. A systematic literature review with meta-analysis," *The International Journal of Oral & Maxillofacial Implants*, vol. 28, no. 6, pp. 1470–1482, 2013.

[52] J. M. Barrachina-Diez, E. Tashkandi, S. Stampf, and W. Att, "Long-term outcome of one-piece implants. Part I: implant characteristics and loading protocols. A systematic literature review with meta-analysis," *The International Journal of Oral & Maxillofacial Implants*, vol. 28, no. 2, pp. 503–518, 2013.

28

Peri-Implant Tissue Adaptation after Implant Rehabilitation with Shoulderless Abutments with 24 Months of Follow-Up

Luca Casula,[1] Alex Gillone,[2] and Davide Musu[3]

[1]*Oral Surgery Resident, Vita Salute University, Milan, Italy*
[2]*Division Director of Periodontology, East Carolina University, Greenville, USA*
[3]*Department of Endodontology, Academic Centre for Dentistry Amsterdam (ACTA), Amsterdam, Netherlands*

Correspondence should be addressed to Davide Musu; davidemusu.dds@gmail.com

Academic Editor: Samir Nammour

An 11-year-old girl presented with agenesis of the maxillary lateral incisors. Orthodontic treatment was performed to close the midline diastema and create adequate space between the central incisors and canines to replace the missing maxillary lateral incisors on both sides. Two-piece implants were placed, and shoulderless abutments were prepared following the "biologically oriented preparation technique" (BOPT) protocol. The soft tissues were allowed to heal directly on the prosthetic emergence profile of the interim crown restorations after implant exposure. Two months later, the gingival tissue adapted to the prosthetic components in a specular manner. No complications were noted at 24 months. The BOPT protocol, originally described for natural teeth, may be applied to dental implants with shoulderless abutments.

1. Introduction

Implant abutment morphology influences marginal bone loss and the biologic width of the peri-implant mucosa [1–5]. Souza et al. [4] reported that an implant abutment design with a wide and more divergent emergence profile induces an apical displacement of the peri-implant biologic width and an increased bone loss compared to an implant abutment with a narrower emergence profile. Agustín-Panadero et al. compared implants with divergent transmucosal collars to those with a convergent collar design and observed that the latter resulted in decreased bone loss [5]. A smaller abutment diameter, relative to the implant platform, seems to reduce the postrestorative crestal bone remodeling, which results in greater bone preservation [6, 7]. However, the role of the abutment design in marginal bone loss and peri-implant soft tissue stability is currently unknown [8, 9]. The crown is usually adapted against the horizontal finish line of the implant-supported cement-retained prosthesis, and together, they form the emergence profile of the implant-supported restoration [10]. The emergence profile of the implant-supported restoration is determined by the contour of the crown as it relates to the adjacent tissues [11]. Similar to natural abutment teeth [12–14], a shoulderless implant abutment has a vertical area without a finish line where the crown margin is placed [15]. The absence of a defined horizontal finish line allows the interim restoration to move in an apical or coronal direction, allowing the tissue to adapt to the emergence profile of the crown restoration in a specular manner [12]. This concept, which was introduced with the biologically oriented preparation technique (BOPT) protocol [12–14], allows for the thickening of the soft tissues in the coronal direction and results in excellent esthetics with both the implants [16–19] and natural teeth [20, 21]. The use of the "adaptation forms and profiles concept" [12] in rehabilitative treatment involving natural teeth [12–14, 20, 21] and implants with shoulderless abutments [16–19] has been well documented; however, the adaptation of the gingiva to the emergence profile of prosthetic crowns has not been reported for the implant-supported cement-retained restorations methodically. This clinical case report describes a patient with agenesis of the maxillary lateral incisors. Orthodontic treatment was performed to create space for implant placement. Two implant-supported cement-retained prostheses were provided, using a protocol similar to the BOPT for natural teeth [12]. The step-by-step gingival movement toward the crown emergence profile during tissue maturation is described up to two years after crown delivery.

2. Case Report

An 11-year-old girl was referred to the Department of Dentistry at the San Raffaele Hospital in Milan, Italy. The patient expressed dissatisfaction with smile, due to misaligned teeth and spaces between the anterior teeth. Radiographic examination revealed the agenesis of the maxillary lateral incisors (Figure 1(a)). A multidisciplinary treatment plan was formulated, which included orthodontic treatment for the midline diastema closure, focusing on creating adequate space between the central incisors and the canines to replace the missing maxillary lateral incisors on both sides. Two implant-supported cement-retained prostheses were planned at the end of the peak of adolescent growth for replacing the lateral incisors [22].

After orthodontic treatment, the patient wore a removable retainer to maintain the space gained for replacement of the lateral incisors with implants (Figure 1(b)). The maxillary implant surgery was performed with the aid of cone beam computed tomography (CBCT) when the patient was 19 years old. Two 3.3 mm diameter implants (Win-Six Biosafin, Italy) were placed in the area of the lateral incisors, with the implant platform positioned at the buccal crest level and with an insertion torque of 30 Ncm.

Immediate loading was avoided, and the patient wore a removable retainer during osseointegration of the implant [23] . Four months after implant placement, two periapical radiographs were taken confirming that the implant platforms were at the level of the bone crest (Figure 2(a)). After confirmation, we proceeded to the second stage of maxillary surgery. First, the two alginate impressions were made, and wax interocclusal records in maximal intercuspation were taken and sent to the dental laboratory for fabrication of the interim complete crown restorations. The gingival thickness at the implant site was determined to be 4 mm by inserting a K-file with an endodontic stop at the center of the edentulous ridges. Subsequently, the implants were exposed by raising a minimal full-thickness flap and moving the occlusal keratinized tissue to the buccal aspect.

The impression copings (Win-Six Biosafin, Italy) were connected to the implants, and an impression was made with vinyl polysiloxane material (Putty and Light Elite HD, Zhermack, Italy), using a perforated custom tray. Two implant analogs were connected to the copings inside the impression, and the cast was immediately poured using the type 4 dental stone. Two modifiable cylindrical shoulderless implant abutments (MF, Win-Six Biosafin, Italy) were connected to the analogs and adjusted (prepared without a finish line) directly on the cast to achieve the appropriate inclination for placement of the temporary crowns. The shoulderless abutments were prepared in the same manner as the natural abutment teeth in the BOPT protocol [12–14] (Figure 2(b)), and the interim complete crown restorations were directly relined over the implant abutments on the implant cast, resulting in an augmented emergence profile (Figure 2(c)) [12]. The interim restorations were placed 3 mm coronally from the analogs that corresponded to the implant platforms (bone crest level), based on the previously measured gingival thickness (4 mm). This ensured that the adequate space remained for biologic width formation (Figure 2(c)) [24]. The temporary abutments were fixed to the implants, and the interim restorations were cemented using a temporary cement (Temp Bond, Kerr, USA). The keratinized mucosa taken from the occlusal space was supported by the overcontoured emergence profile [11] of the crown during the healing process on the buccal aspect (Figure 3).

After the interim restoration placement, the patient returned to the dental department periodically for 2 months during the healing process, which was documented using photographs. Four days after interim restoration placement, the keratinized tissue appeared inflamed and was in a more coronal position (Figure 3(c)) than before (Figure 3(b)). During the one week follow-up, the keratinized tissue appeared swollen, reddened, and more coronally elongated compared to that during the previous appointment (Figure 3(d)). During the second week of follow-up, the redness and swelling disappeared, and the keratinized tissue appeared to recede more apically (Figure 4(a)). At the 1-month follow-up, the gingival tissue appeared healthy and had adapted to the prosthetic emergence profile of the interim restoration in a specular manner (Figure 4(b)). At the 2-month follow-up, the interdental spaces were completely filled by the interdental papillae, and the crown margins were located 1 mm subgingivally (Figure 4(c)). The tissue appeared pink and healthy, even in the transmucosal area. On the occlusal view, the rounded profile of the gingiva was appreciable and specular to the emergence profile [11] of the interim crowns (Figure 5(a)). The adaptation of the tissue against the overcontoured emergence profile of the crowns was clearly appreciable on the lateral view (Figure 5(b)). After the previously described 2 months of tissue maturation, the patient visited the department for final impressions. The temporary restorations and analogs were removed, and the height of the transmucosal soft tissue was determined, with a dental probe placed between the implant platform and the gingival margin, to be 4 mm for both implants. The bone impression copings (Win-Six Biosafin, Italy) were connected to the implants, and an impression was made with vinyl polysiloxane material (Putty and Light Elite HD, Zhermack, Italy) using a perforated custom tray. An alginate impression of the mandibular arch and interocclusal record in maximal intercuspation were obtained and sent to the dental laboratory for the fabrication of two definitive implant abutments with a single zirconia framework for each. The dental technician was instructed to prepare wax patterns and cast customized titanium abutments without a finish line. The dental technician was also instructed to place the margins of the final crowns 1 mm subgingivally, according to the conditioned soft tissue during the interim stage. A reinforced collar was fabricated by the dental technician, to strengthen the feather-edged margin (Figure 5(c)) [10]. Thus, the ceramic

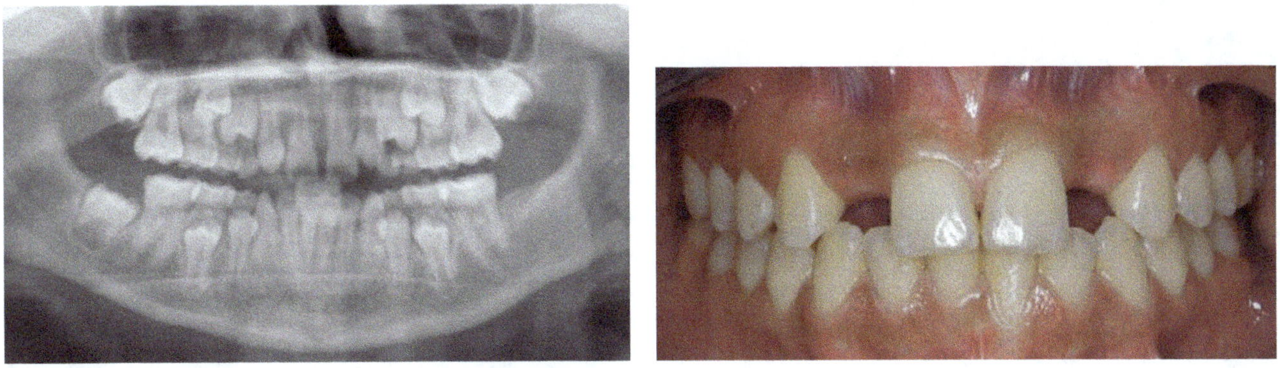

(a) (b)

FIGURE 1: (a) Panoramic radiograph showing agenesis of both maxillary lateral incisors. (b) Facial view at the end of the orthodontic treatment showing the space maintained with the removable orthodontic retainer.

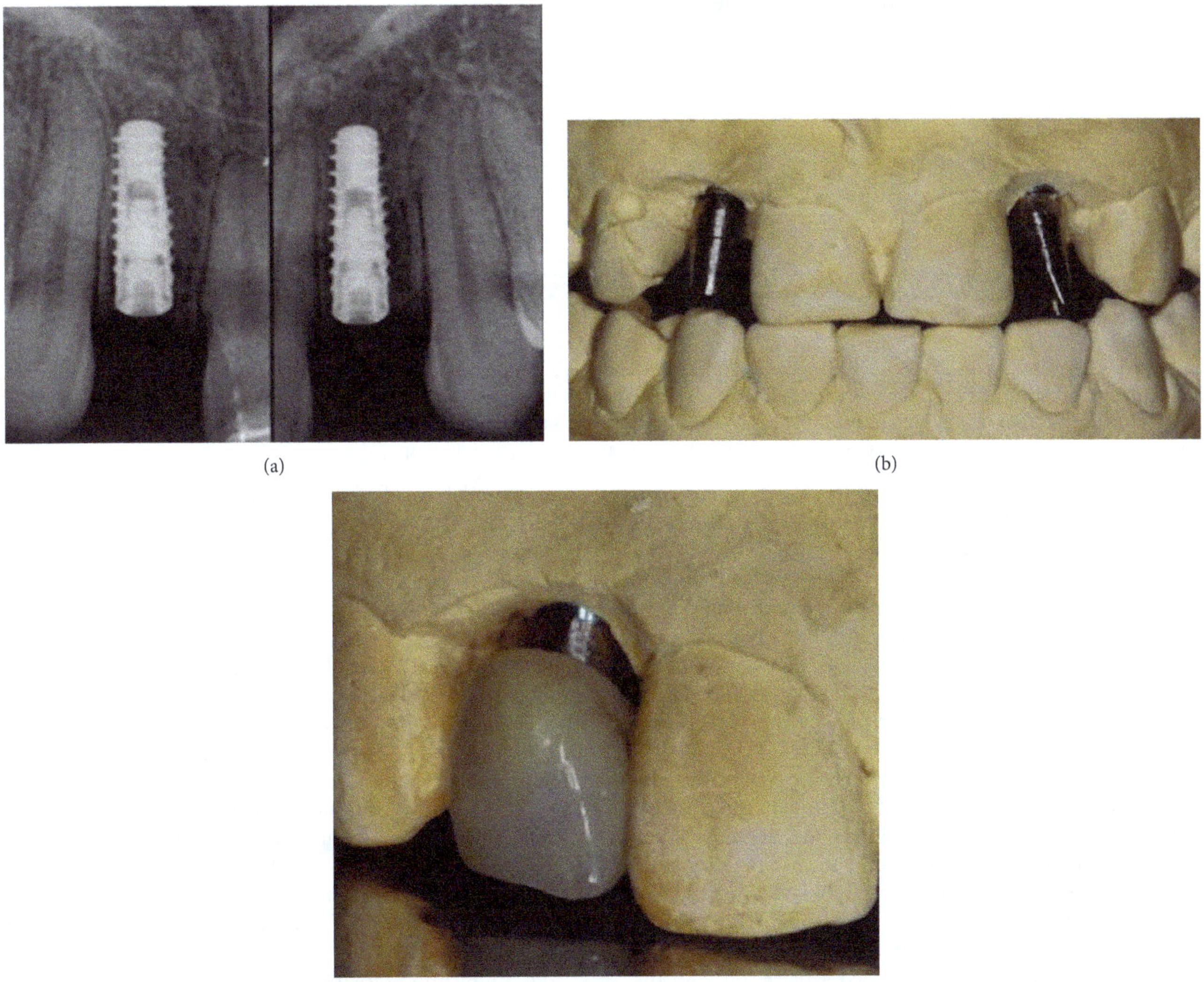

(a) (b)

(c)

FIGURE 2: (a) Implants on lateral incisors positioned 4 months after placement. (b) The shoulderless abutments directly adjusted on the master cast. (c) The crown was placed 3 mm away from the analog (3 mm from the bone crest).

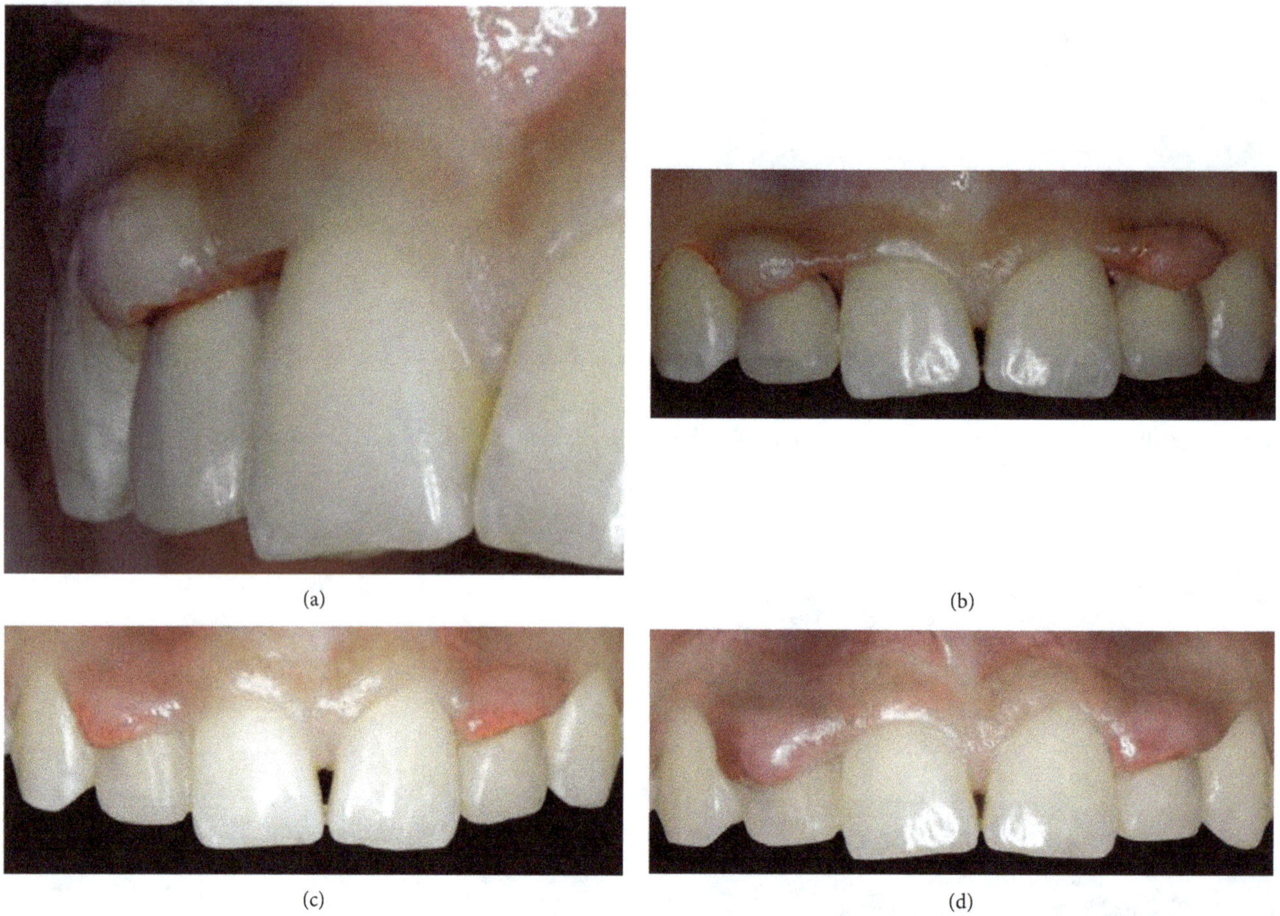

Figure 3: (a) The keratinized tissue moved from the occlusal side and was sustained by the augmented emergence profile of the crown. (b) Peri-implant mucosa formation and gingival adaptation along with the emergence profile of the crown restoration: inflammatory phase with the soft tissues sustained by the immediately placed crowns. (c) Soft tissues at four days of follow-up with minimal inflammation. (d) Soft tissues appeared inflamed and elongated in a more coronal position at one week of follow-up.

layering of the framework was performed along the reinforced collar of the chamfer, to prevent the fabrication of a crown with a thin ceramic margin.

At the following clinical visit, the abutments and zirconia frameworks were evaluated, and new interocclusal wax in maximal intercuspation was made to check the occlusion again. The accuracy of the framework's fit was confirmed clinically with dual-cured paste (Fit Checker Advanced, Gc Corporation, Japan). A framework transfer impression with polysiloxane material (Putty and Light Elite HD, Zhermack, Italy) was made, to capture the framework-soft tissue relationship. The impression was sent to the dental technician with a request that the final restorations be shaped in a manner that allowed the emergence profile to sustain the mature soft tissues. The final restorations were clinically checked and sent for the final glaze. At the final appointment, the finished crowns were cemented with temporary cement (Temp Bond, Kerr, USA), and the patient expressed satisfaction with the esthetics.

At the 24-month follow-up visit, no biological or technical complications were noted, and the gingiva appeared thick, pink, healthy, and completely adapted to the definitive restoration (Figure 6). The papillary filling was achieved in the interdental spaces. At the 24-month follow-up, minimal bone remodeling of approximately 0.5 mm was detected, which was attributed to abutment installation and initial loading (Figure 6) [25].

3. Discussion

The healthy coexistence of dental restorations and the peri-implant structures is essential and is the primary goal of a prosthodontist. The peri-implant tissues should not bleed on probing, and a tight seal should exist between the peri-implant mucosa and the transmucosal component [25]. The abutment design for natural teeth and implants presents a well-defined horizontal finish line or a vertical area without a finish line for the crown margin [10, 26]. A vertical preparation without a finish line in natural abutment teeth [12] results in the formation of an overcontoured cervical portion of the prosthetic crown [27] and has been suspected to have serious implications for the periodontal health of the supporting tissues [28]. The BOPT protocol includes a prosthetic subgingival preparation of the natural abutment teeth without a finish line [12–14] and ensures a good periodontal condition [20, 21]. The "adaptation forms and profiles concept" [12] applied to the natural abutment teeth treated with BOPT [12–14] is applicable for implant-supported cement-retained

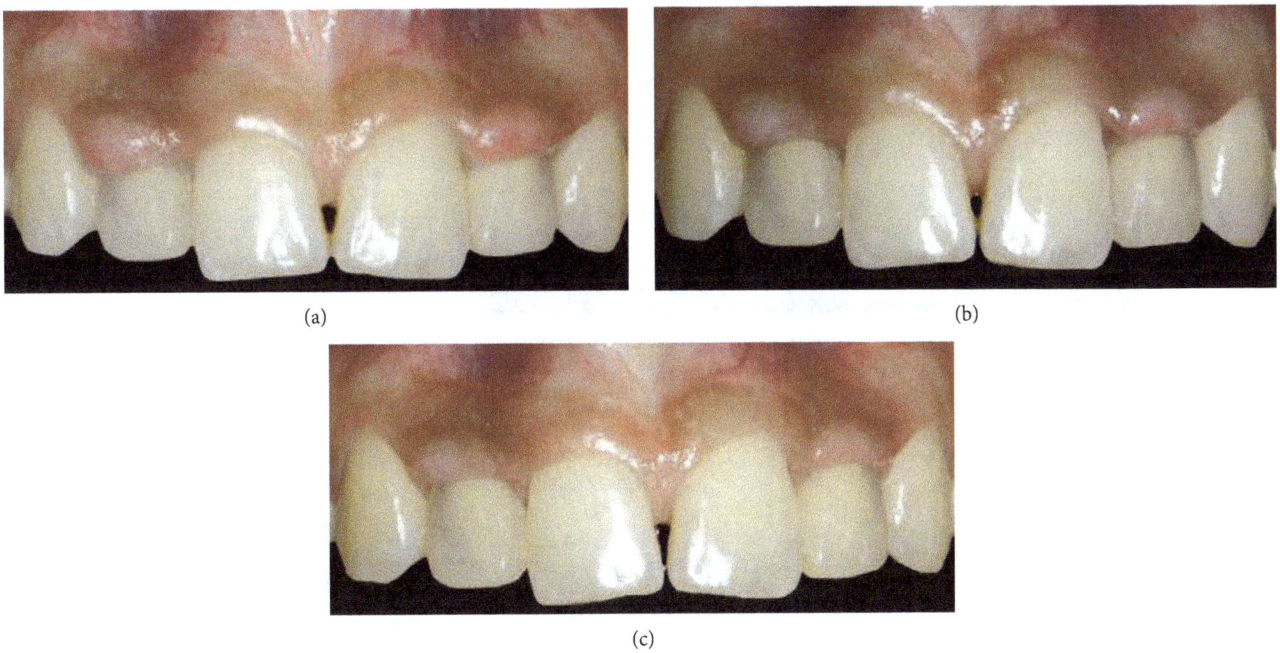

FIGURE 4: Peri-implant mucosa formation and gingival adaptation along with the emergence profile of the crown restoration: adaptation phase. (a) Soft tissues at two weeks of follow-up receded in an apical position and appeared without inflammation. (b) Soft tissues at 1 month of follow-up were adapted along the emergence profile of the crowns. (c) Soft tissues at 2 months of follow-up were stable, and the interdental spaces were completely filled by the interdental papillae.

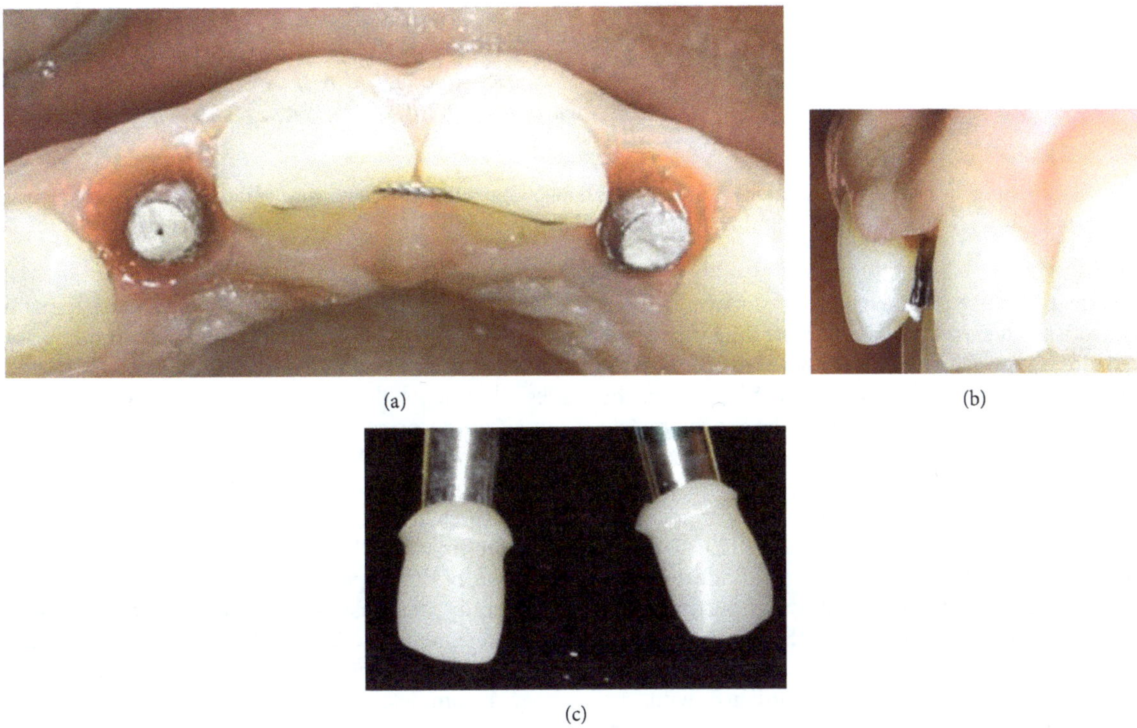

FIGURE 5: (a) Occlusal view of the peri-implant mucosa 2 months after interim restoration placement. (b) Lateral view showing that the keratinized gingiva adapted and conformed to the prosthetic emergence profile of the interim restoration in a specular way. (c) The definitive restoration frameworks with the reinforced collars that allowed a thick layer of ceramic at the margin of the crown.

restorations [11] if shoulderless abutments are used [16–19]. In this case report, the interim restorations were shaped with an augmented contour [12–14] and placed on the shoulderless abutments immediately after flap elevation, while waiting for peri-implant mucosa formation around the restorative components (Figure 3). The positions of the prosthetic

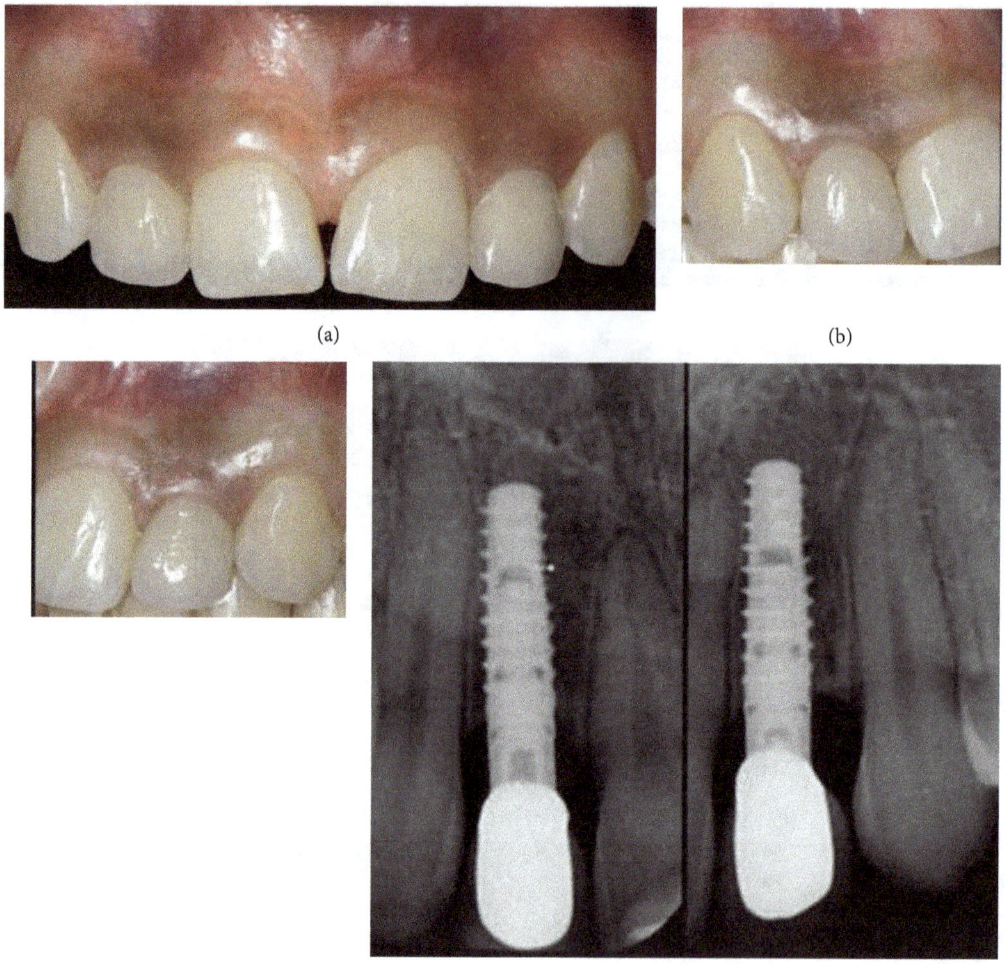

(a) (b) (c) (d)

Figure 6: (a) Facial view of the definitive restorations at the 24-month follow-up. (b) Right lateral view of the definitive restorations at the 24-month follow-up. (c) Left lateral view of the definitive restorations at the 24-month follow-up. (d) Periapical radiographs at the 24-month follow-up.

crowns and their distance from the bone crest (4 mm at both sites) were clinically determined based on the thickness of the keratinized gingiva, measured at the center of the edentulous ridges before flap elevation. In the scientific literature, the peri-implant mucosal height is reported to be approximately 3 to 4 mm [29], and minimal bone remodeling is expected after the initial loading [25]. Therefore, we placed the interim restorations 3 mm from the bone crest, leaving adequate space for the peri-implant biologic width [23, 29, 30] (Figure 3(c)). Two months after implant loading, the peri-implant mucosa appeared pink, healthy, and completely adapted to the emergence profile [11] of the interim restorations. The healing stages of the peri-implant mucosa documented in this case report are in accordance with the healing stages in animal studies [29]. The first week was characterized by low-grade inflammation of the peri-implant mucosa, which healed and stabilized at the 1-month follow-up [30] and reached complete maturation with a pink and healthy appearance at the 2-month follow-up [29, 30]. The influence of abutment morphology on peri-implant mucosa formation has not been properly elucidated [8, 9, 29, 31], and currently, there are no studies comparing the implant abutments with a finish line with the shoulderless abutments. Nevertheless, the horizontal finish line in implant abutments acts as a vertical stop for seating the crown [10]. In shoulderless abutments, the crown restoration may instead be moved in an apical or coronal direction without invading the biologic width [12–19]. Therefore, the emergence profile and the crown margin can be modified until healthy and stable soft tissues are achieved if the inflammation occurs during the interim stage [16–19].

The BOPT approach used for implant rehabilitation in this study demonstrated a good clinical outcome in the esthetic zone at the 24-month follow-up, with healthy peri-implant mucosa, pink and stippled gingiva, and interdental spaces completely filled by the interdental papillae. The interim crowns were not positioned according to the healed soft tissue, but the soft tissue was allowed to adapt itself against the prosthetic components during the healing stage. The position of the crown was predetermined and was based on the gingival tissue thickness and biologic width dimension. A limitation is apparent in cases in which the gingival thickness is not sufficient to ensure adequate space for the biologic width. Moreover, the technique is time consuming because the interim abutments must be adjusted by the dentist during the second stage surgery, which requires ample experience. The technique has not been backed by scientific literature, and long-term clinical studies are still required to understand the role of the abutment design in peri-implant mucosa formation and to better evaluate, both clinically and scientifically, the outcomes of shoulderless implant abutments.

Consent

Informed consent was obtained from the patient, and the San Raphael Hospital ethic committed approved this clinical study.

References

[1] Z. Chen, C. Y. Lin, J. Li, H. L. Wang, and H. Yu, "Influence of abutment height on peri-implant marginal bone loss: a systematic review and meta-analysis," *The Journal of Prosthetic Dentistry*, vol. 122, no. 1, pp. 14–21.e2, 2019.

[2] R. Patil, R. van Brakel, K. Iyer, J. H. Slater, C. de Putter, and M. Cune, "A comparative study to evaluate the effect of two different abutment designs on soft tissue healing and stability of mucosal margins," *Clinical Oral Implants Research*, vol. 24, no. 3, pp. 336–341, 2013.

[3] R. Judgar, G. Giro, E. Zenobio et al., "Biological width around one- and two-piece implants retrieved from human jaws," *BioMed Research International*, vol. 2014, Article ID 850120, 5 pages, 2014.

[4] A. B. Souza, A. Alshihri, P. W. Kämmerer, M. G. Araújo, and G. O. Gallucci, "Histological and micro-CT analysis of peri-implant soft and hard tissue healing on implants with different healing abutments configurations," *Clinical Oral Implants Research*, vol. 29, no. 10, pp. 1007–1015, 2018.

[5] R. Agustín-Panadero, N. Martínez-Martínez, L. Fernandez-Estevan, J. Faus-López, and M. F. Solá-Ruíz, "Influence of transmucosal area morphology on peri-implant bone loss in tissue level implants," *International Journal of Oral and Maxillofacial Implants*, vol. 34, pp. 947–952, 2019.

[6] L. Canullo, G. Pellegrini, C. Allievi, L. Trombelli, S. Annibali, and C. Dellavia, "Soft tissues around long-term platform switching implant restorations: a histological human evaluation. Preliminary results," *Journal of Clinical Periodontology*, vol. 38, no. 1, pp. 86–94, 2011.

[7] R. J. Lazzara and S. S. Porter, "Platform switching: a new concept in implant dentistry for controlling postrestorative crestal bone levels," *International Journal of Periodontics and Restorative Dentistry*, vol. 26, no. 1, pp. 9–17, 2006.

[8] S. Bishti, J. R. Strub, and W. Att, "Effect of the implant–abutment interface on peri-implant tissues: a systematic review," *Acta Odontologica Scandinavica*, vol. 72, no. 1, pp. 13–25, 2013.

[9] E. Rompen, "The impact of the type and configuration of abutments and their (repeated) removal on the attachment level and marginal bone," *The European Journal of Oral Implantology*, vol. 5, pp. S83–S90, 2012.

[10] R. Cocchetto and L. Canullo, "The "hybrid abutment": a new design for implant cemented restorations in the esthetic zones," *International Journal of Esthetic Dentistry*, vol. 10, no. 2, pp. 186–208, 2015.

[11] I. K. Aidsman, "The glossary of prosthodontic terms," *The Journal of Prosthetic Dentistry*, vol. 94, no. 1, pp. 10–92, 2005.

[12] I. Loi and A. Di Felice, "Biologically oriented preparation technique (BOPT): a new approach for prosthetic restoration of periodontically healthy teeth," *The European Journal of Esthetic Dentistry*, vol. 8, no. 1, pp. 10–23, 2013.

[13] R. Agustín-Panadero, M. F. Solá-Ruíz, C. Chust, and A. Ferreiroa, "Fixed dental prostheses with vertical tooth preparations without finish lines: a report of two patients," *Journal of Prosthetic Dentistry*, vol. 115, no. 5, pp. 520–526, 2016.

[14] R. Agustín-Panadero and M. F. Solá-Ruíz, "Vertical preparation for fixed prosthesis rehabilitation in the anterior sector," *Journal of Prosthetic Dentistry*, vol. 114, no. 4, pp. 474–478, 2015.

[15] L. Canullo, R. Cocchetto, F. Marinotti, D. O. Oltra, M. P. Diago, and I. Loi, "Clinical evaluation of an improved cementation technique for implant-supported restorations: a randomized controlled trial," *Clinical Oral Implants Research*, vol. 27, no. 12, pp. 1492–1499, 2016.

[16] L. Canullo, M. Menini, U. Covani, and P. Pesce, "Clinical outcomes of using a prosthetic protocol to rehabilitate tissue-level implants with a convergent collar in the esthetic zone: a 3-year prospective study," *The Journal of Prosthetic Dentistry*, vol. 123, no. 19, pp. 246–251, 2020.

[17] M. F. Solá-Ruiz, J. Del Rio Highsmith, C. Labaig-Rueda, and R. Agustín-Panadero, "Biologically oriented preparation technique (BOPT) for implant-supported fixed prostheses," *Journal of Clinical Experimental Dentistry*, vol. 9, no. 4, pp. 603–607, 2017.

[18] G. Cabanes-Gumbau, A. Pascual-Moscardó, D. Peñarrocha-Oltra, B. García-Mira, J. Aizcorbe-Vincente, and M. Peñarrocha-Diago, "Volumetric variation of peri-implant soft tissues in convergent collar implants and crowns using the biologically oriented preparation technique (BOPT)," *Medicina Oral Patologia Oral y Cirugia Bucal*, vol. 24, no. 5, pp. 643–651, 2019.

[19] L. Canullo, M. Tallarico, G. Pradies, F. Marinotti, I. Loi, and R. Cocchetto, "Soft and hard tissue response to an implant with a convergent collar in the esthetic area: preliminary report at 18 months," *The International Journal of Esthetic Dentistry*, vol. 12, no. 3, pp. 306–323, 2017.

[20] R. Agustín-Panadero, B. Serra-Pastor, A. Fons-Font, and M. F. Solá-Ruíz, "Prospective clinical study of zirconia full-coverage restorations on teeth prepared with biologically oriented preparation technique on gingival health: results after two-year follow-up," *Operative Dentistry*, vol. 43, no. 5, pp. 482–487, 2018.

[21] B. Serra-Pastor, I. Loi, A. Fons-Font, M. F. Solá-Ruíz, and R. Agustín-Panadero, "Periodontal and prosthetic outcomes on teeth prepared with biologically oriented preparation technique: a 4-year follow-up prospective clinical study," *Journal of Prosthodontic Research*, vol. 63, no. 4, pp. 415–420, 2019.

[22] L. A. Loomba-Albrecht and D. M. Styne, "Effect of puberty on body composition," *Current Opinion in Endocrinology, Diabetes, and Obesity*, vol. 16, no. 1, pp. 10–15, 2009.

[23] M. Tallarico, A. Vaccarella, G. Marzi, A. Alviani, and V. Campana, "A prospective case-control clinical trial comparing 1- and 2-stage Nobel Biocare TiUnite implants: resonance frequency analysis assessed by Osstell Mentor during integration," *Quintessence International*, vol. 42, no. 8, pp. 635–644, 2011.

[24] C. Tomasi, F. Tessarolo, I. Caola, J. Wennström, G. Nollo, and T. Berglundh, "Morphogenesis of peri-implant mucosa revisited: an experimental study in humans," *Clinical Oral Implants Research*, vol. 25, no. 9, pp. 997–1003, 2014.

[25] S. Renvert, G. R. Persson, F. Q. Pirih, and P. M. Camargo, "Peri-implant health, peri-implant mucositis, and peri-implantitis: case definitions and diagnostic considerations," *Journal of Periodontology*, vol. 45, no. S1, pp. S278–S285, 2018.

[26] G. I. Pardo, "A full cast restoration design offering superior marginal characteristics," *Journal of Prosthetic Dentistry*, vol. 48, no. 5, pp. 539–543, 1982.

[27] J. Abduo and K. M. Lyons, "Interdisciplinary interface between fixed prosthodontics and periodontics," *Periodontology 2000*, vol. 74, no. 1, pp. 40–62, 2017.

[28] C. J. Goodacre, W. V. Campagni, and S. A. Aquilino, "Tooth preparations for complete crowns: an art form based on scientific principles," *Journal of Prosthetic Dentistry*, vol. 85, no. 4, pp. 363–376, 2001.

[29] M. G. Araujo and J. Lindhe, "Peri-implant health," *Journal of Clinical Periodontology*, vol. 45, no. S20, pp. 230–236, 2018.

[30] T. Berglundh, I. Abrahamsson, M. Welander, N. P. Lang, and J. Lindhe, "Morphogenesis of the peri-implant mucosa: an experimental study in dogs," *Clinical Oral Implants Research*, vol. 18, no. 1, pp. 1–8, 2007.

[31] F. Schwarz, J. Derks, A. Monje, and H. L. Wang, "Peri-implantitis," *Journal of Clinical Periodontology*, vol. 45, no. S20, pp. S246–S266, 2018.

29

Application of Recombinant Human BMP-2 with Bone Marrow Aspirate Concentrate and Platelet-Rich Fibrin in Titanium Mesh for Vertical Maxillary Defect Reconstruction prior to Implant Placement

Kamel Alraei,[1] **Jameel Shrqawi**,[2] **and Khawlah Alarusi**[3]

[1]*Department of Oral and Maxillofacial Surgery, Al Noor Specialist Hospital, Mecca, Saudi Arabia*
[2]*Department of Oral and Maxillofacial Surgery, Royal Commission Hospital, Al Jubail, Saudi Arabia*
[3]*General Dentist, Mecca, Saudi Arabia*

Correspondence should be addressed to Kamel Alraei; kalraee@moh.gov.sa and Khawlah Alarusi; khawlah4488@gmail.com

Academic Editor: Jamil Awad Shibli

Recombinant human bone morphogenetic protein 2 (rhBMP-2) is an alternative bone substitute for extensive maxillary bone defects which avoids the disadvantages associated with other grafting materials. This report details a case of a 32-year-old female with a severe vertical and horizontal maxillary bony defect that developed after tumor removal. She underwent two unsuccessful regenerative surgeries with an iliac bone graft. Reconstruction of the maxillary defect was planned by offlabel use of rhBMP-2/absorbable collagen sponge (ACS) combined with a bone marrow aspirate concentrate (BMAC) and allograft in a titanium mesh covered in platelet-rich fibrin (PRF). Clinical and radiographic evaluations showed good quality and quantity of bone formation, and she was rehabilitated with dental implants and prosthodontic treatment. Based on this case, the use of rhBMP-2 as a graft material appears encouraging with a satisfying outcome. The present case is aimed at reporting the clinical and radiographic effectiveness of rhBMP-2/ACS in combination with PRF and a titanium mesh for severe maxillary bone defects. Future investigations will be required to ascertain the long-term survival of implants in areas grafted with rhBMP-2.

1. Introduction

Reconstruction of bone defects after tumor removal or significant trauma is a common practice in maxillofacial surgery; the augmented bone is utilized to house dental implants with subsequent prosthetic rehabilitation. The goal of such a procedure is to maximize both the aesthetic appearance and function [1]. Reconstruction can be achieved by a variety of techniques and materials for bone grafting, including autografts, allografts, and alloplastic grafts. The choice of technique depends on different factors, including the types and degrees of bone loss, surgical prosthetic planning, and the general condition of the patient [2–4].

An autogenous bone graft is considered the ideal grafting material, with the highest success rate due to its osteogenic and osteoinductive capacity. Although it does not trigger an immune response, it is associated with donor site morbidity, poor efficacy for large bone defects, and prolonged recovery time [5, 6].

Allografts are another suitable alternative material for the reconstruction of severely atrophic maxillary bone, with a lower risk of morbidity and shorter recovery time. However, they are associated with an increased risk of infection and require a longer time for graft incorporation [7, 8].

One promising material that has shown successful bone regeneration in maxillofacial defects is recombinant human bone morphogenetic protein 2 (rhBMP-2), which can stimulate angiogenesis and the migration, proliferation, and differentiation of mesenchymal stem cells into bone-forming cells [9]. rhBMP-2 has been used alone or in combination with other graft types with clinical success [10–12]. rhBMP-2 and the absorbable collagen sponge (rhBMP-

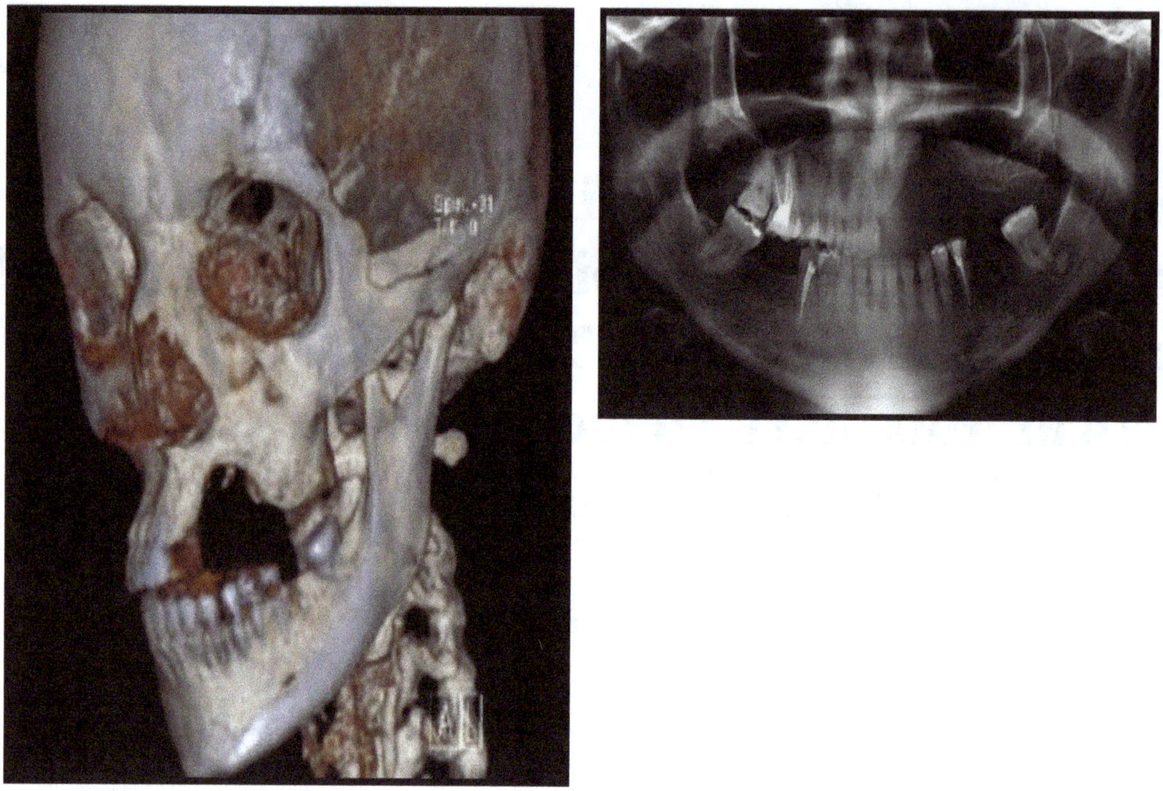

(a) (b)

Figure 1: (a) Three-dimensional computed tomography showing partial bony defect of the left maxillary bone. (b) Preoperative panoramic radiography showing a large radiolucent area at the left side of the maxilla.

2/ACS), when used in combination with an allograft, produce bone similar to an autogenous graft and can even be used in large vertical bone augmentation without the need for harvesting a donor bone. This combination can overcome the drawbacks of an autogenous bone graft [13]. Furthermore, platelet-rich fibrin (PRF) is reported to have a positive effect in soft tissue healing and bone formation.

The present case report is aimed at evaluating the clinical and radiographic effectiveness of rhBMP-2/ACS in combination with PRF and titanium mesh in a case of severe maxillary bone defect.

2. Case Presentation

2.1. Preoperative Examination. A 32-year-old female presented to the Oral and Maxillofacial Clinic at Al Noor Specialist Hospital seeking dental implants, with a complaint of absent left upper teeth and jaw, which developed after the removal of a giant cell tumor 1 year previously. The patient had two failed surgeries 1 year previously in which iliac crest bone grafts were used. She was healthy, with no medications, chronic illness, or allergies. Clinical and radiological examinations (3D computed tomography [CT], orthopantomogram [OPG]) revealed a left maxillary bone defect, extending from the left upper central incisor to the left first molar and vertically to the floor of the maxillary sinus (Figure 1). These findings dictated the necessity for bone grafting before the placement of dental implants.

Reconstruction of the maxillary defect was planned with rhBMP-2 combined with bone marrow aspirate (BMA) concentrate (BMAC) and allograft. Titanium mesh was to be used as a carrier and to protect the bone graft component. The mesh was prepared on a study cast to estimate the required size and shape and was sent for sterilization. To overcome the negative impact of the mesh on the oral mucosa, we decided to cover the mesh with PRF. The treatment plan was discussed with the patient, and informed surgical consent was obtained.

2.2. Surgery. Under general anesthesia, the patient was placed in the prone position after routine draping and scrubbing of the posterior iliac crest. We aspirated 600 cc of BMA, which was collected into a blood donation bag containing the anticoagulant sodium citrate. The BMA was centrifuged and BMAC was prepared by separating the plasma from the blood (Figure 2(a)).

The patient was then moved to the supine position. After administration of local anesthesia (xylocaine) with 2% adrenaline, an incision was performed 4 mm from the crest towards the palatal side along the maxillary defect, with two releasing incisions vertically extended to the maxillary sulcus. A mucoperiosteal flap was elevated to expose the defect. The recipient area was perforated using a small round burr to increase blood perfusion to the grafting area.

rhBMP-2 (Infuse Bone Graft, 8 cc; Medtronic, Minneapolis, MN) was prepared according to the manufacturer's

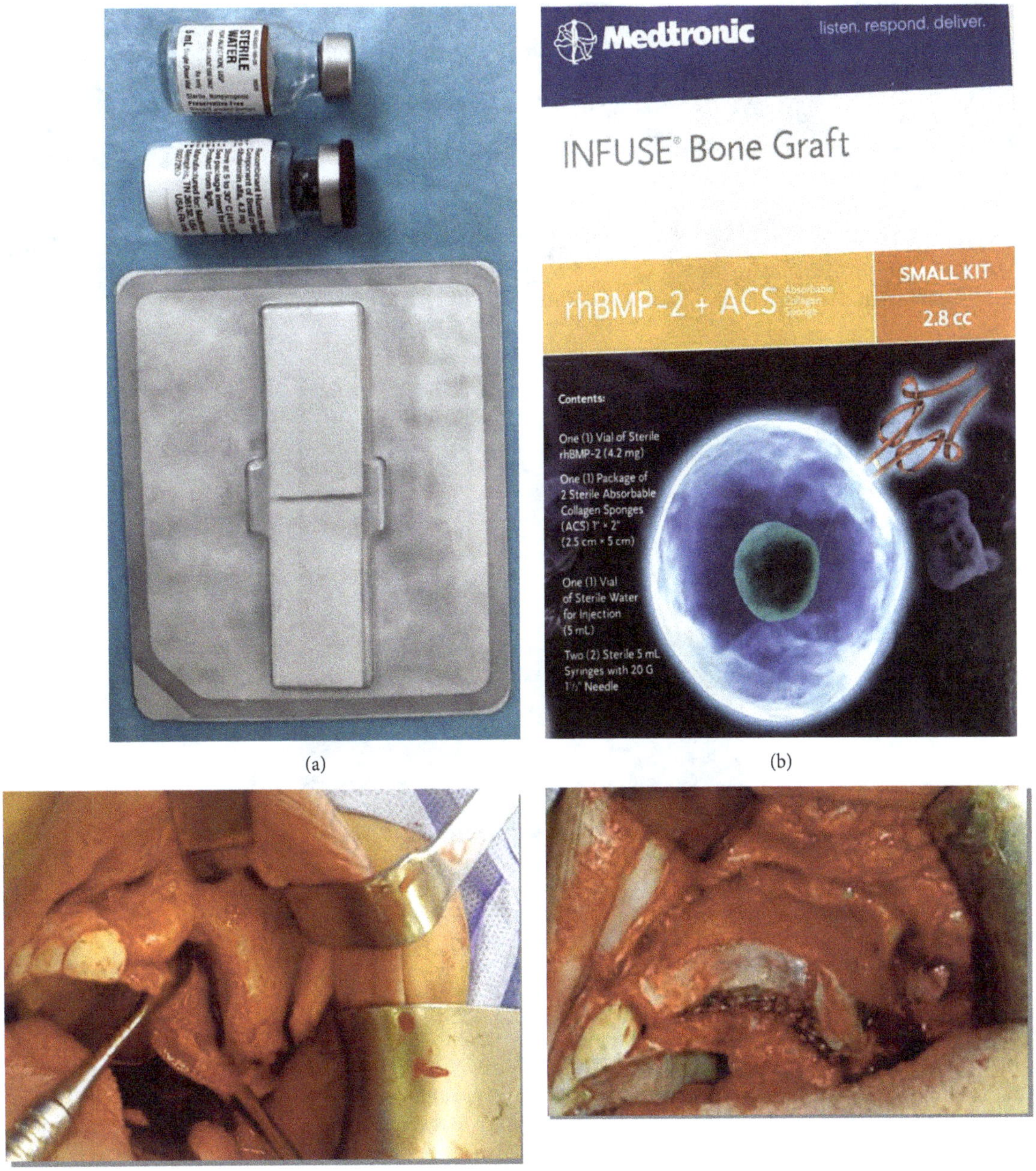

(a) (b) (c) (d)

FIGURE 2: (a) Bone marrow aspirate concentrate. (b) Recombinant human bone morphogenetic protein 2 (rhBMP-2). (c) Maxillary extraosseous vertical ridge defect. (d) rhBMP-2, allograft, and bone marrow aspirate concentrate condensed inside prepared mesh covered by the platelet-rich fibrin.

recommendations (Figure 2(b)). ACS was cut into small pieces and mixed with 15 cc of freeze-dried cancellous allograft and BMAC. All these materials were gently condensed inside the previously prepared mesh. Finally, the mesh was adapted to the recipient area and fixed to the maxillary bone from the buccal side with two screws (Figures 2(c) and 2(d)). To protect the thin mucosa from being torn by the mesh, PRF was prepared by collecting four 6 mL tubes of blood. Blood was centrifuged at 3000 rpm for 12 min and condensed in a PRF condenser kit. A PRF membrane was placed over the mesh (Figure 3). The mucoperiosteal flap at the periosteum was scored in advance to achieve tension-free closure.

The patient was administered 1200 mg augmentin (intravenous [IV], 8 h/day for 5 days), 1000 mg paracetamol (IV, 8 h/day for 5 days), and 8 mg dexamethasone (IV, 8 h/day for 3 days).

After 5 days, the patient was discharged with weekly follow-up for the first month, then monthly follow-up for 6 months. There was no wound dehiscence or mesh exposure during this time (Figure 4(a)).

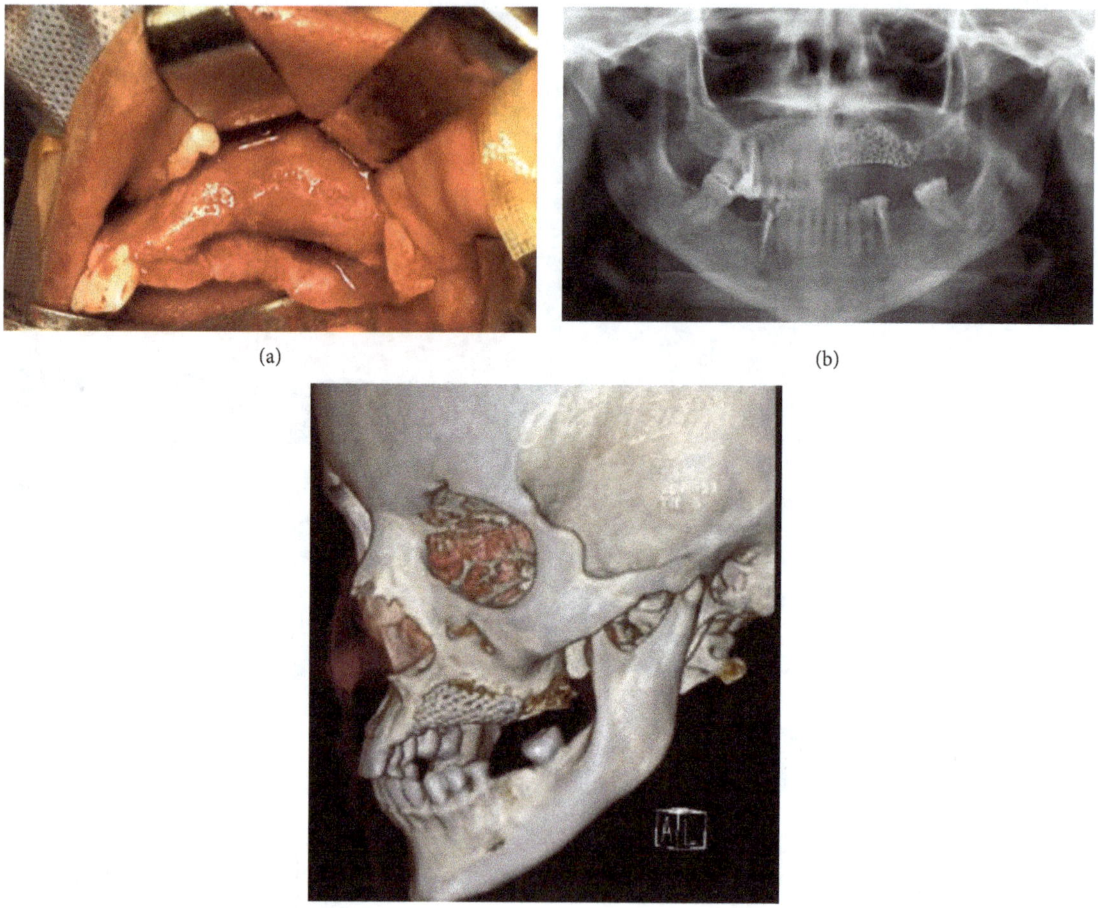

(a) (b) (c)

FIGURE 3: (a) Photographs showing the postoperative view of the maxillary defect. (b, c) Postoperative computed tomography and radiographic evaluation.

2.3. Implant Placement, Abutment Connection, and Bridge Delivery. An OPG and CT scan was performed 6 months later to evaluate bone formation. CT revealed a good quantity of bone formation for the accommodation of four implants.

The mesh was exposed and removed under general anesthesia using the same incision. Using a two-stage protocol, four implants (Biomet 3; Palm Beach Gardens, FL) were placed in the left maxilla (3.25 mm × 10 mm, 4 mm × 10 mm, 5 mm × 8.5 mm, 5 × 8.5 mm) and one implant (4 mm × 10 mm) in the left mandible (Figures 4(b) and 4(c)).

Five months later, osseointegration was successful with 35 N/cm of torque, and the prosthetic part was completed.

2.4. Follow-Up. Three years after bone augmentation and implant placement, a satisfactory quantity of bone around the implants was visible in a follow-up X-ray.

The patient reported normal function and was satisfied with her cosmetic appearance (Figures 4(d) and 4(e)).

3. Discussion

One of the most significant challenges in oral and maxillofacial surgery is the reconstruction of osseous defects, especially in cases of vertical bone augmentation. This is due to the limited osseous walls surrounding the defect, which negatively affect blood supply, graft stability and soft tissue coverage, and the lack of osteoprogenitor cells [14].

For regenerative surgeries, many graft materials have been developed with variable properties. One relatively new material is rhBMP-2, a member of the transforming growth factor-β superfamily, which plays an important role in the modulation and differentiation of mesenchymal cells into osteoblasts [15, 16].

rhBMP-2 is the most investigated growth factor for oral and maxillofacial applications that has shown a high success rate in bone defect reconstruction [17]. In 2008, the US Food and Drug Administration approved the clinical use of rhBMP-2 in sinus lifting and localized alveolar ridge defects associated with extraction sockets [16]. Many studies have reported offlabel uses of rhBMP-2 in the reconstruction of maxillary bone defects [14, 16, 18]. Moreover, it has become an alternative to autogenous bone and other bone grafts, as it can overcome the complications associated with harvesting bone from the iliac crest or other donor sites [19]. Furthermore, the new bone induced by rhBMP-2/ACS was found to be similar to autogenous bone and demonstrated good osseointegration [13].

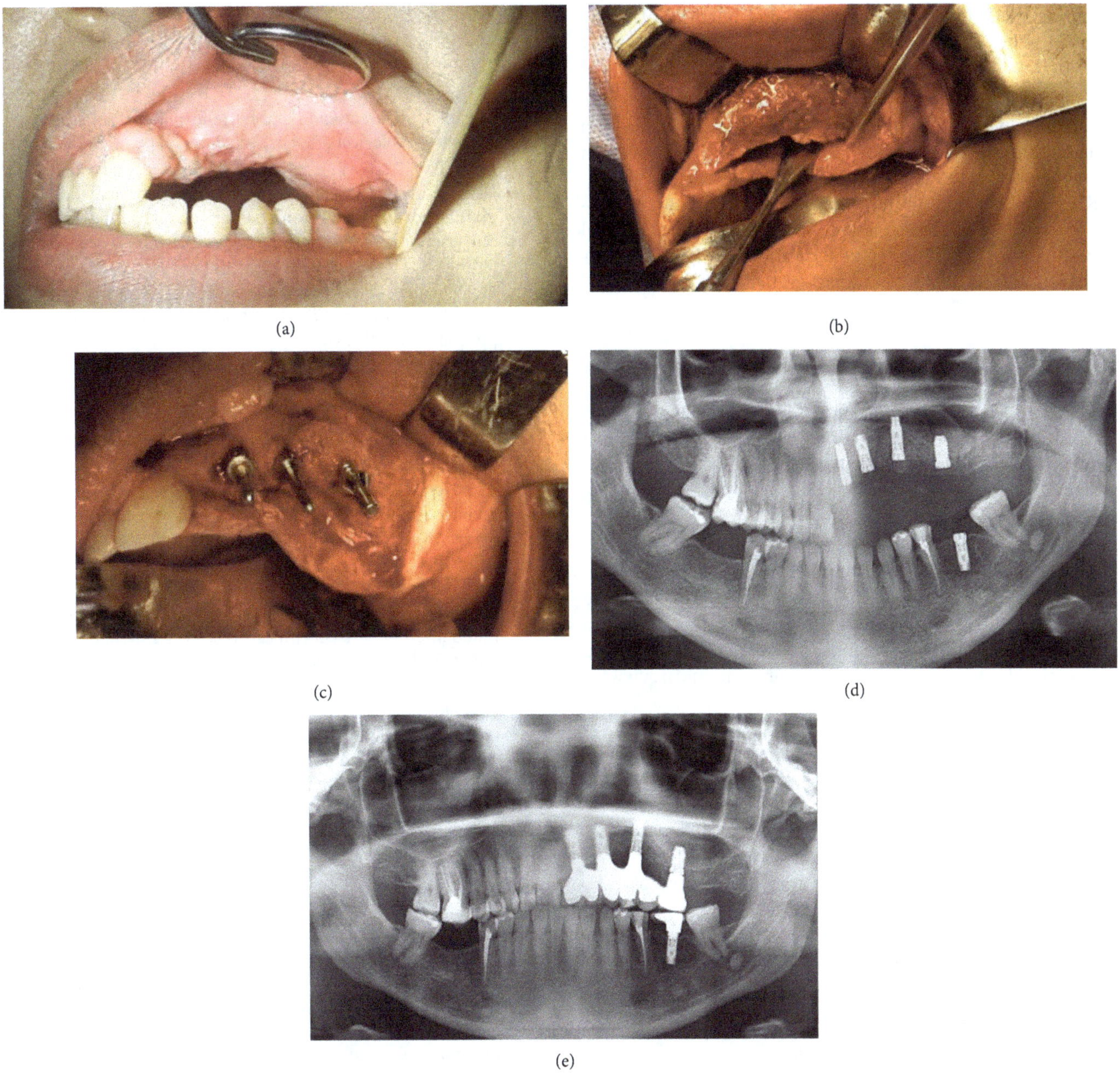

FIGURE 4: (a) Six months postoperation. (b) Exposing and removing the mesh. (c) Implant placement. (d) Radiograph of bone graft at 8-month follow-up. Note: the significant increase in bone augmentation of the maxilla and implant rehabilitation. (e) Complete regeneration in 3 years following reconstruction of the maxillary defect.

However, rhBMP-2/ACS does not provide enough space for bone formation, especially in vertical and lateral alveolar ridge defects, due to soft tissue compression. Thus, a titanium mesh has become an interesting alternative material [12]. Its first use in oral surgery for bone augmentation was reported by Boyne et al. in 1985 [20]. The advantages of using a titanium mesh with rhBMP-2/ACS are that it can support the soft tissue and prevent it from collapsing into the regenerative site, permitting adequate bone formation. Furthermore, it acts as a scaffold to hold the graft in place [21–23].

However, a titanium mesh has some disadvantages. A second surgery is needed to remove it, and it is associated with a high rate of infection [24]. To prevent wound dehiscence in the present case, in addition to decreasing wound closure tension by adequate scoring of the periosteum, the PRF and collagen membrane was added to cover the titanium mesh as a soft layer between the mesh and oral mucosa to counteract the harmful effects of the mesh on the oral mucosa. Growth factors released from platelets also play a role in healing by attracting undifferentiated stem cells to the site of injury. In addition, PRF plays a role in osteogenesis and angiogenesis [25]. PRF enables a slower release of growth factors leading to better healing [26]. Ozdemir et al. concluded that the use of PRF in conjunction with a titanium mesh increased the quality and quantity of newly formed bone [27].

The case described in this study shows that it is possible to achieve successful augmentation of a maxillary defect and rehabilitation with dental implants by using rhBMP-2 in combination with allografts in a titanium mesh covered by PRF, leading to both graft osteoinduction and osteoconductivity. Additional research is necessary to determine the ideal combination of grafting materials and to ascertain the long-term survival of implants in areas grafted with rhBMP-2.

Consent

We discussed our treatment plan with the patient. We also discussed the risks and potential complications and obtained informed consent from the patient.

Authors' Contributions

Kamal Alraei conceptualized the study and collected the data. Kamal Alraei and Khawlah Alarusi contributed to data analysis and writing the manuscript. Jameel Shrqawi and Khawlah Alarusi contributed to the drafting and review of the manuscript.

References

[1] Y.-S. Jung, H. J. Kim, S. W. Choi, J. W. Kang, and I. H. Cha, "Regional thickness of parietal bone in Korean adults," *International Journal of Oral and Maxillofacial Surgery*, vol. 32, no. 6, pp. 638–641, 2003.

[2] C. Maiorana, M. Beretta, D. Rancitelli, G. B. Grossi, M. Cicciù, and A. S. Herford, "Histological features and biocompatibility of bone and soft tissue substitutes in the atrophic alveolar ridge reconstruction," *Case Reports in Dentistry*, vol. 2016, Article ID 3608602, 7 pages, 2016.

[3] M. Cicciù, "A window view from the orient on trauma involving the inner maxillofacial Region," *The Journal of Craniofacial Surgery*, vol. 27, no. 1, p. 6, 2016.

[4] L. Laino, G. Iezzi, A. Piattelli, L. Lo Muzio, and M. Cicciù, "Vertical ridge augmentation of the atrophic posterior mandible with sandwich technique: bone block from the chin area versus corticocancellous bone block allograft—clinical and histological prospective randomized controlled study," *BioMed Research International*, vol. 2014, Article ID 982104, 7 pages, 2014.

[5] M. Cicciù, A. Scott, D. Cicciù, R. Tandon, and C. Maiorana, "Recombinant human bone morphogenetic protein-2 promote and stabilize hard and soft tissue healing for large mandibular new bone reconstruction defects," *The Journal of Craniofacial Surgery*, vol. 25, no. 3, pp. 860–862, 2014.

[6] R. Margonar, P. L. dos Santos, T. P. Queiroz, and E. Marcantonio, "Rehabilitation of atrophic maxilla using the combination of autogenous and allogeneic bone grafts followed by protocol-type prosthesis," *The Journal of Craniofacial Surgery*, vol. 21, no. 6, pp. 1894–1896, 2010.

[7] A. S. Herford, R. Tandon, T. W. Stevens, E. Stoffella, and M. Cicciu, "Immediate distraction Osteogenesis," *The Journal of Craniofacial Surgery*, vol. 24, no. 4, pp. 1383–1387, 2013.

[8] G. Chen, C. Deng, and Y.-P. Li, "TGF-β and BMP signaling in osteoblast differentiation and bone formation," *International Journal of Biological Sciences*, vol. 8, no. 2, pp. 272–288, 2012.

[9] U. M. E. Wikesjö, Y. H. Huang, G. Polimeni, and M. Qahash, "Bone morphogenetic proteins: a realistic alternative to bone grafting for alveolar reconstruction," *Oral and Maxillofacial Surgery Clinics of North America*, vol. 19, no. 4, pp. 535–551, 2007.

[10] H. Dym and J. Pierse, "Advanced techniques in bone grafting procedures," *Dental Clinics of North America*, vol. 55, no. 3, pp. 453–460, 2011, vii.

[11] K. Wada, A. Niimi, K. Watanabe, T. Sawai, and M. Ueda, "Maxillary sinus floor augmentation in rabbits: a comparative histologic-histomorphometric study between rhBMP-2 and autogenous bone," *The International Journal of Periodontics & Restorative Dentistry*, vol. 21, no. 3, pp. 252–263, 2001.

[12] A. S. Herford, "rhBMP-2 as an option for reconstructing mandibular continuity defects," *Journal of Oral and Maxillofacial Surgery*, vol. 67, no. 12, pp. 2679–2684, 2009.

[13] R. E. Marx, L. Armentano, A. Olavarria, and J. Samaniego, "rhBMP-2/ACS grafts versus autogenous cancellous marrow grafts in large vertical defects of the maxilla: an unsponsored randomized open-label clinical trial," *The International Journal of Oral & Maxillofacial Implants*, vol. 28, no. 5, pp. e243–e251, 2013.

[14] C. M. Misch, O. Jensen, M. Pikos, and J. Malmquist, "Vertical bone augmentation using recombinant bone morphogenetic protein, mineralized bone allograft, and titanium mesh: a retrospective cone beam computed tomography study," *The International Journal of Oral & Maxillofacial Implants*, vol. 30, no. 1, pp. 202–207, 2015.

[15] S. Annibali, M. P. Cristalli, D. Dell'Aquila, I. Bignozzi, G. la Monaca, and A. Pilloni, "Short dental implants: a systematic review," *Journal of Dental Research*, vol. 91, no. 1, pp. 25–32, 2012.

[16] C. Fortes Ferreira, J. da Escóssia, T. Pessoa Tabosa e Silva, A. Luiz Zétola, and R. Nunes Tavares, "Reconstruction of severely atrophic pre-maxilla using Rhbmp-2 and titanium mesh for dental Implants," *Journal of Dentistry And Oral Implants*, vol. 1, no. 1, pp. 15–20, 2014.

[17] R. M. Lustosa, L. C. Iwaki, S. Tolentino Ede, M. Chicarelli da Silva, R. de Oliveira Lazarin, and L. Iwaki Filho, "Mandible reconstruction using rhBMP-2: case report and literature review," *Quintessence International*, vol. 45, no. 10, pp. 869–874, 2014.

[18] A. L. Zétola, T. Verbicaro, S. Littieri, R. Larson, A. F. Giovanini, and T. M. Deliberador, "Recombinant human bone morphogenetic protein type 2 in the reconstruction of atrophic maxilla: case report with long-term follow-up," *Journal of Indian Society of Periodontology*, vol. 18, no. 6, pp. 781–785, 2014.

[19] E. Ahlmann, M. Patzakis, N. Roidis, L. Shepherd, and P. Holtom, "Comparison of anterior and posterior iliac crest bone grafts in terms of harvest-site morbidity and functional outcomes," *JBJS*, vol. 84, no. 5, pp. 716–720, 2002.

[20] P. J. Boyne, M. D. Cole, D. Stringer, and J. P. Shafqat, "A technique for osseous restoration of deficient edentulous maxillary ridges," *Journal of Oral and Maxillofacial Surgery*, vol. 43, no. 2, pp. 87–91, 1985.

[21] S. A. Jovanovic, R. K. Schenk, M. Orsini, and E. B. Kenney, "Supracrestal bone formation around dental implants: an experimental dog study," *The International Journal of Oral & Maxillofacial Implants*, vol. 10, no. 1, pp. 23–31, 1995.

[22] M. Simion, P. Trisi, and A. Piattelli, "Vertical ridge augmentation using a membrane technique associated with osseointegrated implants," *The International Journal of Periodontics & Restorative Dentistry*, vol. 14, no. 6, pp. 496–511, 1994.

[23] U. M. E. Wikesjo, G. Polimeni, and M. Qahash, "Tissue engineering with recombinant human bone morphogenetic protein-2 for alveolar augmentation and oral implant osseointegration: experimental observations and clinical perspectives," *Clinical Implant Dentistry and Related Research*, vol. 7, no. 2, pp. 112–119, 2005.

[24] P. J. Louis, "Vertical ridge augmentation using titanium mesh," *Oral and Maxillofacial Surgery Clinics of North America*, vol. 22, no. 3, pp. 353–368, 2010.

[25] S. Kevy, M. Jacobson, L. Blasetti, and A. Fagnant, "Preparation of growth factor enriched autologous platelet gel," in *In proceedings of the 27th annual meeting of service biomaterials*, pp. 15–18, 2001.

[26] D. M. Dohan, J. Choukroun, A. Diss et al., "Platelet-rich fibrin (PRF): a second-generation platelet concentrate. Part II: platelet-related biologic features," *Oral Surgery, Oral Medicine, Oral Pathology, Oral Radiology, and Endodontology*, vol. 101, no. 3, pp. e45–e50, 2006.

[27] H. Ozdemir, S. Ezirganli, M. Isa Kara, A. Mihmanli, and E. Baris, "Effects of platelet rich fibrin alone used with rigid titanium barrier," *Archives of Oral Biology*, vol. 58, no. 5, pp. 537–544, 2013.

30

A Possible Relationship between Peri-Implantitis, Titanium Hypersensitivity and External Tooth Resorption: Metal-Free Alternative to Titanium Implants

Andrea Enrico Borgonovo[1] **Rachele Censi,**[2] **Virna Vavassori**[1] **Mauro Savio,**[1] **and Dino Re**[3]

[1]*Unit of Esthetic Dentistry, Istituto Stomatologico Italiano, University of Milan, Milan, Italy*
[2]*Unit of Periodontology, Istituto Stomatologico Italiano, University of Milan, Milan, Italy*
[3]*Head, Unit of Esthetic Dentistry, Istituto Stomatologico Italiano, Department of Biomedical, Surgical and Dental Sciences, University of Milan, Milan, Italy*

Correspondence should be addressed to Virna Vavassori; virna.vavassori@hotmail.it

Academic Editor: Miguel de Araújo Nobre

Titanium dental implant surface does not remain unaltered but may corrode and release ions or particles which trigger soft and hard tissue damage. Titanium may induce clinically relevant hypersensitivity in patients chronically exposed. A 56-year-old female patient presented peri-implantitis around a single titanium implant positioned three years earlier. Despite nonsurgical therapy, a rapid bone loss associated with pain and swelling occurred, and adjacent teeth presented external resorption. Compromised teeth were removed, and three titanium implants were inserted. Six months later, the patient complained about high mucosa sensitivity and implant exposure. At clinical and radiographic examinations, tissue inflammation and vertical bone loss involved the new implants and the process of external resorption affected the teeth. The blood test confirmed titanium hypersensitivity. Titanium implants were removed, and 5 zirconia implants were placed. No sign of bone loss or tooth resorption was recorded at clinical and radiographic control during 18 months of follow-up.

1. Introduction

Extraction of permanent teeth is carried out for several reasons, including caries, periodontal disease, fractures, orthodontic/prosthetic purpose, and extensive internal or external tooth resorption. Pathologic resorption of teeth has a multifactorial etiology although many aspects remain unclear and can lead to tooth loss [1].

The use of dental implants has become a predictable strategy for replacing missing teeth, and the satisfactory results reported by numerous clinical studies have determined an enormous development of implantology [2]. Currently, the success rate of implants is around 95% in the maxilla and 97% in the mandible after 10 years of follow-up period [3, 4].

However, the increase in the demand for implants is associated with a growing need for longer term results, and, despite the high success rates, implant failures may occur due to biological or biomechanics complication [5].

Among the biological complications, peri-implantitis plays an important role. The American Academy of Periodontology defines peri-implantitis as an inflammatory process around an osseointegrated implant, including both soft tissue inflammation and progressive loss of supporting bone beyond biological bone remodeling [6]. Clinically, peri-implantitis sites exhibit signs of inflammation and, in particular, increased probing depths and/or recession of the mucosal margin, bleeding on probing and/or suppuration, and radiographic bone loss [7, 8].

The prevalence of peri-implantitis has grown enormously over the last decades: recent data report a percentage of implant exhibiting peri-implantitis around 15%-20% after 10 years [9]. Considering the clinical relevance of this disease,

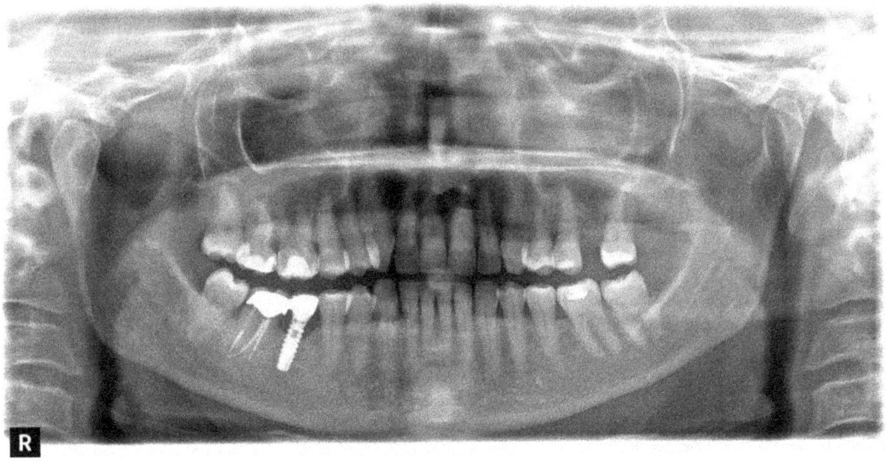

FIGURE 1: Implant 4.6 with initial signs of peri-implantitis.

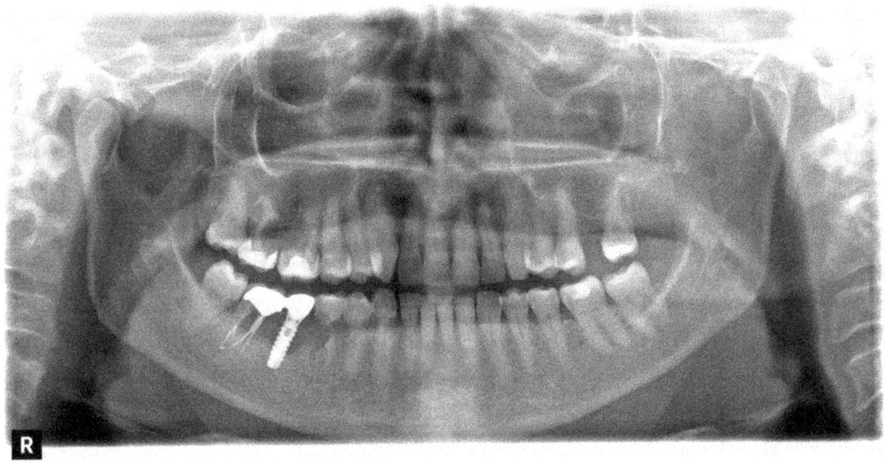

FIGURE 2: Tooth resorption and worsening of peri-implantitis.

research activity has been addressed to identify the etiopathogenesis of peri-implantitis in order to recognize effective protocols for prevention and treatment. Nowadays, there is a lack of consensus on the exact etiology of peri-implantitis and subsequent pathological process [10, 11], although many studies describe different potential mechanisms for peri-implant bone loss, including the microbial biofilm and metal ion/particle release [12]. Titanium degradation products in the form of microparticles or ions may infiltrate the peri-implant tissues and peri-implant bacterial plaque and trigger an inflammatory response with bone resorption, suggesting implications on the pathogenesis of peri-implantitis [13]. Moreover, the literature shows that allergic reactions and hypersensitivity to metal are not uncommon findings; in fact, delayed-onset T-cell-mediated metal hypersensitivity is reported in 12% to 17% of the general population [14].

The emerging limits of titanium have prompted the research to focus on alternative materials. Among the new generation of ceramics in the dental field, zirconia presents excellent aesthetic characteristics [15], a low tendency of plaque adhesion on implant surface [16], excellent biocompatibility [17], good osseointegration, and biomechanics [18]. In addition, zirconia implants have characteristics similar to those of titanium and are frequently used in implant-prosthetic rehabilitations.

The aim of this case report is to describe and analyze the failure of two implant-prosthetic rehabilitation with titanium implants due to a synergy between peri-implantitis and titanium hypersensitivity and the success of a metal-free implant prosthetic rehabilitation in the same patient. In association with implant failure, pathologic external resorption in adjacent teeth was identified.

2. Case Presentation

A 56-year-old female patient presented at the Department of Esthetic Dentistry, Istituto Stomatologico Italiano, University of Milan, Italy, after being treated in a private clinic. She came to our attention with a partial edentulism in the mandible, consequent to multiple implant failures. Thanks to her medical record, it was possible to reconstruct her history. The patient went to the private clinic for pain and swelling around the implant positioned in zone 4.6 three years earlier. She had a medical history of hypertension, treated with a β-blocker therapy and allergies to pollen and dust.

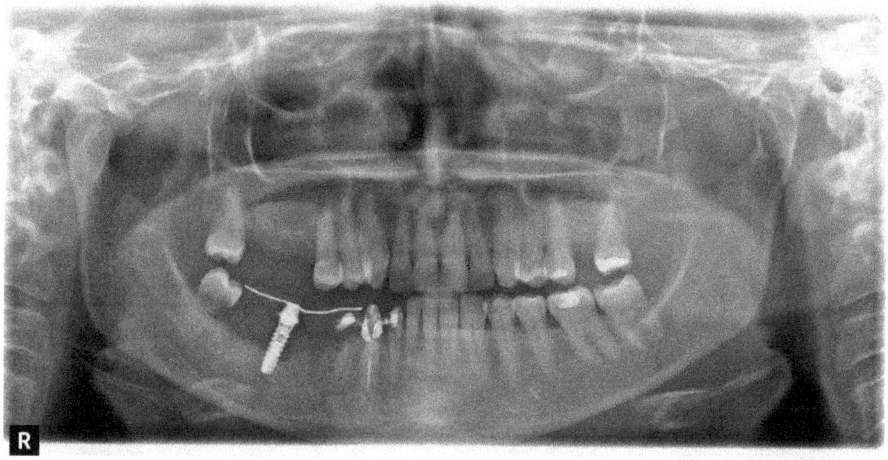

FIGURE 3: After extraction of compromised teeth, a provisional prosthesis was positioned.

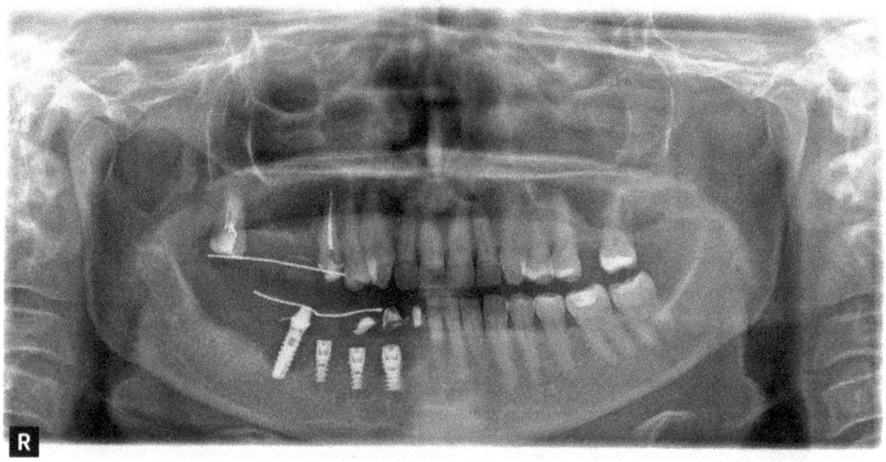

FIGURE 4: Insertion of three titanium implants.

The patient denied any history of tobacco smoking and alcoholism. The last dental check-up visit was done about two years ago. Even if the patient had many restorative and prosthetic treatments, no previous history of periodontitis was detected. At clinical evaluation, peri-implant mucosa appeared swelling and redness and the probing revealed bleeding and a probe depth of 6 mm, buccally and 5 mm, lingually. The radiographic image (OPT) showed a bony defect with a crater-like shape around implant 4.6 and cervical decay on teeth 2.6 and 2.7 (Figure 1). A diagnosis of peri-implantitis was supposed, and the patient was treated with nonsurgical laser therapy. Moreover, she was recommended to maintain excellent oral hygiene standards, attend regular professional maintenance, and treat the decay.

Some months later, the problem has not been solved; the patient returned with pain and swelling around implant 4.6. The orthopantomography showed an increased bone loss which resulted in a deep vertical bony defect. Moreover, at an X-ray picture, a severe resorption of the teeth close to the implant in both of the jaws was observed (Figure 2). The compromised teeth were extracted but the implant was temporarily maintained to support a provisional fixed prothesis (Figure 3). Four months after dental extractions, three new titanium fixtures were inserted and loaded with a fixed prothesis. The patient denied implant 4.6 removal because it was stable and no longer symptomatic (Figure 4).

Six months later, the patient complained about high mucosa sensitivity and implant exposure. At clinical and radiographic examinations, tissue inflammation and vertical bone loss involved the new implants and the process of external resorption affected the teeth up to the 3.3 (Figure 5).

A biopsy was performed taking a sample of cortical and medullary bone to check for bone disorder. The result did not show any kind of bone lesion or disease and even the bacterial culture was negative. The patient was referred from the private clinic to the Department of Esthetic Dentistry for clinical assessment. Medical tests were programmed in order to investigate her condition. Standard blood tests revealed an increased number of eosinophils and so titanium intolerance was supposed. The MELISA (Memory Lymphocyte Immunostimulation Assay) test was performed and confirmed titanium hypersensitivity. It was decided to remove all the

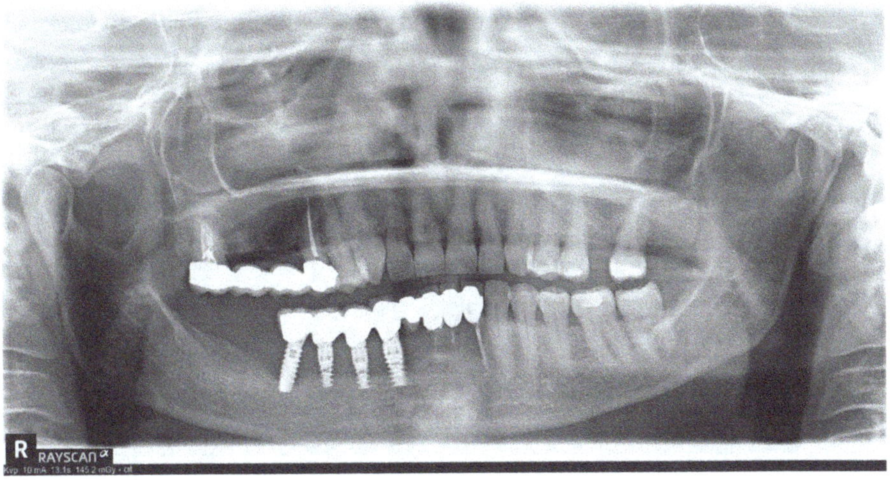

FIGURE 5: Six months after implant surgery: peri-implantitis affects new implants and tooth resorption involved the teeth up to the 3.3.

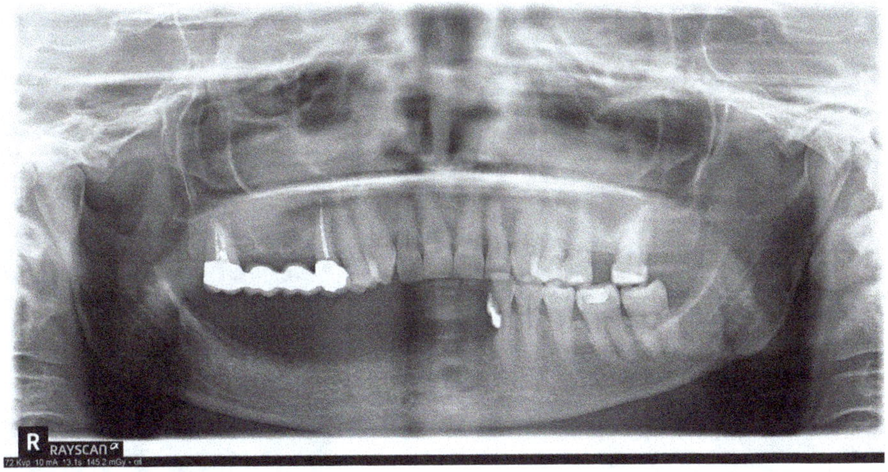

FIGURE 6: MELISA confirmed titanium hypersensitivity: implants were removed.

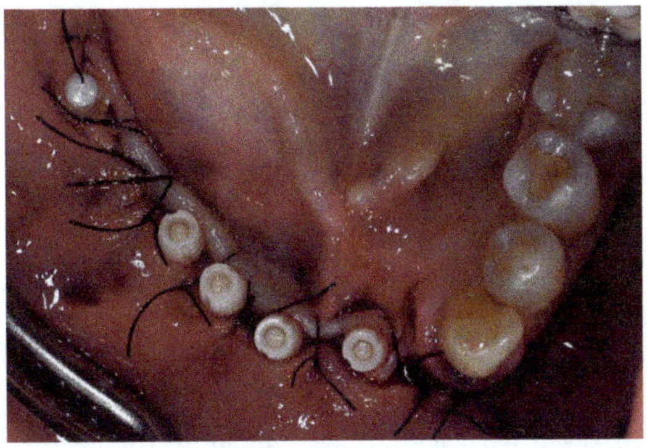

FIGURE 7: Surgical phase: five one-piece zirconia implants were placed.

titanium fixtures and the problematic teeth. Despite the removal of the titanium implant, the patient referred to high mucosa sensitivity for a long period (Figure 6). Subsequently, after nine months, when algic symptoms disappeared, five one-piece zirconia implants were inserted, four in the anterior jaw and 1 in the right molar region (Straumann PURE Ceramic Monotype, Straumann) (Figures 7 and 8). Although a submerged healing was advisable, one-piece zirconia implants were chosen because in the anterior area the bone volume was reduced, and two-piece zirconia implants are available in diameters from 4.1 mm. On the other hand, the one-piece ceramic system offers narrow-diameter zirconia implants (3.3 mm). The posterior implant was lost two months after the loading and then substituted with a two-piece zirconia fixture (Straumann PURE Ceramic, Straumann) (Figure 9). The fixtures were loaded with a fixed metal-free prosthesis made of modified PEEK (Biohpp, Bredent medical, Senden Germany) (Figures 10 and 11). During the follow-up period, the patient did not refer to any symptoms of peri-implantitis or other problems, and after 18 months from surgery, the clinical-radiographic exams showed the success of the metal-free implant prosthetic rehabilitation. In particular, peri-implant tissues appeared healthy, and the X-ray pictures confirmed the absence of marginal bone loss around implants and no sign of tooth resorption (Figure 12).

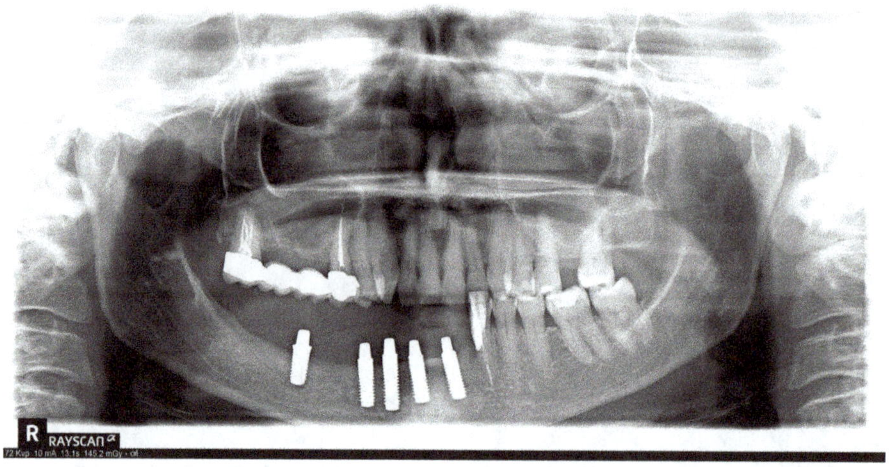

FIGURE 8: OPT after implant insertion.

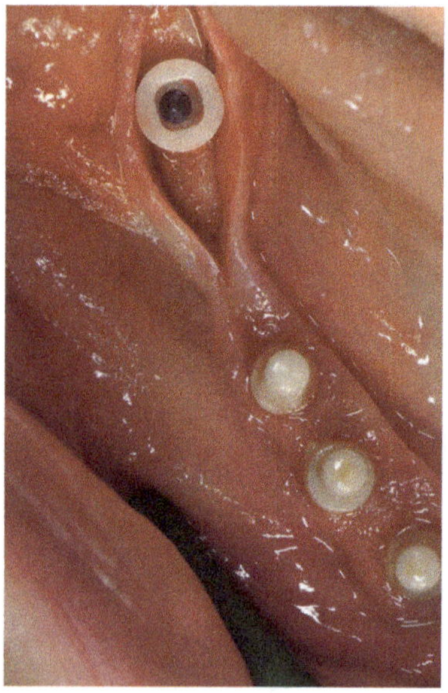

FIGURE 9: Placement of a two-piece zirconia in the posterior area after implant failure.

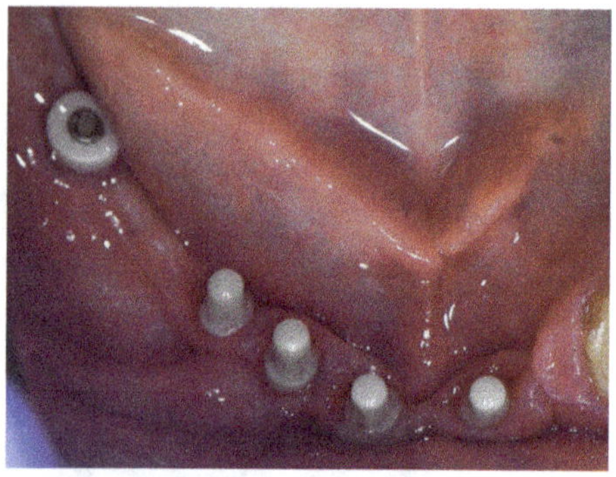

FIGURE 10: Clinical view before prosthesis positioning.

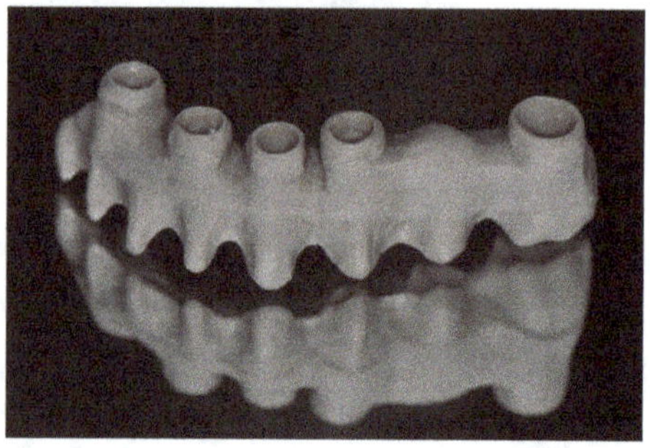

FIGURE 11: Modified PEEK framework.

3. Discussion

Modern implantology is based on the concept of osseointegration proposed by Branemark in 1977 [19]. Osseointegration refers to a direct structural and functional connection between living bone and the surface of a "load-bearing" (titanium) implant [20]. This phenomenon begins with implant placement into alveolar bone and takes up to several weeks. During this period, a cascade of healing events occurs resulting in direct bone contact with the implant surface. If initially, the interest was mainly addressed to the interactions that the bone had around the implant; recently, the attention was directed to the possible influence of metal ions or particle release from implant surface into surrounding tissues [21]. Moreover, in the last decades, an increase in the number of peri-implantitis has required investigations about its causes and risk factors.

In literature, many studies have detected the release of titanium ions and particles from the implant surface with the consequent activation of an inflammatory response [22, 23]. Dissolved particles can accumulate in the peri-implant tissues or can be released into the blood and lymphatic circulation and found in regional lymph nodes and internal organs [24]. Several hypotheses have been proposed about the release mechanisms. According to mechanical theory, titanium particles can be released from implant-abutment connection or during implant insertion or decontamination [25]. The chemical mechanism involves saliva, bacteria, and chemicals that potentially dissolve the titanium oxide layer of implants and trigger a process defined as biocorrosion

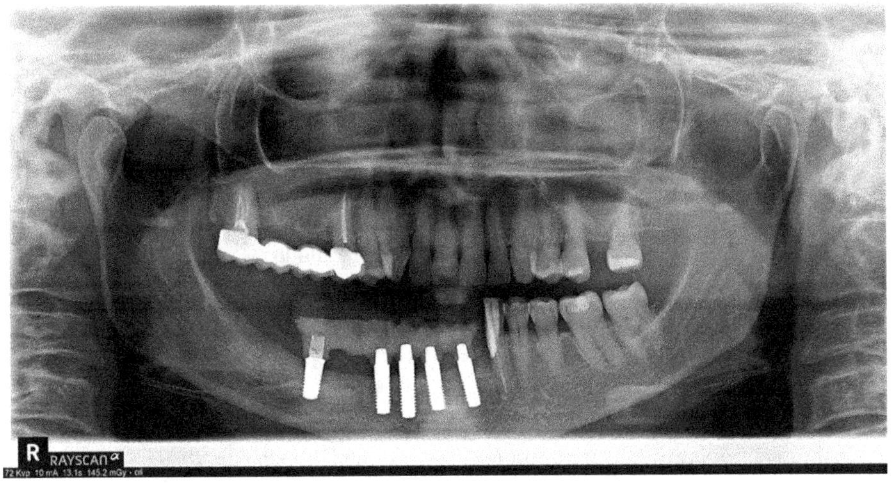

FIGURE 12: Rx control at 18 months of follow-up.

[26]. Recent studies report high levels of dissolved titanium in submucosal plaque of implants with peri-implantitis compared with healthy implants, suggesting a relation between titanium release and peri-implantitis [27]. Reports suggest that peri-implantitis bacteria trigger an inflammatory response and cause electrochemical alteration of the titanium surfaces that include disruption of the titanium oxide layer and release of titanium particles and ions, influencing the pathogenesis of peri-implant bone loss. Moreover, corrosion may be enhanced by some everyday chemical agents, such as acid fluoride solutions [28].

The metal particles and ions released from implant surfaces act as foreign bodies and stimulate inflammatory reactions through the activation of a number of mediators. In particular, phagocytic cells (macrophages and multinucleate giant cells) phagocytize metal particles and promote an immune response through the release of proinflammatory cytokines and grown factors that induce inflammatory reaction and osteoclastogenesis with consequent bone resorption [29]. Titanium ions influence the expression of RANKL (Receptive Activator of Nuclear factor Kappa-B Ligand) and osteoprotegerin (OPG) in osteoblastic cells, promoting osteoclast activity.

This immune response is also strictly connected with titanium hypersensitivity even if the exact cellular pathway involved has not yet been clarified. Probably, metal ions bind to native proteins and form haptenic antigens that trigger the degranulation of mastocytes and basophiles and develop type IV hypersensitive reactions [30].

Hypersensitivity to metal in the general population is frequent, affecting up to 15% of patients, and nickel is the biggest offender, followed by cobalt and chromium [31]. However, recent data suggest an increased incidence of hypersensitivity to titanium for patients with dental implant and orthopedic arthroplasties. Diagnostic technique for type IV sensitivity reaction to potential allergens is commonly based on patch testing, but in the case of titanium, hypersensitivity is not predictable [32].

Titanium hypersensitivity is detected with MELISA that measures lymphocytic proliferation after antigen-specific activation. From a general point of view, the confirm of type IV hypersensitivity requires the avoidance of responsible agent and, for this reason, in the field of implantology, patients with clinical symptoms of hypersensitivity and elevated MELISA levels may undergo surgical removal of titanium implants and alternative material, such as ceramics, must be considered for rehabilitation of edentulous areas.

Oliva et al. describe a case report of a full-mouth oral rehabilitation with zirconia implants in a titanium allergy patient. No complications were recorded after 3 years of follow-up [33].

The presented case may be an example of titanium hypersensitivity probably potentiated by peri-implantitis, even if the report presents some limits that might act as possible cofactors in implant failure. It is well-known that there are several problems connecting a tooth with an implant, including tooth intrusion with consequent loss of crown retention. Moreover, exposed implant surface and continued contamination can lead to peri-implantitis [34].

The medical history of the patient suggested allergies to dust and pollen but not to metals. However, it is known that an allergy can develop at any time in life. Probably, the first single titanium implant rehabilitation and the development of peri-implantitis that commonly affect implants have triggered immune response and consequent hypersensitivity. After implant failure, three titanium implants were placed developing a more intensive allergic reaction. The peculiarity of this case resided not only in the implant failure consequent to titanium hypersensitivity but also in the phenomenon of external resorption of the adjacent teeth. Pathologic tooth resorption is associated with an abnormal stimulation of the RANKL system which is present not only in osteoblasts but also in odontoblasts, cementoblasts, and ameloblasts [35]. As reported, the release of titanium particles and ions influence RANKL expression, suggesting a connection between titanium hypersensitivity and external tooth resorption.

However, after the second implant failure, it was decided to proceed with a metal-free rehabilitation positioning 5 zirconia implants. Zirconia implants appeared well integrated without marginal bone loss, and no sign of pathological tooth resorption was detected at 18 months of follow-up.

Zirconia has some advantages over titanium implants: although the success and survival rates of zirconia and titanium implants are similar, some studies have reported that zirconia has more biocompatibility as compared to titanium, as the latter produces corrosion products at the implant site [36]. However, further investigations about titanium release and its connections with peri-implantitis, hypersensitivity, and tooth resorption are recommended.

Patients detected with hypersensitivity by MELISA should be treated with zirconia implants and metal-free prosthesis. For this reason, zirconia implants may represent a valid alternative to titanium even if further studies are still needed [37].

References

[1] M. Fernandes, I. De Ataide, and R. Wagle, "Tooth resorption part I-pathogenesis and case series of internal resorption," *Journal of conservative dentistry*, vol. 16, no. 1, pp. 4–8, 2013.

[2] D. Schwartz-Arad, R. Herzberg, and L. Levin, "Evaluation of long-term implant success," *Journal of Periodontology*, vol. 76, no. 10, pp. 1623–1628, 2005.

[3] L. W. Lindquist, G. E. Carlsson, and T. Jemt, "A prospective 15-year follow-up study of mandibular fixed prostheses supported by osseointegrated implants. Clinical results and marginal bone loss," *Clinical Oral Implants Research*, vol. 7, pp. 329–336, 1996.

[4] D. Buser, R. Mericske-Stern, K. Dula, and N. P. Lang, "Clinical experience with one-stage, non-submerged dental implants," *Advances in Dental Research*, vol. 13, no. 1, pp. 153–161, 1999.

[5] J. Lindhe, J. Meyle, and on behalf of Group D of the European Workshop on Periodontology, "Peri-implant diseases: consensus report of the sixth European workshop on periodontology," *Journal of Clinical Periodontology*, vol. 35, Supplement 8, pp. 282–285, 2008.

[6] P. Rosen, D. Clem, D. Cochran et al., "Peri-implant mucositis and peri-implantitis: a current understanding of their diagnoses and clinical implications," *Journal of periodontology*, vol. 84, no. 4, pp. 436–443, 2013.

[7] M. Sanz and I. L. Chapple, "Clinical research on peri-implant diseases: consensus report of working group 4," *Journal of clinical periodontology*, vol. 39, Supplement 12, pp. 202–206, 2012.

[8] J. Costerton, L. Montanaro, and C. R. Arciola, "Biofilm in implant infections: its production and regulation," *The International Journal of Artificial Organs*, vol. 28, no. 11, pp. 1062–1068, 2005.

[9] S. D. Ferreira, G. L. M. Silva, J. R. Cortelli, J. E. Costa, and F. O. Costa, "Prevalence and risk variables for peri-im- plant disease in Brazilian subjects," *Journal of Clinical Periodontology*, vol. 22, no. 12, pp. 929–935, 2006.

[10] L. Canullo, M. Tallarico, S. Radovanovic, B. Delibasic, U. Covani, and M. Rakic, "Distinguishing predictive profiles for patient-based risk assessment and diagnostics of plaque induced, surgically and prosthetically triggered peri-implantitis," *Clinical Oral Implants Research*, vol. 27, no. 10, pp. 1243–1250, 2016.

[11] M. Tallarico, L. Canullo, H. Wang, D. Cochran, and S. Meloni, "Classification systems for peri-implantitis: a narrative review with a proposal of a new evidence-based etiology codification," *The International Journal of Oral & Maxillofacial Implants*, vol. 33, no. 4, pp. 871–879, 2018.

[12] Montegrotto Group for the Study of Peri-implant Disease, L. Canullo, M. Schlee, W. Wagner, and U. Covani, "International brainstorming meeting on etiologic and risk factors of peri-implantitis, Montegrotto (Padua, Italy), August 2014," *The International Journal of Oral & Maxillofacial Implants*, vol. 30, no. 5, pp. 1093–1104, 2015.

[13] T. Fretwurst, K. Nelson, D. P. Tarnow, H. L. Wang, and W. V. Giannobile, "Is metal particle release associated with peri-implant bone destruction? An emerging concept," *Journal of Dental Research*, vol. 97, no. 3, pp. 259–265, 2017.

[14] M. Schultzel, C. M. Klein, M. Demirjian, C. Blout, and J. M. Itamura, "Incidence of metal hypersensitivity in orthopedic surgical patients who self-report hypersensitivity history," *The Permanente Journal*, vol. 24, article 19.091, 2019.

[15] A. E. Borgonovo, R. Censi, V. Vavassori, O. Arnaboldi, C. Maiorana, and D. Re, "Zirconia implants in esthetic areas: 4-year follow-up evaluation study," *International journal of dentistry*, vol. 2015, Article ID 415029, 8 pages, 2015.

[16] M. Degidi, L. Artese, A. Scarano, V. Perrotti, P. Gehrke, and A. Piattelli, "Inflammatory infiltrate, microvessel density, nitric oxide synthase expression, vascular endothelial growth factor expression, and proliferative activity in peri-implant soft tissues around titanium and zirconium oxide healing caps," *Journal of Periodontology*, vol. 77, no. 1, pp. 73–80, 2006.

[17] T. ALBREKTSSON, H. HANSSON, and B. IVARSSON, "Interface analysis of titanium and zirconium bone implants," *Clinical materials*, vol. 6, no. 2, pp. 97–101, 1985.

[18] F. P. Koch, D. Weng, S. Krämer, S. Biesterfeld, A. Jahn-Eimermacher, and W. Wagner, "Osseointegration of one-piece zirconia implants compared with a titanium implant of identical design: a histomorphometric study in the dog," *Clinical Oral Implants Research*, vol. 21, no. 3, pp. 350–356, 2010.

[19] P. I. Brånemark, B. O. Hansson, R. Adell et al., "Osseointegrated implants in the treatment of the edentulous jaw. Experience from a 10-year period," *Scandinavian Journal of Plastic and Reconstructive Surgery. Supplementum*, vol. 16, pp. 1–132, 1977.

[20] S. Parithimarkalaignan and T. V. Padmanabhan, "Osseointegration: an update," *The Journal of Indian Prosthodontic Society*, vol. 13, no. 1, pp. 2–6, 2013.

[21] M. Noronha Oliveira, W. V. H. Schunemann, M. T. Mathew et al., "Can degradation products released from dental implants affect peri-implant tissues?," *Journal of Periodontal Research*, vol. 53, no. 1, pp. 1–11, 2018.

[22] M. Franchi, B. Bacchelli, D. Martini et al., "Early detachment of titanium particles from various different surfaces of endosseous dental implants," *Biomaterials*, vol. 25, no. 12, pp. 2239–2246, 2004.

[23] R. M. Urban, J. J. Jacobs, M. J. Tomlinson, J. Gavrilovic, J. Black, and M. Peoc'h, "Dissemination of wear particles to the liver, spleen, and abdominal lymph nodes of patients with hip or knee replacement," *The Journal of Bone and Joint Surgery. American Volume*, vol. 82, p. 45, 2000.

[24] T. Pinheiro, J. Pallon, L. C. Alves et al., "The influence of corneocyte structure on the interpretation of permeation profiles

of nanoparticles across skin," *Nuclear Instruments and Methods in Physics Research Section B*, vol. 260, no. 1, pp. 119–123, 2007.

[25] S. B. Goodman, "Wear particles, periprosthetic osteolysis and the immune system," *Biomaterials*, vol. 28, no. 34, pp. 5044–5048, 2007.

[26] L. M. Safioti, G. A. Kotsakis, A. E. Pozhitkov, W. O. Chung, and D. M. Daubert, "Increased levels of dissolved titanium are associated with peri-implantitis - a cross-sectional study," *Journal of Periodontology*, vol. 88, no. 5, pp. 436–442, 2017.

[27] H. J. Cruz, J. C. M. Souza, M. Henriques, and L. A. Rocha, "Tribocorrosion and bio- tribocorrosion in the oral environment: the case of dental implants," in *Biomedical Tribology*, J. Paulo Davim, Ed., pp. 1–33, Nova Science Publishers, Inc., New York, 2011.

[28] A. Mombelli, D. Hashim, and N. Cionca, "What is the impact of titanium particles and biocorrosion on implant survival and complications? A critical review," *Clinical Oral Implants Research*, vol. 29, Supplement 18, pp. 37–53, 2018.

[29] G. A. Obando-Pereda, L. Fischer, and D. R. Stach-Machado, "Titanium and zirconia particle-induced pro-inflammatory gene expression in cultured macrophages and osteolysis, inflammatory hyperalgesia and edema *in vivo*," *Life Sciences*, vol. 97, no. 2, pp. 96–106, 2014.

[30] M. Goutam, C. Giriyapura, S. K. Mishra, and S. Gupta, "Titanium allergy: a literature review," *Indian Journal of Dermatology*, vol. 59, no. 6, p. 630, 2014.

[31] T. Schäfer, E. Böhler, S. Ruhdorfer et al., "Epidemiology of contact allergy in adults," *Allergy*, vol. 56, no. 12, pp. 1192–1196, 2001.

[32] S. Bernard, M. Baeck, D. Tennstedt, V. Haufroid, and V. Dekeuleneer, "Chromate or titanium allergy - the role of impurities?," *Contact Dermatitis*, vol. 68, no. 3, pp. 191-192, 2013.

[33] X. Oliva, J. Oliva, and J. D. Oliva, "Full-mouth oral rehabilitation in a titanium allergy patient using zirconium oxide dental implants and zirconium oxide restorations. A case report from an ongoing clinical study," *The European Journal of Esthetic Dentistry*, vol. 5, no. 2, pp. 190–203, 2010.

[34] D. French, H. Larjava, and M. Tallarico, "Retrospective study of 1087 anodized implants placed in private Practice," *Implant Dentistry*, vol. 27, no. 2, pp. 177–187, 2018.

[35] Z. Wang and L. K. McCauley, "Osteoclasts and odontoclasts: signal pathway development and disease," *Oral Disease*, vol. 17, pp. 129–142, 2011.

[36] H. Tschernitschek, L. Borchers, and W. Geurtsen, "Nonalloyed titanium as a bioinert metal–a review," *Quintessence International*, vol. 36, no. 7-8, pp. 523–530, 2005.

[37] K. Sivaraman, A. Chopra, A. I. Narayan, and D. Balakrishnan, "Is zirconia a viable alternative to titanium for oral implant? A critical review," *Journal of Prosthodontic Research*, vol. 62, no. 2, pp. 121–133, 2018.

Permissions

All chapters in this book were first published by Hindawi Publishing Corporation; hereby published with permission under the Creative Commons Attribution License or equivalent. Every chapter published in this book has been scrutinized by our experts. Their significance has been extensively debated. The topics covered herein carry significant findings which will fuel the growth of the discipline. They may even be implemented as practical applications or may be referred to as a beginning point for another development.

The contributors of this book come from diverse backgrounds, making this book a truly international effort. This book will bring forth new frontiers with its revolutionizing research information and detailed analysis of the nascent developments around the world.

We would like to thank all the contributing authors for lending their expertise to make the book truly unique. They have played a crucial role in the development of this book. Without their invaluable contributions this book wouldn't have been possible. They have made vital efforts to compile up to date information on the varied aspects of this subject to make this book a valuable addition to the collection of many professionals and students.

This book was conceptualized with the vision of imparting up-to-date information and advanced data in this field. To ensure the same, a matchless editorial board was set up. Every individual on the board went through rigorous rounds of assessment to prove their worth. After which they invested a large part of their time researching and compiling the most relevant data for our readers.

The editorial board has been involved in producing this book since its inception. They have spent rigorous hours researching and exploring the diverse topics which have resulted in the successful publishing of this book. They have passed on their knowledge of decades through this book. To expedite this challenging task, the publisher supported the team at every step. A small team of assistant editors was also appointed to further simplify the editing procedure and attain best results for the readers.

Apart from the editorial board, the designing team has also invested a significant amount of their time in understanding the subject and creating the most relevant covers. They scrutinized every image to scout for the most suitable representation of the subject and create an appropriate cover for the book.

The publishing team has been an ardent support to the editorial, designing and production team. Their endless efforts to recruit the best for this project, has resulted in the accomplishment of this book. They are a veteran in the field of academics and their pool of knowledge is as vast as their experience in printing. Their expertise and guidance has proved useful at every step. Their uncompromising quality standards have made this book an exceptional effort. Their encouragement from time to time has been an inspiration for everyone.

The publisher and the editorial board hope that this book will prove to be a valuable piece of knowledge for researchers, students, practitioners and scholars across the globe.

List of Contributors

Saleh N. Almohammed and Duaa D. Ailabouni
Department of Prosthodontics, Jordan University of Science and Technology, Irbid, Jordan

Reem S. Abdel-Hafez
Department of Preventive Dentistry, Jordan University of Science and Technology, Irbid, Jordan

Paula Bernardon, Carlos Estevão Lagustera, Danielle Shima Luize and Rolando Plumer Pezzini
West State University of Parana, No. 1618 Universitária St., Cascavel, PR 85819-110, Brazil

Luiz Roberto Coutinho Manhães Junior and Bruno de Castro Figuêiredo
São Leopoldo Mandic College-SP, No. 13 Dr. José Rocha Junqueira St., Campinas, SP 13045-755, Brazil

George Borja de Freitas
Integrated College of Patos- (FIP-) PB, Horácio Nóbrega St., S/N, Belo Horizonte, Patos, PB 58704-000, Brazil

José Luiz Cintra Junqueira
Faculdade São Leopoldo Mandic-SP, No. 13 Dr. José Rocha Junqueira St., Campinas, SP 13045-755, Brazil

Rafał Flieger
Private Dental Healthcare, ul. Nacławska 11, 64-000 Kościan, Poland

André Moreira
Private practice, Implantology Institute, Lisboa, Portugal

Filipe Freitas
Private practice, Implantology Institute, Lisboa, Portugal
Department of Oral Surgery and Oral Medicine, Faculdade de Medicina Dentária da Universidade de Lisboa, Lisbon, Portugal

Duarte Marques
Private practice, Implantology Institute, Lisboa, Portugal
Department of Morfo-Functional Sciences, Faculdade de Medicina Dentária da Universidade de Lisboa, Lisbon, Portugal

João Caramês
Private practice, Implantology Institute, Lisboa, Portugal
Department of Oral Surgery and Implant Dentistry, Faculdade de Medicina Dentária da Universidade de Lisboa, Lisbon, Portugal

Yuri Sedov and Anatoly Avanesov
Department of General and Clinical Dentistry, RUDN University, Medical Institute, Moscow, Russia

Oleg Mordanov and Kamil Khabiev
Private Practice, Moscow, Russia

Sergei Grigoriev
Private Practice, Cheboksary, Russia

R. Al Sadhan, R. Al Shagroud and M. U. Zaman
Department of Oral Medicine and Diagnostic Sciences, College of Dentistry, King Saud University, Riyadh, Saudi Arabia

A. Alosaimi
Dental University Hospital, King Saud University Medical City, King Saud University, Riyadh, Saudi Arabia

M. S. Allahyani
Department of Oral and Maxillofacial Surgery, Al Noor Hospital, Makkah, Saudi Arabia

Rolando Crippa
Department of Oral Pathology, Italian Stomatological Institute, Milan, Italy

Riccardo Aiuto, María Peñarrocha-Diago and Miguel Peñarrocha-Diago
Department of Oral Surgery, University of Valencia, València, Spain

Mario Dioguardi
Department of Clinical and Experimental Medicine, University of Foggia, Italy

Francesca Angiero
Department of Medical Sciences and Diagnostic Integrated, S. Martino Hospital, University of Genoa, Genova, Italy

Manfred Nilius
Niliusklinik, Londoner Bogen 6, D-44269 Dortmund, Germany
Universitätsklinikum, Carl Gustav Carus, Technische Universität Dresden, Fakultät für Zahn, Mund-und Kieferheilkunde, Dresden, Germany

Jörg Winterhoff
Niliusklinik, Londoner Bogen 6, D-44269 Dortmund, Germany

Yury Georgievich Sedov and Anatoliy Mikhailovich Avanesov
Department of General and Clinical Dentistry, RUDN University, Medical Institute, Moscow, Russia

Kamil Nail'evich Khabiev, Vasiliy Stanislavovich Tarasuk, Vitaliy Georgievich Pantsulaya and Irina Gennad'evna Sedova
Private Dental Practice, Moscow, Russia

Zulfiya Iltuzurovna Yarulina
Department of Orthopedic Dentistry, Kazan State Medical University of the Ministry of Health of Russia, Kazan, Russia

Nikolay Ivanovich Sergeev
Scientific Centre of Roentgenoradiology and Russian National Research Medical University, n.a. N.I. Pirogov, Moscow, Russia

S. Di Carlo, V. Valentini, E. Grasso, F. De Angelis, L. Piccoli, A. Quarato, S. Jamshir and E. Brauner
Dipartimento Scienze Odontostomatologiche e Maxillo Facciali, Università degli Studi di Roma La Sapienza Facoltà di Medicina e Odontoiatria, Rome, Italy

Elio Minetti
Department of Biomedical, Surgical, and Dental Science, Università degli Studi di Milano, Milan, Italy

Silvio Taschieri and Stefano Corbella
Department of Biomedical, Surgical, and Dental Science, Università degli Studi di Milano, Milan, Italy
IRCCS Istituto Ortopedico Galeazzi, Milan, Italy
Federal State Autonomous Educational Institution of Higher Education I.M. Sechenov First Moscow State Medical University of the Ministry of Health of the Russian Federation (Sechenov University), 8-2 Trubetskaya St., 119991 Moscow, Russia

M. M. Figliuzzi, L. Parentela, A. Forte and D. Aiello
Health Sciences Department "Magna Graecia", University of Catanzaro, Catanzaro, Italy

Graziele Parize, Yeon Jung Kim and Debora Pallos
University of Santo Amaro, São Paulo, Brazil

Samy Tunchel, Alberto Blay and Eduardo Felippe Duailibi-Neto
Private Office, São Paulo, Brazil

Roman Volberg
Private Practice, Moscow, Russia

Oleg Mordanov
Department of Prosthodontics, Central Research Institute of Dental and Maxillofacial Surgery, Moscow, Russia

Won-Pyo Lee, Sang-Joun Yu and Byung-Ock Kim
Department of Periodontology, School of Dentistry, Chosun University, 309 Pilmun-daero, Dong-gu, Gwangju 61452, Republic of Korea

Jae-Heung Choi
Department of Preventive and Public Health Dentistry, School of Dentistry, Chosun University, 309 Pilmun-daero, Dong-gu, Gwangju 61452, Republic of Korea

Igor Ashurko, Svetlana Tarasenko and Sabina Mekhtieva
Department of Surgery Dentistry Institute of Dentistry, Federal State Autonomous Educational Institution of Higher Training I.M. Sechenov First Moscow State Medical University of the Ministry of Health of the Russian Federation (Sechenov University), 8- 2 Trubetskaya St., 119991 Moscow, Russia

Artem Trofimov
Dental Clinic(Rio-Stom), 9 Veliyaminovskaya St., 105318 Moscow, Russia

Keisuke Seki
Implant Dentistry, Nihon University School of Dentistry Dental Hospital, Tokyo, Japan
Department of Comprehensive Dentistry and Clinical Education, Nihon University School of Dentistry, Tokyo, Japan

Yoshiyuki Hagiwara
Implant Dentistry, Nihon University School of Dentistry Dental Hospital, Tokyo, Japan

Ronald Younes
Department of Oral Surgery, Faculty of Dental Medicine, Saint Joseph University of Beirut, Beirut, Lebanon
Craniofacial Research Laboratory-Division of Oral Biology, Saint Joseph University of Beirut, Faculty of Dental Medicine, Beirut, Lebanon

Carla Maria Khairallah
Department of Oral Surgery, Faculty of Dental Medicine, Saint Joseph University of Beirut, Beirut, Lebanon

Andrea Rodríguez Moreno, Mariné Ortiz Magdaleno, Marissa Muñoz Islas, María del Pilar Goldaracena Azuara, Everardo Ruiz Cruz and Gabriel Fernando Romo Ramírez
Autonomous University of San Luis Potosí, Specialty in Aesthetic, Cosmetic, Restorative, and Implantological Dentistry, Faculty of Stomatology, Av. Dr. Manuel Nava #2, Zona Universitaria, 78290 San Luis Potosí, Mexico

Jorge Armando Villar Mercado
Autonomous University of San Luis Potosí, Specialty in Periodontics, Faculty of Stomatology, Av. Dr. Manuel Nava #2, Zona Universitaria, 78290 San Luis Potosí, Mexico

Márcio de Carvalho Formiga, Magda Nagasawa and Jamil Awad Shibli
Department of Periodontology and Oral Implantology, Dental Research Division, University of Guarulhos, Sao Paulo, Brazil

Vincent J. J. Donker, Gerry M. Raghoebar and Arjan Vissink
University of Groningen, University Medical Center Groningen, Department of Oral and Maxillofacial Surgery, Groningen, Netherlands

Henny J. A. Meijer
University of Groningen, University Medical Center Groningen, Department of Oral and Maxillofacial Surgery, Groningen, Netherlands
University of Groningen, University Medical Center Groningen, Department of Implant Dentistry, Groningen, Netherlands

Ali Robaian Alqahtani
Department of Conservative Dental Sciences, College of Dentistry, Prince Sattam Bin Abdulaziz University, Alkharj, Saudi Arabia

Khalid Gufran
Department of Preventive Dental Sciences, College of Dentistry, Prince Sattam Bin Abdulaziz University, Alkharj, Saudi Arabia

Fred Silva
Department of Periodontics, Texas A & M College of Dentistry, Dallas, TX 75246, USA

Mateus Garcia Rocha
Center for Dental Biomaterials, Division of Operative Dentistry, Department of Restorative Dental Sciences, College of Dentistry University of Florida, USA

Jia Chang
Department of Periodontology, College of Dentistry, University of Florida, USA

Igor Ashurko, Nataliia Blagushina, Anisa Borodiy and Mary Magdalyanova
Department of Oral Surgery, E.V. Borovsky Institute of Dentistry of I.M. Sechenov First Moscow State Medical University (Sechenov University), Mozhaisky Val, 11 Moscow, Russia

Carlo Maiorana, Susanna Ferrario, Pier Paolo Poli and Mattia Manfredini
Fondazione IRCCS Ca' Granda Ospedale Maggiore Policlinico, Implant Center for Edentulism and Jawbone Atrophies, Maxillofacial Surgery and Odontostomatology Unit, University of Milan, Via della Commenda 10, 20122 Milan, Italy

Angélica Letícia Reis Pavanelli, Luiz Antônio Borelli Barros-Filho, Joni Augusto Cirelli and Rafael Scaf de Molon
Department of Diagnosis and Surgery, São Paulo State University (UNESP), School of Dentistry, Araraquara Sao Paulo, Brazil

Erica Dorigatti de Avila and Francisco de Assis Mollo Junior
Department of Dental Materials and Prosthodontics, São Paulo State University (UNESP), School of Dentistry, Araraquara Sao Paulo, Brazil

Luiz Antônio Borelli Barros
Department of Social Dentistry, São Paulo State University (UNESP), School of Dentistry, Araraquara Sao Paulo, Brazil

Manon Rey Lescure
Unit of Oral Surgery and Implant Dentistry, Department of Oral and Maxillofacial Surgery, University Hospital of Geneva, 1205 Geneva, Switzerland

Nicola Alberto Valente
Department of Stomatology, Faculty of Dentistry, University of Seville, 41009 Seville, Spain

Sibylle Chatelain
Department of Oral and Maxillofacial Surgery, Lausanne University Hospital (CHUV), 1011 Lausanne, Switzerland

Chiara Cinquini and Antonio Barone
Department of Surgical, Medical, Molecular and of Critical Area Pathologies, Complex Operative Unit of Stomatology and Oral Surgery, University-Hospital of Pisa, University of Pisa, 56126 Pisa, Italy

Gunar Wagner
Department of Restorative Dentistry and Periodontology, University Medical Center Leipzig, 04103 Leipzig, Germany

Dieter Hartung
Dental Practice, 37213 Witzenhausen, Germany

Luca Casula
Oral Surgery Resident, Vita Salute University, Milan, Italy

Alex Gillone
Division Director of Periodontology, East Carolina University, Greenville, USA

Davide Musu
Department of Endodontology, Academic Centre for Dentistry Amsterdam (ACTA), Amsterdam, Netherlands

Kamel Alraei
Department of Oral and Maxillofacial Surgery, Al Noor Specialist Hospital, Mecca, Saudi Arabia

Jameel Shrqawi
Department of Oral and Maxillofacial Surgery, Royal Commission Hospital, Al Jubail, Saudi Arabia

Khawlah Alarusi
General Dentist, Mecca, Saudi Arabia

Andrea Enrico Borgonovo, Virna Vavassori and Mauro Savio
Unit of Esthetic Dentistry, Istituto Stomatologico Italiano, University of Milan, Milan, Italy

Rachele Censi
Unit of Periodontology, Istituto Stomatologico Italiano, University of Milan, Milan, Italy

Dino Re
Head, Unit of Esthetic Dentistry, Istituto Stomatologico Italiano, Department of Biomedical, Surgical and Dental Sciences, University of Milan, Milan, Italy

Index

www.ingramcontent.com/pod-product-compliance
Lightning Source LLC
LaVergne TN
LVHW082222200926
848484LV00008B/2289
9798887406442